MY BODY— MY DECISION!

What You Should Know About the Most-Common Female Surgeries

Lindsay R. Curtis, M.D.
Glade B. Curtis, M.D.
Mary K. Beard, M.D.

Illustrations by Paul Farber

❤ THE BODY PRESS

Notice: The information in this book is true and complete to the best of our knowledge. This book is intended only an as informative guide for those wishing to know more about these operations. In no way is this book intended to replace, countermand or conflict with the advice given to you by your doctor.

There are many variables to any illness or surgical condition. Your doctor knows your symptoms, signs, allergies, general health and the many other variables that challenge his/her judgment in caring for you as a patient.

The ultimate decision concerning any surgery or treatment should be made between you and your doctor, and we strongly recommend that you follow his/her advice. The information in this book is general and is offered with no guarantees on the part of the authors or HPBooks. The authors and publisher disclaim all liability in connection with the use of this book.

Note: Because we have strived for consistency, readability and understandability of material, we have used the pronoun "he" when referring to the doctor and the baby. This in no way reflects a preference for sex in a doctor or child. We hope we have not offended any reader with this practice.

Publisher: Rick Bailey
Executive Editor: Randy Summerlin
Editor: Judith Schuler
Art Director: Don Burton
Design and Assembly: Leslie Sinclair
Typography: Cindy Coatsworth, Michelle Carter
Director of Manufacturing: Anthony B. Narducci

Published by The Body Press,
a division of HPBooks, Inc.
P.O. Box 5367
Tucson, AZ 85703
(602) 888-2150
ISBN: 0-89586-385-5
Library of Congress Catalog Card Number: 85-81397
©1986 HPBooks, Inc.
Printed in U.S.A.
1st Printing

Medical-Technical Consultants:
Boyd Burkhardt, M.D., Plastic Surgeon
Henry Hess, M.D., Ph.D., Obstetrician-Gynecologist
Charles M. Rolle, M.D., Obstetrician-Gynecologist

TABLE OF CONTENTS

Special Thanks

Without the willing help of Mark Meldrum, Director of the Medical Library at the McKay-Dee Hospital in Ogden, Utah, our task would have been far more time-consuming. The skillful typing of Mary Reeve and Terrill Eldredge transformed illegible notes into the accurate accounts you read in this book.

Russell V. Young, M.D., a practicing plastic surgeon in Salt Lake City, Utah, wrote the material on plastic surgery and mammaplasty. We thank him for making the information accurate and understandable.

Before Your Surgery

Most lawsuits and misunderstandings between patients and their doctors do not occur because of poor surgery or even poor results. They usually occur because of poor communication and misunderstood expectations.

It is *your* body that is undergoing surgery and you're paying for it, so you have a right to know as much as you can about your condition. You will be more at ease and will be a happier, more-satisfied post-operative patient if you fully understand why your condition requires surgery. A wise surgeon will give you the time, and encourage you, to ask any questions you may have.

We discuss the most common female operations in lay terms, stressing the questions our own patients have asked most frequently. We understand you are concerned about the risk involved, how completely your symptoms will be relieved and how long it will take to fully recover. We have attempted to answer these questions in a general manner. We encourage you to ask the same questions of your doctor and surgeon, so you will receive answers that are particular to your case.

We hope this book serves as an opener for an enlightened dialogue between you and your doctor. One of our goals in writing this book is to make you a *participant,* not a recipient, in your medical care!

THE FEMALE ORGANS AND SURGERY

According to the *Socio-Economic Factbook for Surgery 1985,* published by the American College of Surgeons, 6 of the 10 most common surgeries are

female surgeries. These surgeries include:
- biopsy (first)
- D&C (second)
- Cesarean section (third)
- hysterectomy (fifth)
- tubal ligation (sixth)
- surgery for ovarian cysts (ninth)

These are the surgeries that are performed most often—and you stand a good chance of having one of these procedures some time in your life. So you need to be prepared!

Every woman needs to know, and be familiar with, her own female organs before she can make knowledgeable decisions about surgeries that involve her body. To be a more-aware consumer of surgery, which is what you really are as a patient, you need to know about your body and be informed enough to participate in your medical care.

In this section, we discuss the organs that are directly involved in the female reproductive system—ovaries, Fallopian tubes, uterus, cervix, vagina, vulva and breast. See illustrations below and on the following pages. With the exception of the plastic surgeries, the surgical procedures we deal with will focus on these organs.

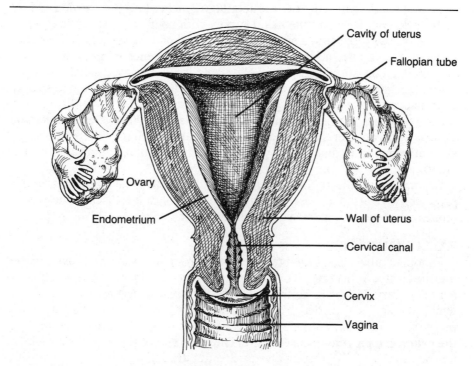

Front view of female internal organs.

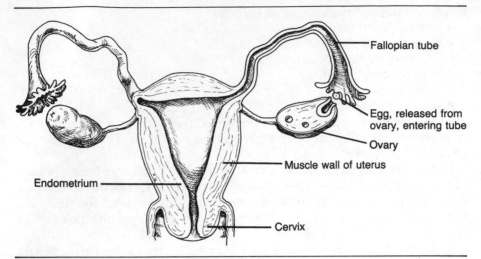

Normal uterus, ovary and tubes show egg released from ovary and entering Fallopian tube.

OVARIES

Your almond-shaped ovaries are about 1 to 2 inches long, 1 inch wide and 1/2 inch thick. Ovaries share the blood supply with your Fallopian tube on each side. Along with the tissue surrounding these blood vessels, cordlike structures (ligaments) extend from the abdominal walls, which support the ovaries and their blood supply. If your Fallopian tube is removed, such as in an ectopic pregnancy, the surgeon must be careful to preserve the blood supply to your ovary.

Although each ovary may contain as many as 250,000 eggs when a female child is born, an average ovary releases only about 200 to 300 eggs during a normal woman's lifetime. Both ovaries share the task of releasing an egg each month.

Beginning at puberty, ovaries may begin to release one egg a month and produce two hormones, estrogen and progesterone. We discuss these hormones when we talk about your menstrual cycle. See page 12.

FALLOPIAN TUBES

Fallopian tubes, also called *oviducts,* lead from the abdominal cavity to the uterine cavity. At the time of ovulation, the open end of your Fallopian tube is near the ovary. It is believed the end of the Fallopian tube covers the site from which the egg is extruded from the ovary. It's possible that the fingerlike projections (fimbria) on the ends of your tubes sweep the area surrounding the ovary, causing the released egg to enter the end of the tube for its 4-inch journey to the cavity of your uterus. See illustration above.

Fertilization of the egg by sperm is believed to occur in the Fallopian tube after the egg travels about 1/3 of the distance from the outer end of the tube toward the uterine cavity. Cilia propel the egg toward your uterus but do not

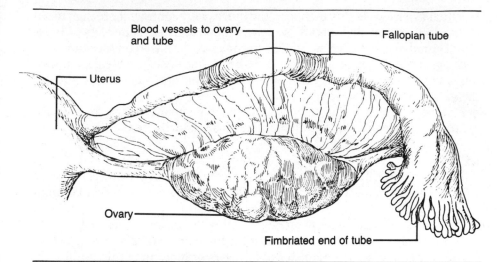

Blood vessels to ovary and tube

Fallopian tube

Uterus

Ovary

Fimbriated end of tube

Ovary and Fallopian tube share the same blood supply.

keep sperm from swimming up the tube, so the two may join. These same cells continue to propel the fertilized egg down toward the uterine cavity.

This journey takes several days. The cells lining your Fallopian tube contain nourishment for the rapidly growing, dividing fertilized egg as it travels. By the time the ball of cells reaches the uterine cavity, it has developed the ability to burrow into the nutrition-filled lining of the uterus, the *endometrium.*

The ball of cells develops into an embryo, which soon outgrows its yolk sac and develops a placenta (afterbirth) within the wall of your uterus. Through the placenta, the embryo obtains nourishment until ready for delivery.

UTERUS

The uterus is a fist-sized organ shaped like an upside-down pear. Although it is hollow, the uterine cavity is almost completely collapsed. Velvetlike tissue (endometrium) lines the entire cavity of your uterus.

The extremely vascular (generous blood supply) endometrium goes through a monthly cycle. In the cycle, it becomes thickened and interlaced with nutritious glands that ready themselves to receive and feed a fertilized egg if it arrives from the Fallopian tube. This meticulously prepared lining permits the fertilized egg to embed itself in the tissue and continue to grow.

If fertilization of the egg does not occur, the thickened outer layers of the lining are shed along with blood that seeps from the blood vessels left open by the shedding. Tissue and blood are called *menstruum* or *menstrual flow*— this is your menstrual period each month. Only the base of the glands remains after shedding has taken place, but the lining quickly heals itself as preparation for embedding a new fertilized egg begins again.

In response to *prostaglandins* (a specific group of hormones or chemicals essential to various body functions), the uterus may contract more than usual to expel the menstruum, and these contractions register themselves as menstrual cramps. Severity of menstrual cramps may be based on the amount of prostaglandin present or the response of the uterine muscle to prostaglandins. Relief from these cramps is often obtained with anti-prostaglandins, such as the generic drug ibuprofen.

In some way that we don't understand, the pregnant uterus at term begins to contract, labor ensues and ultimately the baby is delivered.

CERVIX

The *cervix,* or neck, is the lower part of the uterus that protrudes into your vagina. The cervix is a long, non-contractile segment of the uterus containing a narrow canal.

The cervical canal is large enough to allow only the menstrual flow to escape, yet small enough to keep out most infection. Yet this same cervix is capable of enlarging to a diameter of 5 inches or more to permit a full-term baby to pass through it during birth.

There are some exceptions to this rule. Gonorrhea and other infections have the ability to pass the barrier and continue through the cavity of the uterus, through the Fallopian tubes and into your peritoneal cavity.

Sperm are able to travel from your upper vagina, where they are deposited during intercourse, through the canal of the cervix, across the lining of the body of the uterus and continue out through the Fallopian tube where they may meet a descending egg and fertilize it.

Although your cervix is capable of dilating for labor and delivery at the proper time, under the proper stimulus, its powerful rings of tissue keep the fetus securely inside until it matures and is ready to be delivered. To accomplish this, muscle bands of the cervix must stretch to more than 50 times their normal size.

The cervix contains few nerve endings. It can be cut, sewed, even cauterized with a minimum of pain. It resists stretching except in labor. Forcing it to stretch, as with instrumental dilatation for a D&C, may cause severe discomfort requiring anesthesia. Only rarely are monthly menstrual cramps produced by the cervix.

VAGINA

The vagina is a 5-inch-long tube serving as a passageway. It is part of the birth canal during delivery of a baby, and it serves as the organ of copulation. The vagina leads from the cervix to the outside of the body, called the *introitus* (the entrance to the vagina). See illustration on opposite page.

The vaginal canal remains collapsed until it is stretched by the penis during intercourse, by the gloved fingers of your doctor, by an instrument during a pelvic exam or by the birth of a baby. The vagina seems capable of accommodating itself to any size erect male penis during intercourse, and it is

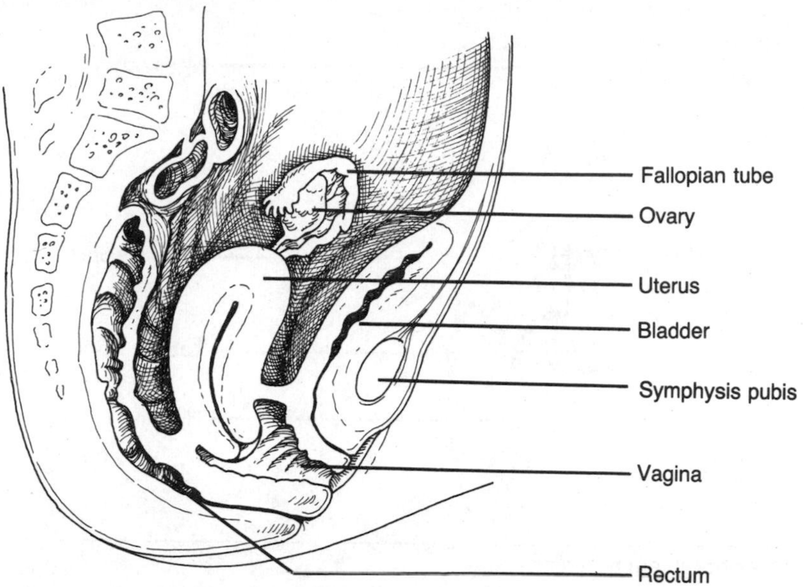
Fallopian tube
Ovary
Uterus
Bladder
Symphysis pubis
Vagina
Rectum

Side view of internal female organs.

capable of stretching to allow an 8- or 9-pound baby to pass through it during delivery.

Although it contains few nerve endings, your vagina responds erotically and sensitively to pressure and friction during intercourse with pleasurable contractions during orgasm. There may be a feeling of pressure and pain in the vagina during delivery that varies in severity with each patient and perhaps in each pregnancy of that patient.

The vagina has its own normal, natural, self-cleansing secretion that also provides lubrication during intercourse. When the vagina is infected or irritated, this discharge may become copious and foul smelling. Normal vaginal secretion may be considerably lower after menopause, even to the point of dryness.

VULVA

Your vulva includes all the female structures that can be seen on the outside of the body leading to the vagina. These include the mons pubis, labia majora and minora, clitoris, hymen and urethral opening from the bladder. See illustration on page 10.

Mons Pubis—The mons pubis is a fat-filled cushion on the bony part of your pelvis in front of your bladder. After puberty, the skin on the mons pubis is covered by curly hair. Distribution of this hair in a female is usually an inverted-triangle shape. On a male, this hair extends upward toward the navel.

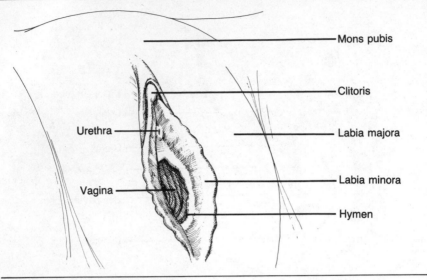

Vulva and external female organs.

Labia Majora and Minora—These are folds of skin that form the outer opening to the vagina. The *majora* consist of rounded folds of fat covered with skin; these extend downward and backward from the mons pubis. The *minora* lie inside the majora and form a covering or hood over the clitoris. The minora contain very sensitive nerve endings.

Clitoris—The clitoris is a small, erectile body located within the folds of the labia minora. It is found above the opening of the vagina and above the urethral opening. The clitoris is about 3/4 inch long and is one of the principal erogenous organs of women.

Hymen—The hymen circles the outer entrance to the vagina. There is great variation among women in the thickness and rigidity of the hymen. The hymenal opening to the vagina can vary from small to no blockage at all. The hymen can be torn or stretched with first intercourse or by internal tampons.

Urethral Opening—The urethral opening lies below the clitoris. It looks like a small slit and serves as the outside opening of the urethra.

BREASTS

The breast, or mammary gland, got its name from "mamma," the Latin word for breast. Your breasts are made up of glandular tissue, supporting tissue and fatty tissue. See illustrations on opposite page.

The breast is located between the second and sixth rib, on top of the pectoralis muscles. Breasts vary in size and shape.

During puberty, breasts enlarge to their adult size under the stimulation of increasing amounts of estrogen. Very often one breast will be slightly larger than the other. During pregnancy, there is an increase in size and weight of breasts. The increase in size will continue during lactation, also called *milk*

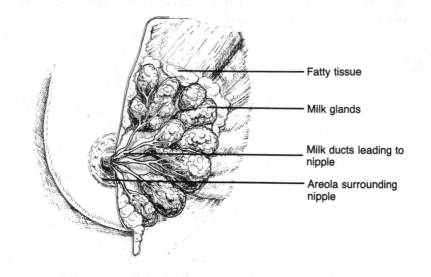

Fatty tissue

Milk glands

Milk ducts leading to nipple

Areola surrounding nipple

Structure of normal breast.

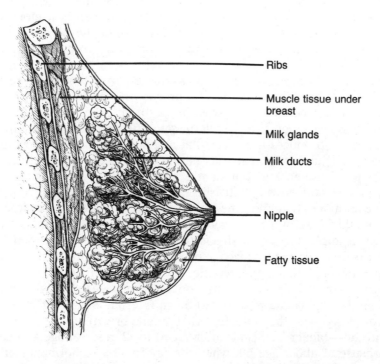

Ribs

Muscle tissue under breast

Milk glands

Milk ducts

Nipple

Fatty tissue

Side view of normal breast structure.

production, due to hormonal stimulation causing the production of milk, which is released in response to suckling by a baby.

The mammary glands consist of a number of small, independent glands. These glands are embedded in fat, which gives the breast its rounded contour. A system of ducts or tubes connects the glands of the breast to the nipple.

The breast includes the nipple, which is surrounded by a pigmented area called the *areola.* The skin covering the breast contains fine hairs and sweat glands. The nipple is a cone-shaped elevation in the center of the breast. Each nipple contains 15 to 25 milk ducts and nerve endings and muscle fibers that react to touch, thermal or sexual stimulation.

Hormonal changes in pregnancy cause significant growth of the duct system, causing considerable breast enlargement. Breasts are further enlarged late in pregnancy by colostrum, which is a secretion from the breasts before breast milk appears. There is a slow decrease in breast size as milk production shuts down after pregnancy.

Menopause, with its loss of estrogen stimulation to the breasts, may leave breasts saggy and flat. The size and contour of breasts may change dramatically after menopause as they become smaller and have less support.

MENSTRUATION

The beginning of menstruation at puberty (10 to 12 years old) is called the *menarche.* The cessation of menstrual periods is called *menopause* and occurs between 48 and 52 years of age. Menstruation is a monthly flow consisting of blood and the discarded tissue from the breakdown of the thickened nutritious lining of the uterus that was prepared to receive a fertilized egg.

It may sound simple, but this process of menstrual flow is the result of a complex, well-integrated, coordinated process that begins in the brain. Hormones first are secreted by an area in the brain called the *hypothalamus.* These hormones react on the *pituitary gland,* the master gland of the body. The pituitary produces hormones that affect growth and development and secretes other hormones that react on the ovaries. The hormones cause the ovaries to release an egg each month.

To protect and provide nourishment for the released egg, your ovaries secrete hormones that affect the endometrium. This hormone-charged lining becomes thickened as glands swell with blood and nutritious fluids preparing to receive, implant and nourish a fertilized egg. If the egg extruded from the ovary does not become fertilized, most of the thickened lining is sloughed off, along with some blood, and becomes the menstrual flow.

The menstrual flow leaves the uterine cavity through the cervix. It continues through the vagina and is absorbed by an internal tampon or by a sanitary napkin placed over the vulva (external female organ).

Menarche—Menarche begins at about 10 to 12 years of age and ceases at menopause at about age 50, when the production of hormones gradually diminishes. These are average ages and vary widely.

Menstrual periods usually occur every 28 days, but it is not uncommon to vary between 24 and 34 days. A period lasts from 1 to 8 days. Ovulation occurs about 14 days before the onset of the next menstrual period, but this may also vary. The most consistent thing about menstrual flow is the inconsistency in the amount, duration and interval of flow among individual women. Each woman develops her own pattern and must not judge her own cycle by the menstrual pattern of someone else.

When we consider a normal woman has from 400 to 600 menstrual cycles during her lifetime, it's surprising menstrual periods remain as regular and normal as they do. In spite of their complex nature requiring close coordination of brain, ovary and uterus, menstrual periods withstand stress and strain fairly well.

YOUR HISTORY AND PHYSICAL EXAM

It's important to find a competent gynecologist, but it's just as important to find one with whom you feel comfortable and can communicate.

Usually, but not always, certification by the American Board of Obstetrics and Gynecology means competency and adequate training. You may want to talk to your family doctor or check with the medical society in your county to select a gynecologist.

On your first visit, you can often determine what your relationship with your doctor will be. Is he too busy to listen? Does he welcome questions and take time to explain what he is doing, what he finds and what it means to you?

Most doctors have a form for you to fill out that provides a medical history that will save time for you and the doctor during your examination. From this information, your doctor knows what your problems are or why you have come to see him. He will elaborate on these as he talks with you.

Be honest with your doctor. Don't be embarrassed or hesitant to talk about very personal matters as they pertain to your condition. You may expect your doctor to be professional and interested in you and your problems for the time he is with you. He must be able to make you feel at ease. If he has biases, hang-ups or is judgmental, you may be wise to seek help from another gynecologist.

Prior to your appointment with your doctor, write down your symptoms and any questions you have. There is nothing wrong with writing down your doctor's answers, his instructions and the medications he gives you. It is to everyone's advantage that you completely understand everything he tells you. If he does prescribe medication, it might be a good idea to look it up in a drug guide so you fully understand what it is, interactions with other medication and substances, and how to take it. An excellent source is *Complete Guide to Prescription and Non-Prescription Drugs* by H. Winter Griffith, M.D., also published by HPBooks.

In this specialized medical age, a gynecologist may be the only doctor a woman sees. She may feel she has had her "annual" physical exam when she has a Pap smear. For this reason, it's important for the doctor to take a relatively complete history and perform a thorough physical examination.

He *should* ask about your eyes, ears, nose, throat, chest and abdomen. Are you having bowel or bladder problems? Do you become short of breath easily? Are you exercising? Any problems with weight control? Most of these areas will be covered in the form you fill out before you see him, but your doctor will pursue any abnormal signs or symptoms you have noticed.

Urinalysis, hematocrit and other blood tests (miniprofile) may be ordered if your doctor feels they are necessary. Even if you bring a urine specimen with you, you'll be asked to empty your bladder so a more thorough pelvic examination can be done.

An unanticipated diagnosis of diabetes for many patients has begun with a routine urinalysis. It doesn't do much good to treat vulvovaginitis locally if it's due to diabetes. It won't clear up until your diabetes is controlled.

Albumin in the urine points toward possible kidney problems. White blood cells in urine on microscopic examination may indicate a urinary-tract infection.

For a complete physical exam, it's necessary to disrobe, although you should be adequately draped to preserve modesty. For example, if you have a malignant melanoma on your back, you want your doctor to discover it, even if he is a gynecologist. There is little excuse to perform *only* a pelvic examination, unless you have just been examined by a referring physician who gave you a complete physical.

It is permissible to have the nurse take your blood pressure and weigh you, but your doctor should perform the remainder of the examination. The nurse will position you and drape you on the examining table. Even though your doctor will examine you very thoroughly, you should not be exposed nude. Hence, the drapes or examining gown.

Your doctor is not an expert on eyes, bones and joints, but he is an M.D., and he should know how to take a complete history and perform a thorough physical. He may begin by inspecting your skin for moles, rashes or other irritation. From this, he may proceed to your eyes, ears, nose, throat—even your tongue and teeth. He can usually tell if you have a goiter in your neck or enlarged glands in your armpits or groin.

His examination of your breasts should be complete, and he should show you how to examine your own breasts. See page 43. He can also listen to your heart and lungs, check for hernias, enlarged liver or spleen, tender areas in your abdomen and kidneys *before* he even begins the pelvic exam.

A complete pelvic examination should take 5 to 10 minutes, including a Pap smear. If he uncovers problems, your doctor may ask for immediate consultation by an office-sharing colleague, or he may refer you to another physician.

A pelvic examination includes inspection of the pubic hair for irritation or even lice and for hair configuration. Some masculinizing tumors of the ovary, for instance, are first indicated by increased pubic hair and a change in the contour of the pubic hairline—it begins to extend toward the navel—plus possible enlargement of the clitoris. A decrease in the amount of pubic hair may be due to vitamin or thyroid deficiency, but most commonly it is due to the aging process.

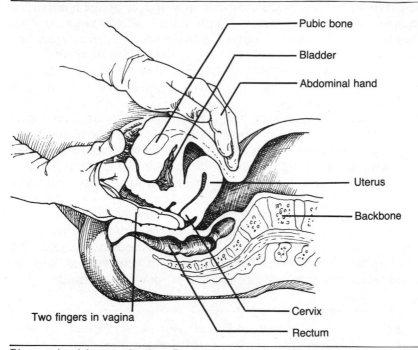

Pubic bone

Bladder

Abdominal hand

Uterus

Backbone

Two fingers in vagina

Cervix

Rectum

Bimanual pelvic examination. Doctor uses pressure from above with his abdominal hand against the two fingers in the vagina to outline pelvic organs and detect abnormalities of size and contour.

Vaginal infections produce irritation of the vulva as their discharge spills onto your perineum and vulva. Sampling and testing of the discharge is reserved until examination of the cervix. Herpes may produce small blisters on the surface of your vulva. Other growths on the vulva could be due to wart viruses.

After thoroughly inspecting your vulva, your doctor will spread the larger lips of the vulva and inspect the vaginal mucous membranes to see if they are healthy, irritated or atrophied (smoothed out due to lack of hormones and aging, usually after menopause).

Before inserting his gloved and lubricated fingers into the vagina, your doctor first gently inserts a speculum of the proper size. A *speculum* is a hinged, bivalved instrument that spreads the walls of the vagina so the doctor can inspect it and the cervix. From the opening of the cervix, he will take a Pap smear to send to the lab where it will be checked for cancer of the cervix.

After he removes the speculum, your doctor will press on the back wall of the vagina (toward the rectum) and ask you to bear down so he can examine the anterior wall of the vagina. He does this to feel for loss of bladder-wall support called *cystocele,* or *urethrocele* if it is under the urethra. He also looks for a loss of urine as you cough. A cystocele is a herniation of the bladder into the vagina and appears as a bulging of the front wall of your vagina.

When a woman bears down, a cystocele may appear or the uterus may descend and actually protrude from the vagina. This is called a *prolapse* of the uterus and is caused from loss of support in the ligaments of the uterus. The decision to operate on prolapse of the uterus depends on its severity, the symptoms it causes and, to some extent, whether other surgery is performed at the same time. The most common symptom of prolapse of the uterus is a feeling of "things falling out."

Your doctor then inserts two gloved, lubricated, fingers into the vagina where he can feel the tip of the cervix. The cervix also has an opening in the center of it. See illustration on previous page. With his other hand pressing on your abdomen, the doctor then outlines the contour of the cervix, uterus, tubes and ovaries. He feels for any enlargement, irregular shape or tenderness.

After completing his vaginal examination, your doctor then inserts one finger in the vagina and one finger in the rectum. See illustration below. He places his other hand on your abdomen. This is called a *rectovaginal exam,* and it enables him to feel certain abnormalities in your rectum, such as polyps, and provides a thorough examination of your pelvic organs.

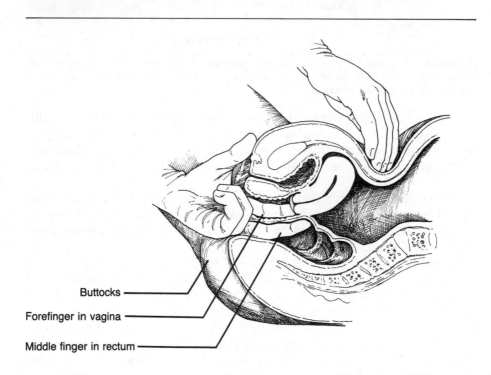

Buttocks

Forefinger in vagina

Middle finger in rectum

Rectovaginal pelvic examination is pelvic exam in which your doctor can feel abnormalities in your rectum (polyps, hemorrhoids, strictures) and feel behind your uterus.

While performing a rectovaginal examination, your doctor also checks to see if there is a herniation of your rectum into the back wall of the vagina. This type of hernia is called a *rectocele*. A rectocele often causes your bowel movement to become "trapped" in the bulge. You may have to help yourself by pressing your finger on the bulge in the vagina to pass a bowel movement.

Cystocele and rectocele can be corrected by surgery through the vagina. Results are often enhanced by vaginal hysterectomy, especially if your uterus has lost its support.

The most common cause of loss of support in pelvic organs is childbirth. The loss of support may be in direct proportion to the number of children a woman has delivered.

Heredity may also play a prominent role in the development of cystocele, rectocele and prolapse of the uterus.

SECOND OPINION

Some patients feel a request for a second opinion about their surgery is an affront to their doctor's good judgment. Others fear their doctor may refuse to take care of them if they question his decision to operate. Many people simply don't realize there may be alternatives to surgery or other types of surgery that may better suit their condition. A second opinion should not be viewed as an affront. You are being careful about getting the best care possible.

All surgery carries some risk, but it is *your* body and *your* life that are subjected to that risk. You have the right to know all about the operation and the *right* to question, to inquire and to be certain before you have an operation. Don't feel guilty about requesting a second opinion.

Many hospitals *insist* on consultation before any major surgery is performed. Some do not. It is possible for a surgeon to reach a status among his colleagues and among the public in which few, if any, will dispute his opinion. But no one is infallible!

Below are a few things that might help you decide if you need a second opinion and how you can obtain it without offending anyone, including your doctor.

• Most conscientious physicians welcome another opinion. Be suspicious of a doctor who resents your request for a second opinion or one who objects to a hospital rule requiring consultation.

• There is often more than one way to handle a medical problem.

• Be suspicious of any doctor who claims he has the "only" way to treat a given condition or if he claims to be the only doctor qualified to perform your operation. This is one sign of quackery. Check him out with your local medical society.

• Doctors do disagree. Honest doctors disagree at times and will not go along with an improper or unjustifiable operation by another doctor. Most hospitals now police their own staff and restrict or remove offenders.

So what's the best way to request a second opinion? Explain to your doctor what your concerns are. Tell him the operation *is* important to you. He should welcome a second opinion to corroborate his findings. Ask him to suggest someone in whom he has confidence to consult with him on your case. Ask the consulting doctor to examine you and discuss his findings with you.

If a second opinion is sought in this manner, you'll rarely find a physician who will take offense. You will already have expressed confidence in him when you ask him to select the consultant.

Not all surgeries require a second opinion, such as emergency, life-saving surgeries, like a ruptured tubal pregnancy, or a non-emergency situation like a tubal ligation. Consultation does cost time and money, especially in an emergency or urgent situation where delay could be foolish and even life-threatening. There may be neither time nor justification for consultation. Elective surgery depends greatly on your desire for the surgery and your reasons for wanting it. A second opinion may still be helpful for elective or cosmetic surgery.

ANESTHESIA

Anesthesia is an integral part of the successful performance of any surgical procedure. Your anesthesiologist is a medical doctor who has specialized in anesthesia, and he is specifically responsible for this important part of your care so your surgeon can devote his attention to your surgery.

The anesthesiologist will probably visit you the night before surgery to talk to you, ask you questions about your general health, previous surgery, allergies, medications you are taking and any drugs you may be allergic to. After the surgery, he will help you awaken by giving you extra oxygen to clear your blood of any gas anesthetic. He will check on you in the recovery room to make certain your vital signs are normal as you awaken.

For all but very minor procedures, in which local anesthesia is used, it's customary for you to have an intravenous solution. This I.V. is an important precaution because it gives you fluid, and it is a ready avenue for emergency medication when needed, as well as transfusions. Through this I.V. needle, your doctor can give you medicine to relax your muscles or even a tranquilizer or pain reliever if you have only a local anesthetic.

There are two major categories of anesthesia—*general* anesthesia (you are asleep) and *regional* anesthesia (you are awake). Regional anesthesia is used for some major surgeries but is more often used for minor, less-involved cases. The three main types of regional anesthesia are spinal, epidural and local. Each has its own application and advantages or disadvantages.

GENERAL ANESTHESIA
General anesthesia is used in most major surgical procedures. The patient is completely asleep, whether due to intravenous medications, inhalation of gas or a combination of the two.

Combinations of drugs often derive the benefits of each medication with a lower dose and fewer side effects. Intravenous medication, such as sodium pentothal, may be used for induction of anesthesia to put you to sleep without the psychological trauma of a face mask. Gas is then given by mask to keep you "under."

After you're asleep, a tube is inserted into your windpipe and further administration of the gas is through this tube rather than by mask. A combination of gases and intravenous medications keeps you safely asleep and relaxed so your surgery can be performed without pain or interference. You usually have no memory of the surgery or the anesthesia. When you awaken, the operation is over.

Advantages of General Anesthesia — In emergency situations, such as ectopic pregnancy or in fetal distress requiring Cesarean section, you can rapidly be put to sleep and the surgery performed at a time when any delay greatly increases the risk.

Many patients are frightened by the prospect of surgery and tolerate the experience better if they are asleep. In some instances, better "relaxation" of abdominal muscles can be obtained by general anesthesia, making surgery easier to perform.

Disadvantages of General Anesthesia — Some patients would rather be awake for various reasons. For some, the worst part of the surgery is their concern about being put to sleep and "losing control." In a Cesarean operation, for instance, some women want to be awake to see their baby immediately and "participate" in the delivery.

With general anesthesia, there is slower recovery time. It may be prolonged after a general anesthetic because all parts of your body are affected, such as your bowel and bladder function. Gas pains and delayed function of your bladder or bowel may result.

Vomiting is more common following general anesthesia. Aspiration of vomit and "aspiration pneumonia" are more common with general anesthesia.

General anesthesia may be more dangerous if you have heart disease. Each case must be considered on its own merits.

Other advantages and disadvantages may apply in individual cases, including allergies to medications. Most patients tolerate general anesthesia very well.

SPINAL

A needle with a syringe full of medication is placed in your back, between vertebrae, and medication is injected into your spinal canal through the needle, which is then removed. The medication acts directly on the spinal cord and its branches. A spinal anesthetic provides anesthesia to specific areas supplied by that segment of your spinal cord. Spinal anesthesia is frequently used for Cesarean deliveries if you want to be awake to see your baby immediately. It is also used in patients with special medical problems, such as lung disease, in which general anesthesia would subject them to greater risk.

Advantages of Spinal Anesthesia — You are awake, and it's safer if you have lung disease or if you are allergic to gas anesthetics. Recovery often is faster, with fewer systemic effects, such as nausea and vomiting. You are not sedated as much.

Disadvantages of Spinal Anesthesia — Even when administered by a skilled anesthesiologist, the result may not provide complete anesthesia. If you still feel pain, you may require general anesthesia to provide complete relief of pain.

The incidence of post-spinal headaches varies and may be influenced by the skill of the anesthesiologist. But headaches do occur occasionally in spite of every precaution. It is believed they are due to leakage of spinal fluid through the needle hole in the covering of the cord after the needle is withdrawn. Headaches may be severe and require strict bed rest for several days.

Damage to the spinal cord is unlikely, but if it occurs, it may be due to sensitivity to the local anesthetic or injury from the spinal needle.

Spinal anesthesia is sometimes the anesthesia of choice and is very effective. Your case will be evaluated by your doctor, who will determine the type of anesthesia best suited for you.

EPIDURAL

Epidural anesthesia is similar to spinal anesthesia in that a needle with a catheter (plastic tube covering the needle) is placed in the back between the

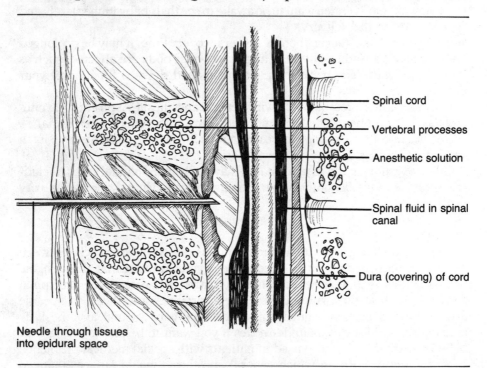

Spinal cord

Vertebral processes

Anesthetic solution

Spinal fluid in spinal canal

Dura (covering) of cord

Needle through tissues into epidural space

Epidural anesthesia. Anesthetic solution is injected through a needle into the epidural space (space that surrounds the dura or covering of the spinal cord).

vertebrae, but the medication is injected outside the spinal canal. The catheter is left in place so medication can be given as many times as is necessary. Risks are lower and benefits are higher with epidural anesthesia as compared to those of spinal anesthesia. Because medication is injected around the spinal-cord roots, the degree of numbness depends on the level of injection. See illustration on opposite page.

Advantages of Epidural—One advantage of epidural over spinal anesthesia is a lower incidence of headaches. However, the anesthesia may be less complete and can cause "spotty" discomfort. But overall, side effects are less than with spinal anesthesia.

Disadvantages of Epidural—A significant disadvantage of epidural (and spinal) anesthesia is that neither can be given rapidly, making them less useful (not even a choice) in an emergency situation. Each method requires at least 15 to 30 minutes for effective anesthesia. An epidural finds greatest application in normal deliveries and in non-emergency Cesarean operations.

PARACERVICAL BLOCK

Paracervical block is a technique that relieves the pain of dilatation or stretching of the cervix and is used for relief of pain in labor. Occasionally it is used also for a D&C or abortion.

This anesthetic is given through the vagina. A long needle is guided by your doctor's fingers to the cervix. The cervix is injected with local anesthetic, such as lidocaine, on both sides. As mentioned, the cervix has few pain fibers, but it is very sensitive to stretch, such as with labor or a D&C. The injection of local anesthetic into the cervix numbs it so it doesn't hurt as it is stretched by the baby's head or by instruments. This technique should be performed only by someone skilled and experienced in this anesthesia. Most obstetricians and some family practitioners can do this.

Relief should be felt within a few minutes because the medication is injected directly along your cervix. Numbness usually lasts for an hour or more. The block can also be repeated, if necessary.

When a paracervical block is used in labor, the baby must be monitored closely for possible side effects. The most common side effect on the baby is a decrease in his heart rate. This is usually transitory and probably will not harm the baby, but it must be watched closely.

Advantages of Paracervical Block — The advantages of using this type of anesthetic include direct placement of medication, fewer systemic side effects, immediate onset of anesthesia, rapid recovery and few complications. An anesthesiologist does not need to be present to administer this anesthetic.

Disadvantages of Paracervical Block — There are some disadvantages to using a paracervical block. These include difficulty in use when large areas are involved, total numbness is not always obtained, occasional drop in blood pressure and possible allergic reaction to the anesthetic.

LOCAL

Local anesthesia is a direct injection of medication into an operative site to provide immediate numbness. A local is sometimes used to perform certain major operations when surgery is so urgent (emergency situations, such as Cesarean section) it can't wait for spinal or epidural anesthesia or when the anesthesiologist is on his way but has not arrived.

Local injections are used most often for minor procedures or biopsies in which a large area of anesthesia is not required.

Advantages of Local Anesthesia — Some advantages include direct placement of medication, fewer systemic side effects, immediate onset of anesthesia, anesthesiologist does not have to be present, rapid recovery and few complications.

Disadvantages of Local Anesthesia — Disadvantages include difficulty in use when large areas are involved — total numbness is not always obtained — and possible reaction to the anesthetic. Discuss with your doctor and anesthesiologist your particular situation and which type of anesthesia they feel is best for the surgery you are having. Don't hesitate to ask questions and express your concerns or fears. Tell them if you prefer to be asleep or awake. They will discuss why a given anesthetic may be best in your particular case.

Feeling comfortable and aware of what is happening and why decreases stress and may improve the final result of your surgery.

QUESTIONS TO ASK YOUR DOCTOR

In each section of this book, we have included many questions that may be raised in your mind and hopefully answered by your doctor. As a patient who wants to receive the best care possible, there are questions you will want to ask your doctor before the surgery is undertaken. Some common general questions you might ask include:

Are there alternatives to surgery for my problem?

Does the surgery need to be done now, or could it wait? Is it dangerous to wait?

What are the specific risks to this particular surgery? What are the risks if I don't have it?

Will you perform the surgery? Do I need to see a specialist? Who else will be there?

How long will I be in the hospital? When can I go back to work?

Will there be consultants on my case?

What can I do to get ready for the surgery? For recovery?

What tests will be performed before the surgery?

What do you do with the tissue removed at surgery?

Many other questions can be raised, and each situation will be different. As we've already said, if you're well-informed about your surgery, the risks, the benefits and the expected outcome, you'll tolerate it better and recover sooner.

If you've been able to communicate your feelings to your doctor, and if he is sympathetic to your feelings, you have the beginning of an excellent doctor-patient relationship.

Abortion

DEFINITION OF ABORTION

Abortion is a method of *electively* terminating a pregnancy. Since the 1973 Supreme Court decision legalizing abortion in the United States, the number of abortions has increased.

ABBREVIATIONS AND OTHER NAMES

Abortion is described by many terms, including AB, termination, therapeutic abortion, TAB, D&C for termination, menstrual extraction, menstrual regulation, dilation and evacuation, D&E and vacutage.

PARTS OF BODY INVOLVED

The parts of your body involved in an abortion include the vagina, cervix and uterus. With an abortion, your mind and emotions may also be involved. This can be a determining factor in how you accept and recover from your surgery.

COMMON REASONS FOR ABORTION

There are two principal reasons you may seek an abortion—medical and social.

MEDICAL

Medical reasons for abortion, as outlined by the American College of Obstetrics and Gynecology, include the following:

● When continuation of pregnancy may threaten your life or seriously impair your health.

- When pregnancy has resulted from rape or incest.
- When continuation of pregnancy is likely to result in the birth of a child with severe physical deformities or mental retardation.

Medical-Maternal Reasons — Illnesses during pregnancy, such as cancer requiring radiation or chemotherapy, or heart disease, may threaten your health. Some illnesses worsen with pregnancy, so each situation must be evaluated individually.

Medical-Fetal Reasons — Your baby may be known to have, or is likely to have, severe mental or physical problems. Modern technology has made it possible for us to diagnose more of these conditions before birth.

The primary method of diagnosis in such instances is amniocentesis. This is the process of removing amniotic fluid from the sac surrounding the baby. Amniocentesis is more likely if you are over 35 years old, have previously given birth to abnormal children, have a family history of birth defects or have been exposed to defect-causing agents (*teratogens)* during early pregnancy.

If you suspect your baby is abnormal, this may be confirmed by amniocentesis as early as 16 weeks of pregnancy. By this time there is sufficient amniotic fluid to remove and examine. Tests require 2 weeks to complete, which gives enough time to perform a safe abortion if necessary.

SOCIAL

After you discover you're pregnant, you may decide the birth of a child cannot be a reality in your life for personal reasons. Whatever your reasons for choosing an abortion, you have the legal right to make that choice.

Guilt or embarrassment may cause you to keep pregnancy and abortion a secret from your friends or relatives. If you are depressed or have other reasons for not wanting a pregnancy, you may find enormous relief when you are given the alternative of abortion.

However, you may not understand the risks of abortion in regard to your health and future fertility. Whatever the reasons, insist on having all of your questions answered *before* you have an abortion.

HOW COMMON IS ABORTION?

Many abortions are performed in the doctor's office or in an outpatient surgery unit and are often unreported. Statistics on abortion are difficult to obtain; at best, they are a guess.

A 1977 survey indicated that 1,079,430 legal abortions were performed that year — a ratio of 325 abortions for every 1,000 live births. These figures are thought to be low, which could mean that nearly 1/3 of all pregnancies might have resulted in abortion.

If spontaneous or unintentional abortions (miscarriages) are included, figures are overwhelming. Estimates for 1981 were 1.3 million legal abortions in the United States. This figure now approaches 2 million abortions a year and may actually be higher.

FUNCTIONS INVOLVED IN ABORTION

Your first indication of pregnancy is a late or missed menstrual period, a suspicion easily confirmed by a pregnancy test. An over-the-counter pregnancy test can be purchased and done at home. Other symptoms, such as morning sickness and breast tenderness and swelling, soon confirm the diagnosis.

With pregnancy confirmed, you must decide how to deal with it. Even though at first you may deny the situation, you must eventually make some decisions. You may consult with your doctor, friends or family about possible options.

HOW ABORTION IS PERFORMED

The method of abortion is, to a great extent, dictated by how far your pregnancy has advanced. Early abortion may be a minor procedure performed in your doctor's office without anesthesia. It also may be a more complicated process, involving general anesthesia and a stay in the hospital. Usually, the earlier the pregnancy, the lower the risk and the less difficult the abortion.

A full-term pregnancy (40 weeks) is divided into trimesters. The first trimester lasts from 1 to 12 weeks, the second from week 13 to 24 weeks and the third from 25 weeks to full term (40 weeks). In most states, abortion can be legally performed up to 20 weeks. In a few states, the procedure is permitted up to 24 weeks.

1 TO 6 WEEKS

Within 14 days after a missed menstrual period, the procedure is often called *menstrual regulation* or *menstrual extraction*. It is usually performed in a doctor's office and requires no anesthesia. It carries minimal risk of complications. Performed in the office under sterile conditions, it may be no more painful than a Pap smear.

After cleansing your cervix and vagina with sterile soap, a small plastic tube is passed through your cervix. The contents of your uterus are suctioned out using a syringe or small vacuum machine. The tube is small, so your cervix does not need to be dilated. The amount of tissue removed is small, so anesthesia is not required. The procedure takes about 30 minutes, after which you will be observed to make sure bleeding is not excessive and there are no other problems.

Bleeding is about the same as a menstrual period, or lighter, and may continue for a week. Pain should be no worse than menstrual cramps, but you may ask for medication if you need it. Usually no medication is required to control bleeding in early abortion.

6 TO 12 WEEKS

This method extends through the first trimester of your pregnancy and requires dilatation of your cervix. Stretching of your cervix is painful and requires anesthesia. The procedure can often be accomplished in a doctor's office or in outpatient surgery.

To dilate a closed cervix, mechanical dilators can be used, or laminaria (narrow strips of dried, sterile Japanese seaweed) are placed in your cervix the day before the procedure. See illustration below. Laminaria absorb fluid and swell, thereby starting the dilating process, which makes surgery safer and easier.

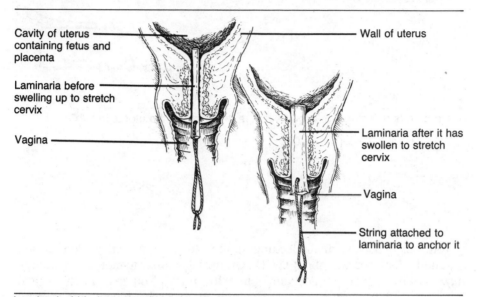

Cavity of uterus containing fetus and placenta

Laminaria before swelling up to stretch cervix

Vagina

Wall of uterus

Laminaria after it has swollen to stretch cervix

Vagina

String attached to laminaria to anchor it

Laminaria (dried seaweed) are inserted into the cervical canal, where they swell and stretch the cervix.

On the day of surgery, your cervix and vagina are cleansed, then a paracervical-block anesthesia is given. If general anesthesia is required, it is used only in an operating room. If laminaria were used, they are removed. Your cervix is dilated further using cervical dilators large enough to accommodate the instruments used to perform your abortion.

When your pregnancy is farther advanced, larger instruments must be used because more tissue is removed. Cervical dilators of increasing caliber are inserted in your cervix until its canal is wide enough to permit passage of the larger instruments.

Once dilated, a suction curette is carefully passed through your cervix, barely into the uterine cavity. When attached to a suction machine, the curette applies a controlled amount of suction that removes the contents of your uterus with gentle action against the uterine walls. In addition to the suction catheter, sharp curettes may be used to ensure no tissue is left to cause bleeding or infection. See illustration on page 28.

After the abortion is complete, you are carefully observed for bleeding or other problems. As soon as your vital signs — blood pressure, pulse and temperature — are normal, you'll be able to go home.

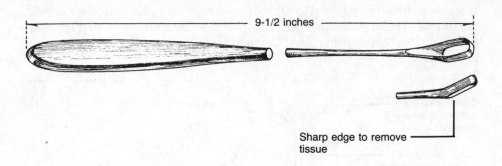

9-1/2 inches

Sharp edge to remove tissue

Sharp curette is instrument used to scrape the lining of the uterus in D&C.

You can expect vaginal bleeding similar to a menstrual period, which gradually disappears in about 1 week. Cramping similar to menstrual cramps may require aspirin or acetaminophen for relief. You may need to take ergotrate tablets every 4 to 6 hours to prevent excessive bleeding. Ergotrate causes your uterus to contract and may produce cramps.

SECOND TRIMESTER
The second trimester is over 12 weeks but less than 24 weeks. Abortions performed after the 12th week of pregnancy are more dangerous and more difficult to perform. This time period may be separated into 12 to 16 weeks, 16 to 20 weeks and 20 to 24 weeks. Methods used in these time periods vary according to the skill and experience of your doctor and your preference.

Most of these methods require hospitalization or a surgical-center setting. Laminaria may be used to start cervical dilatation in any or all of these methods. Anesthesia is required in *all* instances.

12 TO 16 WEEKS (GRAY ZONE)
This is called a *gray zone* because two different techniques can be used — medication or surgery.

Medication — Medication may be used to stimulate contractions of your uterus, causing it to expel its contents and abort your pregnancy. Even if medication is used, there is still no guarantee a D&C may not be necessary. If there is heavy bleeding or if all the uterine contents are not passed, curettage

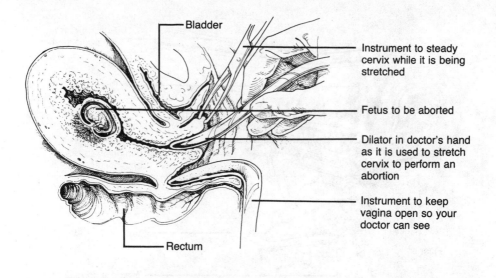

Bladder

Instrument to steady
cervix while it is being
stretched

Fetus to be aborted

Dilator in doctor's hand
as it is used to stretch
cervix to perform an
abortion

Instrument to keep
vagina open so your
doctor can see

Rectum

If medication alone does not expel all the contents of your uterus, the cervix can be
dilated using dilators.

is required to remove the remaining placental tissue. See illustration above.

Medication includes laminaria and substances that cause contractions of
your uterus, such as prostaglandin E2 vaginal suppositories or prostaglandin
F2 injections. Both stimulate contraction of your uterus.

Surgery — The surgical procedure is called a *dilatation and evacuation* or
D&E. General anesthesia and 1-day hospitalization are usually necessary.
After your cervix is dilated, a plastic suction curette and ovum forceps are
used to empty your uterus. The uterine lining is scraped with a sharp curette
to make sure all the tissue has been removed. See illustration on page 30.

Whether D&C or D&E is used, bleeding may be heavy, and you must be
watched closely. Anesthesia and pain medication are required because dilatation of your cervix is painful. For a D&E, general anesthesia may be used. Pain
medications are similar to those used in normal labor. Antibiotics may be
prescribed for any infection.

16 TO 24 WEEKS

At this stage, four methods for termination of pregnancy may be used:
- dilatation and evacuation (D&E). This is described above.
- instilling a salt solution into the amniotic sac.
- instilling a prostaglandin into the amniotic sac.
- hysterotomy.

Concentrated Salt Solution — Hypertonic salt is injected directly through
your abdominal wall and uterus into the amniotic sac. The salt solution causes

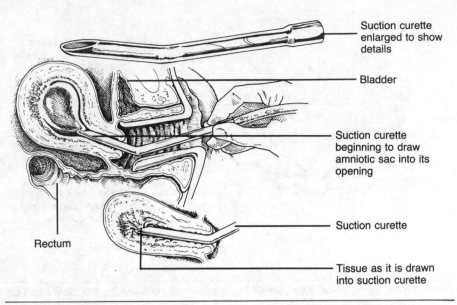

Suction curette enlarged to show details

Bladder

Suction curette beginning to draw amniotic sac into its opening

Suction curette

Rectum

Tissue as it is drawn into suction curette

Early abortion using suction curette. Tissue is being drawn into curette.

uterine contractions and eventual expulsion of the products of the pregnancy (the fetus and placenta).

Pain is due to contractions of the uterus and dilatation of the cervix. Medications may be prescribed to control pain, bleeding and infection.

Prostaglandin — Prostaglandin F2, injected into the amniotic sac, causes the uterus to contract and expel its contents.

Hysterotomy — This is the same as a Cesarean operation, except it is performed early (before the fetus can live on its own outside the uterus) for the purpose of abortion. See illustration on opposite page. General anesthesia is usually required, and surgery is done in an operating room. Epidural anesthesia may be used in some cases.

An incision is made through your lower abdomen, into the uterus. Through this incision, the fetus and placenta are removed. Three or more days of hospitalization and 3 to 4 weeks of recovery are average following a hysterotomy.

Hysterotomy is used as a *last* resort when other methods have failed or when your health is in jeopardy enough to require immediate termination of your pregnancy. When you've had previous Cesarean operations, hysterotomy is also the safest method of abortion at this stage of pregnancy.

In rare cases, a D&E may be done if you are 16 to 24 weeks along, but this may cause profuse hemorrhage, perforation of the uterus and other problems. Much depends on the skill, experience and judgment of your physician.

Hysterotomy is essentially the same as a Cesarean operation, but it is

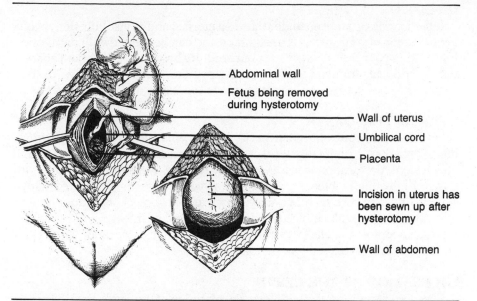

Abdominal wall

Fetus being removed
during hysterotomy

Wall of uterus

Umbilical cord

Placenta

Incision in uterus has
been sewn up after
hysterotomy

Wall of abdomen

Hysterotomy for late abortion is essentially the same as for Cesarean operation except the baby is too premature to survive.

performed before the baby is mature enough to survive. For more information on Cesarean operation, see the section that begins on page 149.

RISKS OF ABORTION

The risks of a properly performed abortion are minimal, although there may be some long-lasting consequences. The chances of dying after an abortion depend on the duration of your pregnancy and the method of abortion.

Death Rate	Method	Rate of Deaths
First trimester	Suction	1.6 per 100,000
Second trimester	Intra-amniotic instillation	22.9 per 100,000
	Hysterotomy	45 per 100,000

The death rate for normal labor and full-term delivery is 10.6 per 100,000.

Complications may be short-term or long-term and vary according to duration of your pregnancy and the method used to terminate it.

BLEEDING

Bleeding is usually light and lasts a few days to a week, but it can be sufficient to require blood transfusion with its attendant risks—AIDS and hepatitis—or even surgery to stop the bleeding. If your blood count was low before your abortion, this risk can be more serious.

INFECTION

Infection can occur even under the most sterile conditions. Infection involving the lining of your uterus is uncommon and can be treated with antibiotics. Infection of your tubes and ovaries may require hospitalization. If an abscess forms, surgical drainage may be necessary. You might even have to have some, or all, of your pelvic organs removed in cases of extreme abscess.

UTERINE PERFORATION

Perforation of your uterus can occur with any instrument used in performing an abortion. A pregnant uterus is very soft and can easily be perforated. If only a small perforation is made, you may require overnight observation for signs of infection or bleeding. However, if your uterus is perforated with a suction or sharp curette, other organs such as your bowel or bladder may be injured, causing profuse bleeding and the chance of infection.

Laparoscopy is usually performed first. If further exploration and repair are required, a laparotomy is performed.

LACERATION OF THE CERVIX

This occasionally occurs with forcible dilatation of the cervix resulting in an incompetent cervix. An incompetent cervix is unable to contain a pregnancy to full term.

ECTOPIC PREGNANCY

An ectopic pregnancy is possible in any pregnant patient, even one seeking an abortion. If tissue sent to a pathologist for exam doesn't show a pregnancy, the actual pregnancy products could still be in your uterus or an ectopic pregnancy could be present and undiagnosed. See page 187 for more information on ectopic pregnancy. If you have an IUD for contraception, you have a greater chance of having an ectopic pregnancy.

FERTILITY

After an abortion, fertility could be a problem. If adhesions (bands of scar tissue) form inside your uterus because of infection or if your uterus is scraped too vigorously, you may have difficulty conceiving and carrying future pregnancies. Adhesions may also block or distort your Fallopian tubes, decreasing fertility and increasing your risk of ectopic pregnancy.

Some abortions require stretching or dilatation of the cervix, and the cervix may be damaged. This results in an incompetent cervix that dilates too easily, will not contain a pregnancy or may dilate before the baby is mature enough to survive.

SPONTANEOUS ABORTION

According to some studies, the number of miscarriages increases in some women after they have an abortion.

PERINATAL MORBIDITY AND MORTALITY
Problems with damage to, or even death of, a fetus or infant increase if you have had a previous abortion. The exact reason for this is unclear, but figures are statistically significant.

EMOTIONAL PROBLEMS
You may experience emotional problems immediately after the abortion, or they may surface years later. Counseling before and after the procedure may be helpful in avoiding feelings of guilt or remorse.

Rh-SENSITIZATION
If you have Rh-negative blood and your husband is Rh-positive, you can become sensitized from an abortion. As an Rh-negative mother, if you have an Rh-positive baby, some Rh-positive blood from your baby may enter your system and cause antibodies to be formed.

These antibodies then attack your Rh-positive baby's blood cells in a subsequent pregnancy, causing serious or fatal complications in your unborn fetus. To protect against this, if you're Rh-negative and you have an abortion, you should receive an injection of Rh-immune globulin immediately following your abortion to prevent sensitization.

ADVANTAGES OF ABORTION
MEDICAL
If you have diabetes or heart disease, your health may be in serious jeopardy with pregnancy. When magnified by the changes due to pregnancy, medical problems can become life-threatening. In such instances, abortion may be considered life-saving.

If you have been exposed to agents or infections that can cause deformity or mental retardation of your baby, abortion may be the best solution. Some medication can damage an unborn fetus. The majority of medications fall into the category "no definite information" or "human studies have not been done." Abortion to avoid a malformed child sometimes becomes an emotional, moral issue with arguments colored by an anti- or pro-abortion stance. Each case must be considered individually.

Mental or emotional strain due to an unwanted pregnancy may be intense. Abortion may be the only relief from a situation you can't handle.

Since abortion became legal, the incidence of infection due to illegal abortions by unqualified physicians and others has decreased drastically. Women seeking abortion are now able to obtain it by qualified people in safe surroundings.

SOCIAL
One major cause of child abuse stems from an unwanted pregnancy. An unwanted infant may be blamed for financial problems or for depriving a woman of doing the things she wanted to do. Unwanted children may feel guilty and unhappy.

The cost for support through social service agencies for unwanted pregnancies is shared by everyone. Some pro-abortionists contend that the cost of an abortion is much less than the cost of care for an unwanted child.

DISADVANTAGES OF ABORTION

LACK OF CHILDREN TO ADOPT
Fifteen percent of all married couples are unable to have children. If abortion was not so easily available, there would probably be more children for adoption by childless couples.

COST
If abortion was not so readily available, people might be more careful about contraception. Contraception is less expensive than abortion.

MORAL ISSUES
Politically, ethically, socially, religiously and in many other ways, abortion is a volatile issue that is viewed differently by each person. Some feel it is their right to have an abortion. Others feel a baby has a right to life.

WHO OPERATES?

In most instances, a doctor who has specialized in obstetrics and gynecology will perform the abortion. In some areas, a general practitioner or family medicine specialist performs abortions.

It's important for the doctor who performs your abortion to be experienced and skilled in various techniques. Complications are fewer when an abortion is performed under ideal circumstances.

Some hospitals do not allow abortions, and some doctors do not perform them. But hospitals and doctors should be willing to refer you to the appropriate facility and personnel for best care.

DIAGNOSTIC TESTS BEFORE, DURING AND AFTER ABORTION

Tests likely to be performed prior to surgery include a pregnancy test, urinalysis, complete blood count, Rh-type determination, gonorrhea culture and a test for exposure to syphilis. If there is a question as to the length of your gestation, ultrasound may be used to help determine this and to dictate the best procedure to use.

If general anesthesia is required, blood-chemistry levels, urinalysis, blood typing and crossmatching for possible blood transfusion precede your surgery.

Regardless of the method used, the tissue removed is sent to the laboratory. The pathologist can verify the pregnancy has been removed (important in ectopic pregnancy) and rule out any abnormality, such as cancer of the endometrium or cancer of the placenta (very unlikely). This cannot be determined by examination with the naked eye and requires a pathologist's special microscopic exam.

With an early abortion, no special tests may be required. If there is significant blood loss, a blood count is done, along with a complete blood count if infection is suspected. Cultures from the cervix or uterus may be obtained if your doctor suspects an infection is present.

WHERE IS SURGERY PERFORMED?

Early abortions (up to 12 weeks of pregnancy) require minimal anesthesia. They are often performed in a doctor's office or a clinic.

When more anesthesia is needed, such as with D&E or D&C, the procedure is performed in an operating room in a hospital or outpatient surgery center. If you need to stay overnight after your abortion, your D&C is usually done in the hospital. If a hysterotomy is performed, it is always done in a hospital.

HOSPITALIZATION AND DURATION

This is determined by the method of abortion and the presence of complications.

12 WEEKS OR LESS
No Anesthesia — Abortions in the first trimester usually do not require an overnight stay in the hospital. Menstrual extraction or regulation requires less than half an hour to perform and is usually performed without anesthesia.

Following your abortion, you are observed for an hour or so to make certain bleeding is not excessive. Your blood pressure and pulse are carefully monitored.

If you have no problems or complications, you can go home. You will probably be able to resume normal activities later that day or the next day. Take it easy for the remainder of the day.
General Anesthesia — If general anesthesia is used, recovery time is longer. A D&C requires about 30 minutes in the operating room. You are in the recovery area about the same amount of time, under close observation. Until you're fully awake, alert and able to walk on your own, you will be under observation. This is usually about 1 to 2 hours of total recovery time. You'll need someone to drive you home.

Rest at home the remainder of the day. You'll probably be able to return to work or other activities the following day.

MORE THAN 12 WEEKS
D&E—The more advanced the pregnancy, the longer the operating time and recovery period. A D&E requires 30 to 60 minutes in the operating room. Recovery is another 60 minutes, and you may need to stay overnight in the hospital.

With D&E, blood loss can be significant. If there are no complications and your blood count is adequate, you may be allowed to return home after recovery in the recovery room. Before resuming routine activities at home, you'll probably want to rest for a couple of days. If complications occur, such as excessive blood loss or infection, your recovery will be longer.

Injection — If labor is induced by injection, it may require hours for delivery and will vary with each patient. For a first pregnancy, 12 or more hours is about average to expel a pregnancy. If you've had previous pregnancies, labor usually goes faster, with expulsion in 4 to 6 hours.

You will be checked for signs of blood loss, infection or other problems during your recovery period. When you're home, you'll probably want to rest for a couple of days before you resume your activities.

Hysterotomy — Hysterotomy is *always* performed in a hospital operating room. Operating time and recovery are similar to a Cesarean operation. Surgery requires from 1 to 1-1/2 hours. Average stay in the recovery room is about 1 hour, then you'll be taken to your hospital room. Average stay in the hospital is 4 days. Recovery at home is gradual and takes 4 to 6 weeks. Plan on taking at least 4 weeks off work.

ANESTHESIA

Anesthesia is usually not required for menstrual extraction because the cervix isn't dilated. Some doctors give analgesics, plus a tranquilizer, before the procedure to help you relax. Analgesics should be unnecessary after the first day of an early abortion and only rarely after a second trimester abortion.

Abortions performed after 6 weeks of pregnancy often require some anesthesia. If done in the doctor's office before 12 weeks of pregnancy, a local or paracervical block may be sufficient. Xylocaine injected around the cervix produces enough anesthesia to permit stretching of the cervix and scraping of the uterine lining. This type of anesthesia can be safely given in the doctor's office and is often used for a D&C in the hospital in combination with pain relievers or tranquilizers.

Although a D&C for abortion can be done with a paracervical block, it really depends on your pain tolerance and how far along your pregnancy is. If a D&C is performed in an operating room, general anesthesia is often administered. General anesthesia requires an anesthesiologist and means you are asleep during the entire procedure. Recovery from the anesthetic is longer and usually means a few extra hours in the hospital.

In special circumstances, such as allergy to general anesthesia, spinal or epidural anesthesia may be used for D&C. These methods require a skilled anesthesiologist.

For a D&E, general anesthesia (either gas or I.V.) is nearly always used because significant relaxation is required for surgery. A D&E often requires more dilatation of your cervix and more manipulation to remove all the products of your pregnancy. For the same reasons, spinal or epidural anesthesia *could* be used, but general anesthesia is preferred by most anesthesiologists.

Hysterotomy is major surgery and requires general anesthesia. Spinal and epidural methods usually are not used.

PROBABLE OUTCOME OF ABORTION

The aim of any abortion is to remove the products of conception — the outcome is termination of a pregnancy. The tissue removed at surgery is always sent to the lab to be certain the entire pregnancy has been removed.

POST-OPERATIVE CARE

Post-operative care after an abortion varies according to the type of procedure done. It's best to have someone drive you home, even after an early abortion. Rest the remainder of the day, and don't plan on returning to work for a day or two. You should be able to return to activities the following day, unless you have a D&E or a hysterotomy. Plan 2 or 3 days for a D&E and 2 to 4 weeks to recover and regain your strength after a hysterotomy.

It's normal to have some bleeding after an abortion. It may begin like a heavy menstrual period but gradually tapers off in the following hours and ceases after a few days. Use sanitary napkins for the first few days, if necessary. Bleeding should not persist or become heavier, and you should not pass clots or tissue after 3 days.

Your next period should start 4 to 6 weeks after an early abortion. The first period may be heavy or light, but it will return to normal over the next few months.

Use contraception as soon as you resume intercourse, unless you wish to conceive again. There is no medical reason you can't conceive (after waiting a few months), if you want to. If you don't want to begin another pregnancy, start birth-control pills or some other type of contraception immediately, in consultation with your doctor. If you choose to use an IUD, wait until after your next period to have it inserted. In the meantime, have your partner use condoms.

Intercourse may be resumed about 1 week after an abortion. If you continue to bleed, you may want to wait until your bleeding stops.

Pain after an abortion should not be severe enough to require more than aspirin or acetaminophen. Ergotrate tablets to control bleeding are occasionally needed. Ask your doctor about resuming medication for any other illnesses you have.

DIET

There is no special diet after an abortion. If you're anemic or have lost much blood with surgery, you may need vitamins with iron.

MISCONCEPTIONS ABOUT ABORTION

Abortions are safe, and there are no risks.

There *are* risks and complications that could influence your life permanently. Most abortions are safe and have no complications or significant aftereffects. However, the possible influence of future decreased fertility and impaired ability to carry a normal pregnancy are realities you can't ignore. If an abortion is to be performed, have it done as early as possible.

It doesn't matter when an abortion is done. It can be done in the office, and you don't have to go to the hospital.

This is not true, and our reasons have been covered in detail. Most doctors can perform abortions in their office or clinic up to 12 weeks of pregnancy. After 12 weeks, they may have to be done in the hospital.

I can have all the children I want later.

This is not always true. Infertility and inability to carry future pregnancies are not common following abortion, but they do occur occasionally.

ALTERNATIVES TO ABORTION

One alternative to abortion is to continue your pregnancy and have the baby. For some, this is not a consideration. For them, abortion is the only choice.

Those who argue against abortion claim if abortion were not so easily available, more women would continue their pregnancy, and there would be more adoptive children available for childless couples. On the other hand, there might be more unwanted children and more child abuse.

Research indicates certain chemicals may be available in the near future to provide a safe, non-surgical method of inducing early abortion. But regardless of the method, abortion is legal and safe in skilled hands. At present, women have a choice to continue their pregnancy or have an abortion.

CALL YOUR DOCTOR IF . . .

1. You have excessive bleeding (more than the heaviest day of your period).
2. You develop chills and fever.
3. You have persistent abdominal pain.
4. You develop any signs or symptoms that cause you concern.

QUESTIONS TO ASK YOUR DOCTOR

How long will the procedure take?

This may vary, but your doctor can give you an idea, depending partly on the duration of your pregnancy.

When can I return to work?
    Usually after a few days, but this depends on the type of work you do, how much blood was lost and your physical condition.

When can I resume having sex?
    Some doctors want you to wait at least a week, others a month. Discuss it with your doctor.

When can I use a tampon?
    Use napkins for about a week, then you can use internal tampons. Ask your doctor.

When can I go swimming?
    If it's an early abortion, you might use an internal tampon and swim after about a week. Many women prefer to wait until their checkup in 2 to 4 weeks. Ask your doctor.

Do I need RhoGam?
    If you are Rh-negative, you will be given Rh-immune globulin to prevent Rh-sensitivity.

Were there any problems or complications with the abortion?
    You may want a written report in case you move before your next pregnancy or before your next visit to a doctor.

Do I need to have my blood count checked?
    Ask this if you lost a lot of blood or if you had a low blood count before your abortion. Your doctor will probably have your blood count checked until it returns to normal.

Is this a procedure you do, or do I need a specialist?
    Some doctors prefer not to perform abortions. If they don't, they will refer you to a competent doctor who will do it.

If this is to be done in your office, will it be painful? Would it be better if I were admitted to the hospital and put to sleep?
    Discuss these questions frankly with your doctor. If you prefer to go to a hospital, tell him why.

Benign Breast Lumps

DEFINITION OF BENIGN BREAST LUMPS

A lump in the breast can be a single cyst (a tissue sac filled with fluid), a solid mass of tissue, a "lumpiness" throughout the breast (as found with fibrocystic disease) or many degrees in between. A cystic mass may become infected and form an abscess.

A lump can be cancerous (malignant) or non-cancerous (benign). A solid tumor may also be surrounded by, or encased in, fluid. See pages 10 and 12 for information on anatomy of a normal breast.

ABBREVIATIONS AND OTHER NAMES

Lumps can be called by many other names, including cyst, mass, tumor, abscess, Ca (abbreviation for carcinoma or cancer), induration, thickening, swelling, enlargement or growth.

PARTS OF BODY INVOLVED

Only the breasts are involved—see illustrations on opposite page—except with an abscess or infection when lymph glands under the arm may be swollen. If your cyst is cancerous, the cancer may spread elsewhere in the body. Spread usually begins with lymph glands under the arm and often spreads to the opposite breast. Cancer may also spread to bones, liver, lungs or the brain. It usually spreads to organs where there is a rich blood supply to support its rapid growth.

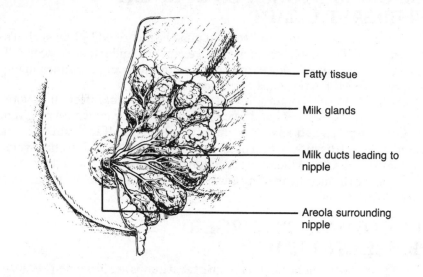

Fatty tissue

Milk glands

Milk ducts leading to nipple

Areola surrounding nipple

Front view of normal breast.

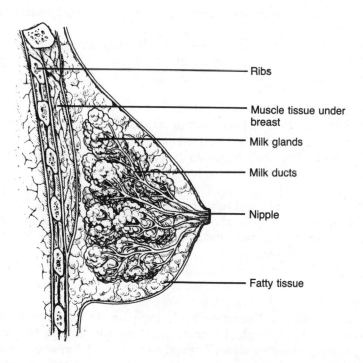

Ribs

Muscle tissue under breast

Milk glands

Milk ducts

Nipple

Fatty tissue

Side view of normal breast.

COMMON REASONS FOR SURGERY FOR BREAST LUMPS

If a mass is discovered in your breast, it must be identified by biopsy. If it's solid, part or all of the mass is removed and examined under a microscope. If the mass is cystic (contains fluid), the fluid is withdrawn and examined in the laboratory to check for presence of cancer cells.

The exception to surgery for a breast lump might be an infection in your breast with redness, soreness and swelling. In this case, you would be given antibiotics, hot packs and analgesics to relieve the pain. If the "lump" is an infection, it should disappear with treatment. Occasionally, an infection walls itself off into an *abscess,* which is a collection of infected tissue and fluid. The abscess must be drained by making an incision through the breast tissue and the wall of the abscess.

HOW COMMON IS SURGERY FOR BREAST LUMPS?

It's difficult to determine how common breast lumps are in women because many lumps are never seen by a doctor. Some cysts are temporary and disappear spontaneously. It's impossible to estimate the number of women seen in a doctor's office for breast lumps. Some estimates indicate up to 25% of all visits to a gynecologist are for breast lumps. These are statistics only from lumps that were biopsied and reported by their doctors. We really don't know how common the surgery is.

During childbearing years, about 2/3 of all breast lumps are benign. About half of the breast lumps are benign around menopause, and the majority of lumps occurring after menopause are cancerous.

DETECTION OF BREAST LUMPS

We know that 90% of all breast lumps are discovered by women themselves, not by their doctors. This places most of the responsibility on you to examine yourself thoroughly and often. Below are some suggestions to help you become proficient at examining your own breasts for lumps.

When?—Examine breasts once a month, preferably right after your menstrual period. Fullness and tenderness are no longer present.

Where?—Do it in the tub or shower because the "wet" feel appears to be more accurate. Fingers slide more easily over wet skin. Or do it lying down. See illustrations on opposite page.

How?—Use the palm of your hand and the flat part of your fingers as you examine each part of each breast with a circular, almost "massaging" motion. See illustration on opposite page.

Examine All of the Breast—Divide each breast into four quadrants—upper, lower, left and right. Examine each quadrant of each breast. Keep in mind the *upper-outer* quadrant (toward your armpit) is most likely to contain cancerous lumps.

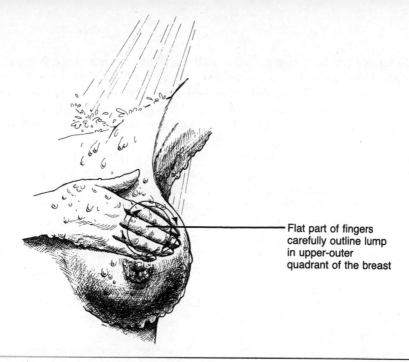

Flat part of fingers
carefully outline lump
in upper-outer
quadrant of the breast

During a shower is a good time to check breasts; touch is more sensitive when skin is wet. The most likely place for cancer is toward the armpit, in the upper-outer quadrant of the breast.

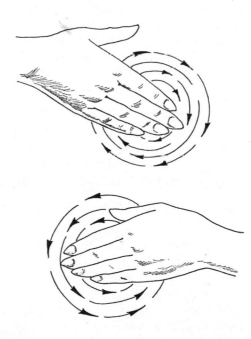

Rotation method of examining breast for lumps. Use flat part of fingers to examine breast, then reverse direction.

Normally you have some small lymph nodes under your arms. If glands are enlarged enough to be easily outlined, check with your doctor. There is a projection of breast tissue that extends under your armpit, which means any lump could be *breast* tissue, rather than an enlarged lymph gland. Infection also causes enlarged lymph nodes in your armpit, including infection anywhere within your arm or your breast.

Mirror Inspection — Stand or sit in front of a mirror, and inspect your breasts. Sometimes cancer causes an obvious bulge. Certain cancers retract tissue and may cause dimpling of the breast.

Look for any lesion that pulls, pushes or distorts the nipple in any way. Any chronically sore nipple that won't heal should be examined by your doctor for *Paget's disease* (cancer of the nipple and surrounding area.)

It's common for one breast to be larger than the other. But if breasts have appeared to be equal in size in the past and now show a discrepancy, check for the presence of a lump in the larger breast.

Examine your breasts when you're standing or sitting. When standing, you may discover something in your breasts that you didn't find when you checked them lying down.

Discharge — There should be no discharge from your nipple, especially a bloody or foul-smelling one. You should not be able to express any discharge from your nipple.

Practice Examining Breasts — Become familiar with the contour, texture and density of your breasts. If you think you feel a lump in one breast, check to see if there is a similar mass in the opposite breast. It's uncommon to have a solitary lump in *each* breast, especially in the same location.

Sleep on Stomach Occasionally — Many women discover a lump in their breast while sleeping face down. They say they feel as if they are lying on a marble or some other object. If you don't sleep on your stomach regularly, do it occasionally to see if you feel any unusual lumps.

WHICH LUMPS ARE IMPORTANT?

All lumps are important and must be diagnosed as to type and cause. If you feel a lump in your breast, don't try to second-guess it. Have it examined immediately by your doctor. The only way to reduce the high number of breast cancers that spread by the time they are detected is to discover them earlier!

MUST ALL LUMPS BE BIOPSIED?

If you discover a lump just before, or during, your menstrual period, watch it to see if it disappears as your period subsides. If it persists, even beyond one menstrual period, have it examined by your doctor.

If you discover a round, regular breast mass, it may be a cyst. Your doctor may decide to try to withdraw fluid from it with a syringe. If he withdraws fluid and the mass completely disappears, it was a cyst, and there is no cause for concern. Aspirated fluid is sent to the lab to be examined for any suspicious cells.

If your doctor can't aspirate any fluid or if there is still a mass, even though it's smaller after he has aspirated all the fluid possible, the remaining lump must be biopsied to rule out cancer. *Don't ignore any breast lump!*

FIBROADENOMA

A *fibroadenoma* is a common, benign breast lump that usually appears in young women and occasionally in adolescents. It's a painless, freely movable, firm tumor that may become large. These masses almost always appear in groups, and often they are found in both breasts. See illustration below.

Perhaps the greatest problem a fibroadenoma causes is your worry that it might be malignant. Because it occurs most often in younger women, and because cancer is rarely found in women under age 25, the worry is usually unwarranted. Under the age of 25, fibroadenomas can be safely observed and do not demand immediate biopsy.

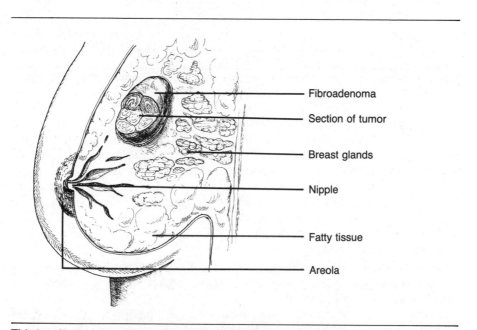

— Fibroadenoma

— Section of tumor

— Breast glands

— Nipple

— Fatty tissue

— Areola

This is a fibroadenoma, a benign tumor often found in young women between 15 and 30. It is not painful and will not turn into cancer.

FIBROCYSTIC DISEASE

Fibrocystic disease means your breast contains many cysts, which can keep you constantly worried about whether any of these "lumps" might be cancerous. See illustration on page 46. In fact, 35 to 50% of all women have fibrocystic disease at some time during their lives.

It is usually found in both breasts and is often in multiples; there may be countless cysts. Sometimes the condition produces a feeling of "lumpiness" in the breasts.

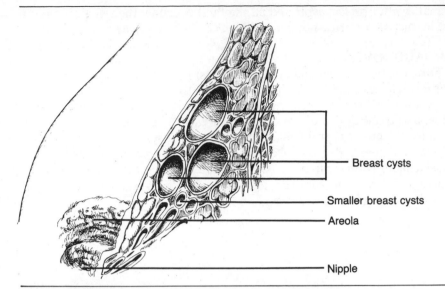

Breast cysts

Smaller breast cysts

Areola

Nipple

Fibrocystic disease of the breast. Cysts are multiple and vary in size. They often enlarge just before a menstrual period and become tender.

Typically, fibrocystic disease produces a dull, heavy pain. It often causes a feeling of fullness and tenderness that increases each month just before the onset of your menstrual period and becomes more tolerable after your period. Cysts become larger and more tender, then decrease in size and tenderness.

These cysts are often easy to locate and outline with your fingers. They are tender to the touch. Deeper clusters of cysts are more worrisome and are more likely to be biopsied, often repeatedly. Usually larger breast cysts can be aspirated with a syringe and needle, but deeper cysts lead to scarred breasts from repeated biopsies.

In some cases, the problem becomes so worrisome that all breast tissue is removed, leaving the skin intact. An artificial breast, made of a silicone-gel envelope, is inserted in its place.

Certain types of fibrocystic disease have no relationship to breast cancer; others are suspect. It requires all your doctor's skill and sometimes several diagnostic methods to be certain.

INTRADUCTAL PAPILLOMA

Another small, benign tumor is called an *intraductal papilloma.* It is found in a milk duct and can produce a clear, milky or bloody discharge from your nipple. Usually, no tumor mass is found.

Only rarely are these tumor masses cancerous, but they are of concern to you. Discharge from your breast should be examined microscopically for cancer cells. A mammogram should also be done.

If your breast discharge persists, the papilloma must be removed because of its nuisance factor. But these tumors are almost always benign.

DUCTAL ECTASIA

Ectasia means blocked, stretched, swollen or dilated breast ducts. Ductal ectasia is characterized by a sticky, multicolored discharge from your nipple that causes burning and itching around the nipple and areola.

Along with a drawing, dull pain, you can often feel tender, tubular swellings under the areola. If these swellings increase in size, they may be confused with cancer, although they are definitely benign.

In some cases, all the breast tissue is removed, leaving the skin intact. A silicone-gel envelope is inserted in its place.

FUNCTIONS INVOLVED IN SURGERY FOR BREAST LUMPS

MILK PRODUCTION AND INFECTION OF BREAST

Your breast has an amazing ability to retain its function to produce milk, even if it's infected. For Nature's own reasons, you can usually continue to nurse your baby from an infected breast without the milk or your baby suffering any ill effects.

MILK PRODUCTION AND CANCER OF BREAST

Even a breast that contains cancer, often unknown to you and undiagnosed by your doctor, supplies milk for your baby. There is no evidence cancer is transmitted to your baby, although if cancer is diagnosed, you may be asked to discontinue nursing and begin treatment.

MILK PRODUCTION WHEN ONE BREAST HAS BEEN REMOVED

If a large amount of your breast tissue is removed, it could result in some decrease in the amount of milk you produce. But Nature compensates even for the complete loss of one breast by increasing milk production in the other breast.

MILK PRODUCTION AND BREAST PROTHESIS

There are instances in which all your breast tissue must be removed because of fibrocystic disease; a prosthesis is inserted under the skin of your breast. You cannot produce milk when there is no breast tissue.

A radical dissection of your breast, such as with cancer of the breast, leaves no breast tissue to produce milk. If a prosthesis is inserted for cosmetic reasons, it's usually inserted *under* your breast tissue and does not alter the ability of your breast to produce milk. Breast reduction surgery decreases the amount of breast tissue, but your breast has the ability to produce sufficient milk to nurse your baby.

HOW SURGERY FOR BREAST LUMPS IS PERFORMED

NEEDLE ASPIRATION OF CYSTS

This can be done in a doctor's office, often with only a small amount of local anesthetic. If the mass disappears after withdrawal of the fluid, your problem is solved. See illustration below.

If a mass is still present, it may have to be biopsied. But the doctor first probes with the needle to make certain it isn't another cyst. If the fluid is blood-tinged, it is more suspicious because it may also contain cancer cells from a cancer in the cyst.

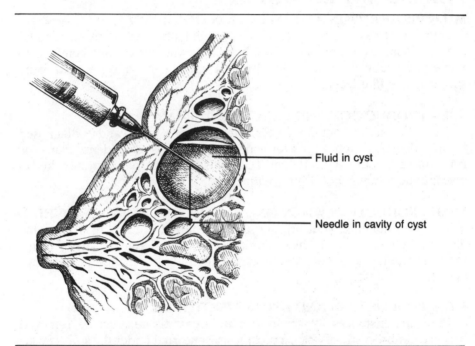

Fluid in cyst

Needle in cavity of cyst

Withdrawal of fluid from breast cyst is a simple way to make a diagnosis. If mass completely disappears after withdrawal of fluid, the problem is solved. If there is still a mass, it must be biopsied.

NEEDLE BIOPSY OF SOLID TUMOR

A special large biopsy needle is inserted into your breast lump. See illustration on opposite page. As the sleeve is advanced over the needle, tissue is trapped and removed for examination and diagnosis in the lab.

BIOPSY BY REMOVING LUMP

In performing this biopsy, an attempt is made to remove the entire lump. Unless the tumor is too far removed from your nipple, a semicircular incision is made in the outer edge of the areola. The mass is cut free, and the incision is

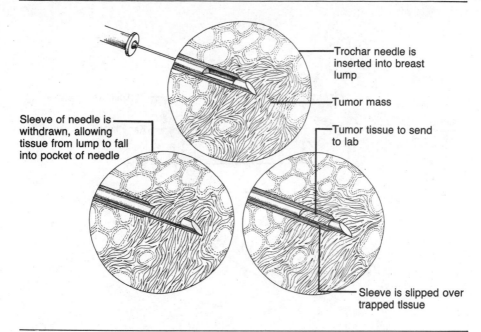

Trochar needle is inserted into breast lump

Tumor mass

Sleeve of needle is withdrawn, allowing tissue from lump to fall into pocket of needle

Tumor tissue to send to lab

Sleeve is slipped over trapped tissue

Detailed view of method of removing breast tissue from breast lump for examination.

closed. See illustration on page 50. The incision is compressed with pressure bandages for several hours after surgery.

The advantage of an incision that follows the border of the areola is that your scar is scarcely visible. Another name for this operation is *lumpectomy*.

BIOPSY BY REMOVING PART OF LUMP
This operation is the same as the biopsy described above, except only a *piece* of the lump is removed for biopsy. This type of biopsy is done when it seems certain your tumor is malignant or if for some other reason it cannot be removed completely in the office or in outpatient surgery.

RISKS OF SURGERY FOR BREAST LUMPS
LOW RISK OF BIOPSY
The risk in surgery of a biopsy or complete removal of breast lumps is very low. A *radical mastectomy* — removal of the breast with wide dissection that includes underlying muscles, overlying skin, removal of lymph nodes under the arm and fatty tissue — is massive and carries significant risks of complications in up to 50% of all cases.

This operation is rapidly being replaced by simple lumpectomy and postoperative radiation. Results with a radical operation have always been severe, hazardous, disabling and disfiguring. By contrast, a lumpectomy is relatively simple, safe and, in many instances, may be as effective for cure as the radical approach when followed by radiation.

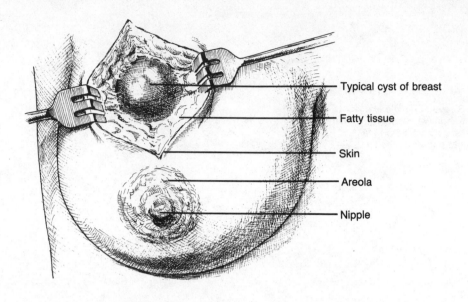

Typical cyst of breast

Fatty tissue

Skin

Areola

Nipple

Typical cyst of the breast, which is benign. It is often seen in fibrocystic disease of the breast.

RISK OF CANCER

The true risk lies not in the surgery but what is found at surgery. Whether your lesion is benign or malignant, immediate healing and recovery seem uneventful. If your lump is malignant, further treatment depends on the type of cancer, whether it can be destroyed by X-ray and whether it has spread to other parts of the body and how extensively.

The risk lies in the possibility and extent of malignancy. Figures vary depending on the population, but 1 in 11 women in the United States develops breast cancer in her lifetime. The majority of tumors are discovered by women themselves. Doctors uncover only 10% of all breast cancers. Of all the major cancers in women (except for lung cancer) only breast cancer has had *no* decrease in mortality in the past 50 years.

When we study these statistics, we quickly realize our greatest hope lies in diagnosing breast cancer earlier. At present, more than 50% of breast cancers have spread beyond local limits by the time they are discovered. This points up the importance and urgency of finding ways to diagnose breast cancer earlier.

CERTAIN WOMEN ARE MORE LIKELY
TO DEVELOP BREAST CANCER

Certain women are more likely to develop breast cancer. If you have had *no* children, you're more likely to have breast cancer. The same applies if you have your first child after age 27. If you have your first child after age 34, you are 4 times as prone to have breast cancer.

Breast-feeding was thought to protect women against breast cancer. Actually, it gives protection *only* if you nurse your baby for over 36 months.

Heredity is a factor in breast cancer. Breast cancer in your mother or sister increases your relative risk 3 times. This risk increases to 5 times if both your mother and your grandmother had breast cancer.

Obesity is thought to increase the risk of breast cancer. When combined with high blood pressure and diabetes, obesity increases the risk 3 times.

In most studies conducted since 1970, it has been concluded that there is no relationship between estrogen and breast cancer, whether the hormone is taken before, during or after menopause, and whether given alone or in combination with other drugs, such as birth-control pills. There is some evidence oral contraceptives may even have a slight *protective* benefit in reducing the risk of breast cancer. One study indicates if oral contraceptives are used for more than 4 years, they may *reduce* your risk of breast cancer by as much as 50%.

If you have had cancer in one breast, you are 5 times as likely to develop cancer in your other breast. Check yourself frequently and have regular exams by your physician, along with mammography.

If you have significant fibrocystic disease of the breast, you are 2 to 4 times more likely to develop cancer of your breast, although not in the cysts. Check your breasts regularly and have regular exams.

MAMMOGRAPHY

At any age, when clinical findings indicate a reasonable suspicion of cancer, you should have a mammogram. Cancer of the breast is infrequent under the age of 35, so you don't need to have mammography unless there is a specific and strong indication of cancer. There is some relationship between cancer and X-ray, so it is wise to avoid exposure to X-ray unless definitely necessary.

Between 35 and 40, have a *baseline* mammogram, with subsequent mammograms to indicate any subtle changes that suggest cancer. There is some difference of opinion among doctors regarding the need or propriety for this baseline mammogram.

Have periodic mammograms if you are at a high risk for cancer of the breast, such as having female relatives with cancer.

The National Cancer Institute suggests that any woman over the age of 50 should have annual or periodic mammograms, even if there are no symptoms. If you had an early onset of menstruation and a late menopause, your risk of getting breast cancer is greater.

ADVANTAGES OF SURGERY
FOR BREAST LUMPS

Most women would rather have several biopsies that showed only a benign mass than to miss the one cancerous mass that could be successfully treated if biopsied early. Your cure rate soars from 46 to over 80% if cancer of the breast is discovered early, *before* it has time to spread.

DISADVANTAGES OF SURGERY
FOR BREAST LUMPS

There are no disadvantages to having a biopsy of your breast. Regardless of the number of benign biopsies, it's worth it to avoid the tragedy of cancer in a breast lump that is observed instead of biopsied. The only possible exception is when you have fibrocystic disease with multiple cysts in each breast. Even these lumps must be aspirated to remove the fluid and make certain no residual mass is present.

On *rare* occasions, if cysts become too numerous, too deep in your breast to examine or too worrisome, it may become necessary to remove all your breast tissue, leaving the skin intact. The diseased breast tissue can be replaced with a silicone-gel implant. This dispels the worry, avoids frequent biopsies and does not disfigure the contour of your breast. This is called *prophylactic subcutaneous mastectomy*. However, this procedure performed on a fibrocystic breast simply to remove the threat of cancer is condemned as unwarranted and unnecessary surgery. If your doctor suggests this operation, obtain a second opinion from a breast center or cancer specialist.

WHO OPERATES?

If a simple biopsy or breast aspiration is anticipated, your family physician, obstetrician or general surgeon may perform the operation. The same might apply for a simple lumpectomy.

If more radical treatment is needed, a general surgeon usually performs the surgery. If all the breast tissue is to be removed because of chronic fibrocystic disease and a prosthesis inserted, a plastic surgeon is the person most qualified to perform your surgery. Before having such an operation, get a second opinion.

DIAGNOSTIC TESTS BEFORE, DURING
AND AFTER SURGERY FOR BREAST LUMPS

There are ways to tell if you have cancer earlier than feeling a lump. The procedure is called *screening for breast cancer*. It is estimated that approximately 25% of all women who see a physician do so because of concern about a breast mass or some other problem with their breasts. About 90% of all breast cancers are initially discovered by women.

By the time a cancer is large enough to be discovered by a woman, enough of the cancer may have spread so only about 50% of the women can hope for a

5-year cure. We must discover breast cancer *before* you can feel it if we hope to improve cure rates.

Statistically, detection of "preclinical" breast cancer by various screening methods can result in 5- and 10-year survival rates in over 90% of the cases.

There are more than a dozen different methods of examining breasts other than by "feeling" or palpitation during a physical exam. Every method cannot, and should not, be used on every woman. Let's discuss them and how they apply to you.

HEAT SENSING TECHNIQUES

The human body gives off electromagnetic waves within the infrared spectrum. These waves are influenced by the temperature of your tissues. Irritated, infected tissue gives off more heat, and so does tissue that contains cancer. Radiation of heat can be measured and recorded like we record an X-ray image. There are various methods, but we'll call all of them *thermography*.

The trouble with thermography in detecting early cancers is it yields too many false-positives and false-negatives. Hopefully, use of the computer may make this method more accurate. At present, we can't rely on thermography when used alone. But one study showed the accuracy of X-ray mammography is increased when combined with thermography on the same patient at the same time.

ULTRASOUND MAMMOGRAPHY

Ultrasound is sound waves "echoed off" tissue of your breast; these sound waves can be recorded. We feel there is little risk with ultrasonography, but its usefulness in screening for breast cancer is minimal at this time. It can help detect benign cysts in your breast that can be drained to rule out breast cancer, but it has very limited use.

LIGHT TRANSMISSION

The medical term is *diaphanography,* but it means shining a very intense, cool light through your breast and noting the shadow it casts. This light can be recorded on film. Light transmission is a helpful tool, but it is not very accurate when compared with X-ray mammography.

NUCLEAR MAGNETIC RESONANCE

Something to watch in the future is *nuclear magnetic resonance* (NMR), also called *nuclear magnetic imaging* (NMI). To simplify the explanation, an entire room is converted into a huge magnet. You are placed in the room, and radiowaves are directed toward the magnetic field. The nuclei of your tissues align themselves temporarily, according to the magnetic field, and form an image that can be recorded. Breast tumors show up well. This is proving to be an effective way to distinguish harmless lumps from those that must be removed.

Equipment for this type of testing costs from half a million dollars to several million dollars. But this method, which in time will become less expensive, simpler and more available, promises to be an extremely sensitive method for early detection of breast cancer.

WHICH IS BEST SCREENING METHOD FOR EARLY DETECTION OF BREAST CANCER?

We often combine methods and variations in methods, but at present, *X-ray mammography* is our best screening tool. In fact, one large study done in 1963 showed the fatality rate from breast cancer was reduced by as much as 33% by mammographic screening. Techniques have improved since then, and mortality rates could be reduced even more using these improvements.

WHO SHOULD HAVE A MAMMOGRAM AND HOW OFTEN?

X-ray mammography offers excellent help in early diagnosis, but its use is individualized. Mammography involves radiation, so it should not be used routinely in young women. It is now recommended annually for asymptomatic women over 50 years of age, with a baseline mammogram done between the ages of 35 and 40. Also, women between the ages of 40 and 50 should have an exam every 2 years; some doctors and researchers recommend it be done every year.

Recommendations are different for younger women with a family history of breast cancer or other high risk factors, as previously discussed. Talk about your concerns with your doctor.

All suspicious lesions that show up on mammograms should be biopsied. Some may be as small as a cantaloupe seed. Other mammograms may show only calcification. Suspicious lesions that persist on mammograms must be biopsied, even though they are probably benign.

This practice may lead to more biopsies of benign lesions, but malignant lesions will be discovered earlier. Your life could be saved by these precautions.

TO INCREASE YOUR CHANCE OF SURVIVAL

Learn how to examine yourself for breast lumps. Make a habit of checking yourself at least once a month, right after your menstrual period.

If you have breast cancer in your immediate family, follow all these recommendations and have a mammogram on a routine basis, depending on your age. The development of nuclear magnetic imaging probably will be a great help in the near future for high-risk women.

If you are over 25, any lump in your breast should be watched unless due to obvious infection, such as a breast abscess. The lump should be biopsied. At the longest, observe it to see if it persists through one menstrual period.

Any mass believed to be a cyst should be aspirated first. If it disappears completely after draining, your problem is solved. If it can't be aspirated, or if part of the lump persists after draining, it should be biopsied as soon as possible.

EXAMINING TISSUE REMOVED FROM BREAST

All tissue removed at surgery should be examined, even if your doctor *thinks* it looks benign. Microscopic examination by a pathologist is required.

A biopsy can be performed in your doctor's office without risk. He will send the tissue to the lab for examination.

WHERE IS SURGERY PERFORMED?

Simple aspiration can be performed in your doctor's office with complete safety. It requires only a small injection of local anesthetic, such as xylocaine. Many physicians perform minor surgery in their offices, and the removal of breast lumps can be done safely. Any surgery beyond this, such as complete removal of all breast tissue, insertion of implants or any other major surgery, requires more equipment and hospitalization.

Most emergency rooms are equipped to aspirate cysts and remove lumps from your breast. Before a radical mastectomy is performed, a complete paraffin exam, also called *permanent fixation and staining,* is done on the biopsied tissue instead of having a frozen biopsy specimen taken. Paraffin exam requires more time, but it is more accurate than a frozen biopsy.

HOSPITALIZATION AND DURATION

Most breast biopsies are outpatient procedures. Even lumpectomies can be performed in a doctor's office, emergency room or in an outpatient surgery department.

It takes only a few minutes in surgery to aspirate a cyst. A biopsy can take about 30 minutes. It takes about 1 hour for a lumpectomy. Removal of all breast tissue and insertion of a breast prosthesis may require 1-1/2 hours or more.

Recovery depends on the amount of sedation or anesthetic you have and the extent of your surgery. Usually your doctor likes to observe you to make certain there is no post-operative hemorrhage in your breast. He may place considerable padding, with pressure, over your breast, along with an elastic adhesive bandage to maintain that pressure. Average recovery-room time is about 1 hour.

Only a radical mastectomy requires a stay in the hospital. Hospital stays average 5 to 7 days.

ANESTHESIA

Only rarely is anything other than local anesthesia required for biopsy of a breast lump. If the surgeon feels relatively certain of spread of cancer to the armpit, and if he prefers a radical mastectomy to lumpectomy and radiation, he will make preparations for a longer procedure. It will require general anesthesia and blood for transfusions.

PROBABLE OUTCOME OF SURGERY
FOR BREAST LUMPS

There is no absolute way your doctor can be certain whether or not your breast lump is malignant without a biopsy. Your physician can suspect malignancy and feel relatively certain the lump is malignant, but he still must biopsy the lump and have it examined under a microscope.

Other than a little scarring, excision of a benign lump causes no aftereffects. Aspiration of a cyst has no aftereffect either. A malignant tumor is usually more widely dissected, so there may be more scarring and tenderness after surgery.

Survival with cancer of the breast depends on whether it has spread when discovered and the type of cancer it is. In general, you can expect an 84% 5-year cure rate if your cancer has not spread beyond the initial site. If spread has occurred, the survival rate drops to about 46%.

POST-OPERATIVE CARE

The only post-operative care you'll need after biopsy or lumpectomy is to keep compression on the incision to avoid hemorrhage. Keep movement to a minimum for a couple of days until your incision has had a chance to heal.

Inspection of your incision by your doctor will detect any infection so treatment can be started. Post-operative infection, if any, is easily controlled with antibiotics.

DIET

There is no special diet after removal of a breast lump. No special diet or fasting is necessary for minor surgery. General anesthesia is not used, so you should not experience nausea or gastric upset. There is a rare chance you'll be sensitive to the local anesthetic used.

If general anesthesia is necessary, you'll be asked to refrain from food and drink for 8 to 12 hours before surgery.

MISCONCEPTIONS ABOUT SURGERY
FOR BREAST LUMPS

Cutting into a tumor makes it spread.
It has never been proved that biopsy caused a tumor to spread or caused it to grow faster. By contrast, if you fail to biopsy the breast lump and choose to observe it or ignore it, it could spread beyond the point of cure.

Tumors come and go.
Breasts become fuller and more congested just before a menstrual period and certain armpit glands also become larger. But if these lumps do not completely disappear after *one* menstrual period, they should be biopsied. Any lump that can be felt by your examining hand (or the doctor's) should be aspirated or biopsied if you are over 25 years old.

Cutting the breast will make nursing impossible.
Cuts heal by scarring, but the amount of scarring due to a biopsy is not enough to interfere with nursing. If you were able to nurse your babies before you had a biopsy, you'll be able to nurse any babies you have after the biopsy.

Having breast augmentation makes it impossible to detect breast lumps.
A prosthesis inserted between the breast tissue and muscle underlying the breast causes breast tissue to be spread or flattened more than usual. As a result, it should be *easier* to examine your breast for lumps *after* augmentation.

ALTERNATIVES TO SURGERY FOR BREAST LUMPS

A breast lump due to inflammation or infection can be treated with antibiotics and usually subsides within a day or two. If the infection becomes an abscess, it may be necessary to cut and drain it.

A cystic mass can be aspirated. But if a mass remains after aspiration, it must be biopsied.

If your lump is small enough, it can be removed completely when it is biopsied. If it's benign, treatment is completed by the procedure. If malignant and the complete tumor mass is removed, the only additional treatment is radiation therapy.

The only situation in which observation of breast lumps is permissible is when your lump is believed to be due to premenstrual engorgement. The lump may be observed for one menstrual period, but if it is still present after that time, it should be biopsied.

CALL YOUR DOCTOR IF . . .

1. You discover a lump in either breast or under either arm.
2. You have persistent pain in one small area of a breast.
3. You notice a puckered area in either breast.
4. You notice a different contour to either breast.
5. You have a bloody discharge from your nipple.
6. You have a persistent puslike or foul-smelling discharge from either nipple.

QUESTIONS TO ASK YOUR DOCTOR

Are you going to biopsy the tumor mass or remove it completely? Why?
This helps you understand if you need another operation to remove your lump.

Are you going to take a frozen section of the biopsy or have a more thorough examination of the tissue, even though it takes longer? Will you wait for the final result before anything more is done?

There are some instances when a frozen biopsy section is necessary, but final diagnosis and treatment should be based on a firm, accurate diagnosis. If it's necessary to wait for this definite diagnosis to be certain, your doctor may elect to depend on a paraffin exam, which requires a few days.

Do you intend to perform only a lumpectomy if the lump is malignant, or do you intend to perform a radical mastectomy?

Most evidence shows lumpectomy, followed by radiation therapy, obtains results that are as good as a radical mastectomy. If your doctor insists on a radical mastectomy, consider a second opinion.

Do you think my lump could be a cyst? Are you going to aspirate the fluid first to see if the mass disappears?

If any of the mass persists after aspiration, a biopsy of the mass is needed to make certain there is no cancer underlying the cyst.

Will you explain to me what the biopsy shows? Is it malignant?

This is a forthright question. It's better to know the truth and deal with it.

What is the course of the disease from here? How soon do we begin therapy? Will it make me ill?

These are some of the questions that may cross your mind. You may have many more. You have a right to know what was found, what further treatment you require and what your outlook is. Don't be afraid to ask these questions. Your doctor will appreciate talking honestly with you.

Benign Ovarian Tumors

DEFINITION OF BENIGN OVARIAN TUMORS

The ovary has the potential of producing more different types of cancer than any other gland or organ of the body. The adult ovary contains "embryonic remnants," which are cells from the earliest stages of life. They are capable of changing into various types of tumors. The monthly growth, enlargement and subsequent regression of cells in the ovary, along with your menstrual cycle, account for most benign growths of the ovaries.

ABBREVIATIONS AND OTHER NAMES

Cyst, mass, functional cyst, follicle cyst, corpus luteum cyst, theca lutein cyst, polycystic ovaries, endometrioma, Stein-Leventhal Syndrome, SLS and tumors are some names for benign ovarian tumors.

PARTS OF BODY INVOLVED

All your female organs may be involved in benign ovarian tumors. Your ovaries lie adjacent to the Fallopian tubes and uterus, so any ovarian enlargement may shift the position of these organs. Rupture of ovarian cysts, ovarian adhesions or ovarian scar tissue may also extend to your tubes and uterus. Ovarian tumors may extend to, and involve, your bowel and bladder, causing pain or malfunction.

Pain due to ovarian tumors may also affect you because it prevents you from performing normal functions and activities. Besides pain, menstrual periods may be irregular, fertility can be affected and intercourse may be painful. Many parts of your body are affected by ovarian tumors.

COMMON REASONS FOR SURGERY FOR BENIGN OVARIAN TUMORS

The treatment of ovarian tumors is primarily surgical to relieve pain or bleeding and exclude malignancy. The likelihood of cancer in ovarian growths is between 15 and 25%. It is even higher in children and in women who are post-menopausal. In fact, an ovarian mass in a child or post-menopausal woman is considered malignant until proven otherwise.

Many enlargements of the ovaries simply represent an exaggeration of normal cystic response of your ovary to regular monthly changes of normal body functions. For example, a tiny cyst may be formed around an egg that is released from your ovaries. The cyst might keep growing. These changes are called *functional cystic enlargements* and are non-cancerous. They do not always require surgery because they usually rupture or resolve spontaneously, and their fluid is absorbed by the body, so they "cure" themselves.

Surgery is often determined by the size of the mass. If a cyst is larger than 5 to 6 centimeters (a new tennis ball has a diameter of about 7 centimeters), surgery is probably necessary.

In addition to size, surgery is often performed because of pain. Immediate, severe pain may be due to "stretching" of the ovary as the cyst enlarges. The enlargement may be due to increasing fluid or from bleeding into the cyst.

If a cyst ruptures, it can cause severe pain similar to a ruptured tubal pregnancy. The sudden pain is a result of a spill of the contents of the cyst, whether blood or fluid, into your abdomen, which irritates your bowel and peritoneum.

If an ovarian mass becomes twisted, it can also cause severe pain if the twisting shuts off blood supply to your ovary. Similar pain results from appendicitis, diverticulitis, tubal pregnancy and pelvic inflammatory disease. Often the only way to diagnose the problem is by surgery. Laparoscopy is often used to confirm the diagnosis and to avoid major surgery if possible. For more information on laparoscopy, see page 237.

Pain from a gradually enlarging ovarian mass may be more chronic in nature. If an ovary enlarges each month in cadence with your menstrual period, then subsides, pain may wax and wane. If your ovary is bound by adhesions from infections or previous surgery, even small changes in position can cause severe pain.

Fertility may be lessened by ovarian cysts because often no egg is produced. Polycystic ovaries are also a cause of anovulation and decreased fertility.

Another urgent reason for surgery on ovarian tumors is to exclude malignancy. Any ovarian mass in a post-menopausal woman should be considered cancerous until proven otherwise. This can't be determined with laboratory tests; it requires surgical removal and examination under a microscope. This procedure is also followed for girls under 16 years of age. Malignancy is also found in women of other ages, but ovarian enlargements in women between 16 and 50 are usually functional and benign.

FOLLICLE CYSTS

These cysts occur when you fail to give off an egg, but the tissue around the egg keeps growing until it becomes a cyst. These cysts are usually less than 2 inches in diameter and contain straw-colored fluid. They rarely cause symptoms unless they become large enough to cause pressure or if they bleed or rupture. See illustration below.

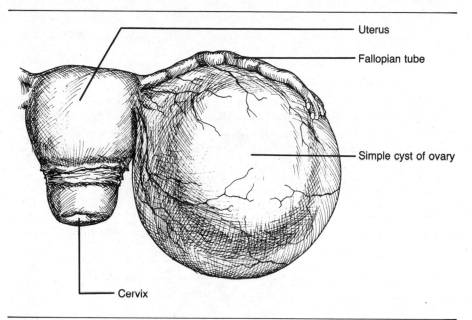

Uterus

Fallopian tube

Simple cyst of ovary

Cervix

Simple cyst of the ovary may rupture by itself and effect a cure. These cysts often rupture when your doctor examines you.

A corpus luteum cyst usually occurs after ovulation but rarely causes symptoms. Normally the area in your ovary that surrounds the egg regresses after ovulation. But when a cyst forms, instead of regression, fluid collects and distends your ovary. Corpus luteum cysts imitate ectopic pregnancy because they produce irregular bleeding or no period at all. The cyst may be mistaken for a pregnancy in the Fallopian tube.

Theca lutein cysts result from the hormone produced in pregnancy — the same hormone that gives a positive pregnancy test. Fertility drugs can cause a "batch" of these cysts in both ovaries. If they become larger than 8 centimeters in diameter, they may produce pain or pressure.

POLYCYSTIC OVARIES

This condition is also called *Stein-Leventhal Syndrome.* It is the result of missed periods (anovulation) and usually involves both ovaries. It occurs most often in young girls and adolescents. It may cause infertility and irregular bleeding. Ovaries are enlarged, have a thick outer coating (capsule) and are often oval. They are full of cysts from lack of periods with continual secretion of hormones that can cause masculinization—growth of hair on the face and body.

ENDOMETRIAL CYSTS

This type of cyst is also called *endometrioma* and may occur in the ovary. It is a collection of endometrial tissue on the ovary that forms a cyst or an enlargement of the ovary.

OTHER OVARIAN TUMORS

There are other types of benign ovarian tumors and other ovarian tumors that are neoplastic. Some examples include germinal inclusion cysts, which can become cancerous, and serous cystadenomas, which are common benign ovarian tumors (15 to 23.5% of all benign ovarian tumors). Often they occur on both sides, and they are usually benign but may become malignant. Mucinous cystadenomas are rarely malignant and may occur during pregnancy. See illustration below.

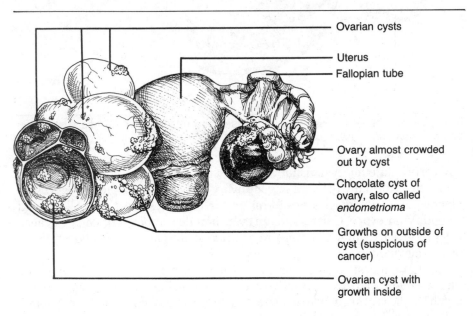

Composite shows endometrial cyst (chocolate cyst) on one side and many cysts on the other side, with growths on the inside and outside of the cyst. When there are growths on the outside of the cyst, it is more suspicious of cancer.

Cystadenofibromas are a slightly different form of serous cystadenomas. Sex-chord tumors are hormone-producing lesions. Granulosa cell tumors produce hormones that cause masculinization; 1/3 are malignant. Theca cell tumors produce estrogen and cause a feminizing effect. A few cause masculinization, but they are rarely malignant.

Connective tissue tumors can become quite large. Ovarian fibroma occurs primarily in women in their 40s. Benign cystic teratomas (dermoids) are fairly common and make up 18 to 25% of all ovarian tumors. These tumors can occur at any age and are almost always benign. It is not known why, but these tumors may contain hair, teeth or bone. See illustration below. Struma ovarii contain thyroid tissue that can produce the thyroid hormone. Gonadoblastomas are nearly always benign, but if they become malignant they are *very* malignant.

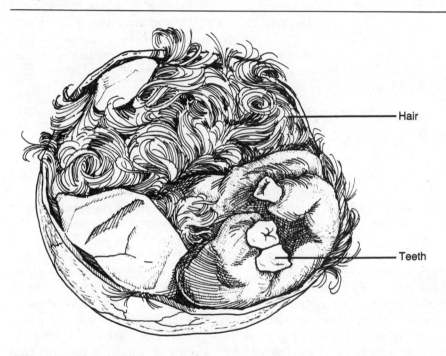

Dermoid cyst of ovary is a benign cyst that has various tissues in it, such as teeth and hair. It can become cancerous.

Tumors of uncertain origin include brenner tumors, which are benign and rare. Adrenal-rest tumors cause masculinizing effects, and 21% of them are malignant. The average age of women affected by this tumor is 32 years. The above descriptions and terms are greatly simplified and give only an indication of the complex nature of the subject of ovarian tumors.

HOW COMMON IS SURGERY
FOR BENIGN OVARIAN TUMORS?

Surgery for ovarian tumors is most common during your reproductive years — age 18 to 40. When any pelvic mass is found, other possibilities must be considered, such as conditions involving bowel tumors or tumors of the uterus. Appendicitis, ectopic pregnancy, pelvic infections and other conditions can cause the same acute abdominal pain that is produced by a ruptured or twisted ovarian mass.

When a pelvic mass is found on routine pelvic exam, even without symptoms, it cannot be ignored. Sometimes the only way to make the diagnosis is with surgery. Laparoscopy and ultrasound may be very helpful in evaluating these masses.

Ovarian tumors discovered in a young child or in a post-menopausal woman should be considered malignant until proven otherwise. This usually requires surgical exploration. However, ovarian tumors have been discovered in women of all ages, including intrauterine female fetuses. Discovery has been accomplished by use of ultrasound or by examination of fetuses that have not survived.

FUNCTIONS INVOLVED IN SURGERY
FOR BENIGN OVARIAN TUMORS

The ovary is one of the most fascinating organs of your body. Your ovary is a dynamic organ that produces and responds to hormones. It is the organ that produces estrogen and other hormones that give you feminine characteristics. To an extent, it controls menstruation and helps prepare your uterine lining for pregnancy. It also helps maintain a pregnancy in its early stages.

To properly treat you when you have an ovarian tumor, your doctor must have a clear understanding of the changes and dynamic nature of the ovary. Some ovarian changes are only a reflection of normal physiology and require no surgery — just a little time. On the other hand, ovarian cancer can be so devastating you must be suspicious of any ovarian tumor until it is diagnosed.

Benign and malignant ovarian tumors may remain symptomless for long periods of time. Symptoms may come from pressure on the bowel or bladder, pain from distention of bowel or bladder, twisting or rupture of the cyst, pain with intercourse, menstrual irregularities or infertility. A large cyst may cause no symptoms, and a small tumor can cause distressing symptoms if it becomes twisted or if it causes masculinizing symptoms.

HOW SURGERY FOR BENIGN
OVARIAN TUMORS IS PERFORMED

The extent of surgery performed may be determined by your age, the desire for further pregnancies and the possible malignancy potential of the tumor as evaluated at the time of surgery. If you're young and want more children, and if your uterus, tubes and ovaries can be saved without leaving malignant lesions, only the cyst may be removed. This leaves the remainder of the ovary. Some cysts, including functional ones, may cause enough destruction so the entire ovary must be removed.

LAPAROSCOPY

Treatment of ovarian tumors is basically surgical — laparoscopy can be diagnostic and therapeutic. When other diagnostic tests, such as X-rays and ultrasound, are unable to determine the cause of a pelvic mass, laparoscopy may provide a direct look at these structures and a biopsy, if desired.

Surgery may consist of making a diagnosis, then no further treatment is necessary. However, if there are adhesions on your ovary or if there is a simple cyst on your ovary, adhesions can be cut or the cyst drained through the laparoscope. Laparoscopy for ovarian tumors is useful to rule out other benign conditions, such as ectopic pregnancy.

MAJOR SURGERY

Some doctors prefer major surgery over laparoscopy for older patients if there is a possibility of cancer or if there is a chance of possible "spill" of cancer into the rest of the abdomen when a cyst accidentally breaks. It may be difficult to obtain an adequate biopsy of certain tumors or cysts, such as polycystic ovaries, because enough tissue may not be obtained in a biopsy through the laparoscope.

After your abdomen has been thoroughly scrubbed with sterile soap and you are asleep, a small 2- to 3-inch incision is made in your lower abdomen. The size and type of incision (midline or bikini) made depends on the reason for your surgery. If malignancy is suspected, a midline incision will usually be made to allow for evaluation of your pelvic and abdominal organs. If a benign tumor is suspected, a bikini incision will be made. The type of incision depends on your age, other studies done (ultrasound or X-ray) and possible laparoscopy—these are all used to evaluate the mass before surgery.

Abdominal and pelvic organs are inspected to evaluate the extent of your ovarian tumor. Your entire ovary can be removed by placing clamps close to the ovary. This can leave your Fallopian tube untouched. Sutures are placed next to these clamps to control bleeding when clamps are removed.

If the cyst is removed and the remainder of your ovary left, your doctor then sews the ovary together to prevent any bleeding.

In some cases of repeated bouts of pain due to ovarian cysts, it may be best to remove your entire ovary at the time of surgery. Discuss this possibility with your doctor *before* surgery.

If there is a high suspicion of malignancy, a biopsy may be done and sent to the pathology lab for immediate microscopic examination while surgery is still underway. The result will determine the extent of surgery that is necessary.

It's important to discuss all the possibilities with your doctor and what your future plans are for having more children. If you have special feelings about having your ovaries removed, let him know! This will help him decide what surgery is best for you.

RISKS OF SURGERY
FOR BENIGN OVARIAN TUMORS

Risks depend on the extent of your surgery. *Laparoscopy* is a low-risk procedure. The risks of *laparotomy* for ovarian cystectomy are similar to those for hysterectomy, but the surgery is shorter and less involved. These are discussed in the section on hysterectomy, beginning on page 218. The risk of bleeding may be higher because your ovary is a very vascular organ, so the risk of bleeding during surgery requires skilled technique by your doctor.

Your ovaries are important in fertility, so every care will be taken to preserve them during surgery. Scar tissue and adhesions often form as a part of the natural healing process of your body, even if you have flawless surgery. These adhesions can cause distortion or blockage of your Fallopian tubes, or they can bind your ovaries, causing infertility or pain in the future.

Other risks include infection, bleeding, damage to other organs and reactions to anesthetic medications.

ADVANTAGES OF SURGERY
FOR BENIGN OVARIAN TUMORS

Advantages of surgery to remove ovarian cysts depend on the findings at surgery. If malignancy is found, the surgery is an essential part of treatment and a possible cure. *Ruling out* malignancy by finding a benign tumor is also essential. Ovarian tissue must be examined under the microscope to determine if a tumor is malignant or not.

Relief of pain is certainly an advantage if an ovarian tumor has been the cause of it. Bleeding problems are also relieved, in some cases, by removing an ovarian tumor. Fertility is often enhanced by removing endometrial implants.

DISADVANTAGES OF SURGERY
FOR BENIGN OVARIAN TUMORS

Removal of an ovarian cyst is a disadvantage only if it did not need to be removed. This might apply to functional cysts, which often cure themselves by spontaneous rupture or regression. A skillful doctor knows when to wait and watch and when to proceed without delay with surgery for a benign ovarian tumor.

Other disadvantages of surgery include the usual complications and risks. However, when you're considering potentially malignant ovarian tumors, follow your doctor's advice.

WHO OPERATES?

In most cases, surgery is performed by a gynecologist with surgical skills. Laparoscopy is performed almost exclusively by specialists and should be done only by those experienced in this type of surgery.

In some areas, a general surgeon is the only person available to perform this surgery. Some family practitioners are also skilled in this type of surgery.

DIAGNOSTIC TESTS BEFORE, DURING AND AFTER SURGERY FOR BENIGN OVARIAN TUMORS

The primary diagnostic test helpful in evaluating ovarian tumors is ultrasound. It may be very helpful in identifying a tumor, its size, location and, in some cases, the nature of the mass. In almost all cases, it is more helpful than X-ray, except in the case of dermoid cysts in which X-ray may show the presence of teeth in your tumor.

Prior to any surgery, a complete blood count and urinalysis should be done. Certain blood chemistries, typing and screening for blood transfusion may be ordered by your doctor. Other tests, such as a cardiogram or chest X-ray, may be necessary if you have heart or lung disease.

If malignancy is suspected, X-ray studies may also be done to evaluate the tumor and other adjacent organs. These X-rays include IVP (intravenous pyelogram, which is an X-ray of the kidneys) or a barium enema, an X-ray of the bowel.

WHERE IS SURGERY PERFORMED?

Surgery for an ovarian tumor is performed in a hospital operating room under sterile conditions. It is not performed in a doctor's office or outpatient surgery facility.

HOSPITALIZATION AND DURATION

Laparoscopy is an outpatient procedure requiring about 1 hour to perform. Recovery after surgery is 1 to 2 hours in the recovery room or a short stay in the outpatient department of the hospital.

Recovery following major surgery for removal of a cyst or an ovary or for a hysterectomy is longer. The approach to surgery for a cyst is similar to that for a hysterectomy. Surgery takes 1 to 2 hours. You will stay in the recovery room for an hour or less, then be taken to your hospital room.

Depending on the extent of your surgery, you will be in the hospital 3 to 7 days. Each day, your diet and activity will gradually be increased. Before you go home, you'll be walking and eating and will have had a bowel movement.

ANESTHESIA

General anesthesia is used in all but very special instances to remove an ovarian tumor. Spinal or epidural anesthesia are used infrequently and only when general anesthesia cannot be used, such as in severe illness like heart disease.

PROBABLE OUTCOME OF SURGERY FOR BENIGN OVARIAN TUMORS

Occasionally a functional cyst may only be drained. Discuss with your doctor the possibility of more extensive surgery. If surgery is done to relieve pain from a ruptured or bleeding cyst, pain should be relieved and bleeding controlled. In many cases, this is an emergency and can even be life-threatening.

When surgery is done for infertility, it takes longer to evaluate the outcome as you attempt to become pregnant. In the case of endometriomas, the surgery should improve fertility.

In instances in which the ovarian tumor is cancerous, surgical removal could be life-saving — an excellent outcome, to say the least.

POST-OPERATIVE CARE

Care and recovery after a laparotomy for an ovarian tumor is comparable to any other abdominal surgery. If you have a simple cyst drained or removed, recovery should be rapid. The day after surgery you should be able to walk with assistance and walk unassisted in the following days. Diet begins with liquids and rapidly progresses to a full diet.

Avoid heavy lifting and exercise until given the go-ahead by your doctor. Most abdominal incisions require at least 4 to 6 weeks to heal before you can resume full exercising. Don't stay in bed. Remain active and gradually increase your activity.

DIET

There is no special diet. For any surgery, avoid eating or drinking anything after midnight the night before surgery. A well-balanced diet is always advised for improved general health.

MISCONCEPTIONS ABOUT SURGERY FOR BENIGN OVARIAN TUMORS

The entire ovary must be removed to remove an ovarian cyst.
This is not always true, particularly if it is caused by a functional cyst. The cyst can be removed, leaving your ovary intact.

If my ovary is removed, I won't be able to get pregnant.
This is untrue unless *both* ovaries are removed. As long as there is even part of an ovary remaining, you may be able to conceive.

Most ovarian cysts are cancerous.
Most ovarian cysts are not cancerous; they are benign.

ALTERNATIVES TO SURGERY FOR BENIGN OVARIAN TUMORS

Alternatives depend on your age and the size and type of tumor you have. Many ovarian tumors are functional, and they can be watched. With a little time, they may become smaller or rupture and go away. If you are of childbearing age, you can afford to wait a month or two to see if the cyst goes away. This may avoid unnecessary surgery.

If your cyst is larger than 3 inches in diameter, it's less likely to go away on its own. The risk of twisting or torsion must be considered. These tumors usually should be removed.

In post-menopausal women or very young girls, surgical exploration should be done to rule out cancer. Laparoscopy may help avoid major surgery.

CALL YOUR DOCTOR IF . . .

1. You have chills or fever.
2. You have severe abdominal pain.
3. Your incision opens or becomes inflamed.
4. You are unable to eat or carry on other normal activities.
5. You have repeated nausea and vomiting.

QUESTIONS TO ASK YOUR DOCTOR

Could the mass be a functional cyst? Could we watch it for a month? Would laparoscopy be of value in evaluating the tumor?
Ask your doctor these questions. Your specific situation should be considered.

Exactly what will you be removing? How will that affect my ability to get pregnant in the future?
You want to know ahead of time if only your ovary will be removed or if there is a possibility of more-involved surgery.

Are there any alternatives to surgery?
Talk to him about medical alternatives, such as chemotherapy or radiation.

Will you be performing conservative surgery to try to save the ovary or part of it?

You will want to know what type of surgery he is planning on performing. Discuss this *before* your surgery.

How soon can I return to work? Get pregnant?

Your doctor will usually ask you to wait for at least 6 weeks after your surgery.

What did the pathology report show from the tissue you removed during surgery?

You will have to wait until 2 or 3 days after surgery before your doctor will have the pathology report back.

Is it cancer or an early form of cancer?

You will want to know whether additional therapy is needed or if the surgery has "cured" you.

Operating on Cancers of Female Organs

This is a book on female surgeries, but a discussion of cancer of the female organs would be incomplete if it were limited to only surgical treatment. Many types of cancer are best treated non-surgically or with a combination of radiation, chemotherapy and surgery.

Cancer is not just one disease but a series of diseases that share certain characteristics. Before we discuss cancer cells, let's talk about normal cells and their typical characteristics.

A normal cell has a nucleus in its center surrounded by substance called *cytoplasm*. A normal cell doesn't change into any other type of cell. A skin cell does not change into a muscle cell or a nerve cell. It only produces skin cells.

Normal cells work together *for* the body and do not harm it. If tissue is injured, cells work together to repair the damage, but they also know when to stop working and repairing.

By contrast, a cancer cell ignores all rules. It allows its nucleus to become larger, darker in color and irregular in shape. The material inside the nucleus becomes jumbled.

A cancer cell does not stay in formation. It does as it pleases and seems to forget what its functions are. It robs other cells of nourishment and oxygen. It grows and reproduces much faster than normal cells. Cancer cells begin to crowd, push and compress normal cells, growing completely out of control.

As cancer cells become overwhelmingly numerous, they take over and cause normal cells to die of starvation and suffocation. Up to this point, the cancer is localized and is called *cancer-in-situ*. At this early stage, it may be easy to cure.

WHAT HAPPENS NEXT?

As cancer cells continue to grow and multiply at rapid speed, they break through natural barriers and begin to spread to tissues around them. When they break through barriers, the cancer becomes *invasive*. Spread confined to just one organ is called *local extension*. When cancer breaks through the capsule of the organ and spreads to surrounding organs, it is called *direct extension*.

Eventually, the cancer penetrates the walls of blood vessels or lymph channels, which are part of the body's immune system. The cancer cells are transported to other organs of the body, which is called *distant spread*. In general, cancer cells tend to settle in organs that have the best blood supply, such as the liver, brain, bone marrow, lungs and lymph nodes. These sites of spread produce additional cancer nests called *metastases*.

When distant spread has taken place, surgery plays only a partial role in treatment. We must also use chemotherapy or radiation therapy to help treat larger areas of the body.

Only the most common cancers of the female organs, such as cancer of the breast, cervix, endometrium and ovary, are discussed in this book. Cancers of the vulva, vagina and Fallopian tube occur much less frequently, so we only briefly mention their treatment.

TREATMENT OF FEMALE CANCERS

The treatment of cancer in males or females is not only by surgical means. Today, combinations of methods are used to achieve the best possible result — cure or pain relief of the disease. The methods of treatment available include surgery, chemotherapy and radiation therapy or a combination of these.

Your care is usually directed by more than one doctor; it is usually "orchestrated" by a team of experts. This includes your doctor, a gynecologist (if your primary doctor is not one), a cancer specialist (oncologist), a radiation oncologist, you and your partner and possibly a specialist in internal medicine (internist).

TREATMENT PLANS

Studies and research are constantly being done to evaluate methods of treatment for all cancers. This includes combinations of several drugs and radiation and surgery. Information is pooled by a group called the Gynecologic Oncology Group (GOG), which evaluates treatment plans used across the country.

Treatment plans are designed using combinations of treatment methods (surgery, radiation, chemotherapy), and results are collected. As a part of this study, different drugs are used in combinations to obtain the best result. This is called *combination chemotherapy*. If one combination is found to be better than another, that combination is used for treatment of all cases but continues to be re-evaluated.

SURGERY

Surgery is discussed at length in the individual sections on surgery for female cancers. Surgery may be used for removal of the cancer, evaluation of the extent of disease, called *staging,* and for relief of pain. All cancers are staged, with or without surgery. Staging allows evaluation of the extent of spread of disease so the best treatment plan can be chosen.

CHEMOTHERAPY

Chemotherapy means the application of chemical agents (drugs) in an attempt to kill cancer cells without harming normal cells. Chemotherapy has been used as an effective treatment method for female cancers for more than 25 years. The drugs attack the growth process of the cancer cell. There are no well-defined, unique metabolic steps in cancer cells, so there are adverse side effects on normal cells in the body.

Combinations of medications are used in an attempt to minimize side effects and to take advantage of good effects, which are the destruction of cancer cells. This is based on two principals of chemotherapy:

● differences between cancer cells and normal cells in metabolic steps.

● cancer drugs in combinations have an "additive" (two better than one) effect of killing more cancer cells with fewer side effects. Giving cancer drugs in cycles allows normal cells an opportunity to recover.

Not all cancer patients can be treated with drugs. At least three important criteria are considered—the type of cancer; the extent of spread of cancer; and the ability to tolerate the drugs, including their side effects.

Cancers respond to chemotherapy in varying degrees. The investigational trials by the GOG seek to identify the most effective combinations for each cancer.

Currently, chemotherapy is often used for cancer that has spread, and surgery and radiation are used more often for cancer that has not spread. But this is a generalization and may not apply to your particular circumstances.

In most cases, chemotherapy is an attempt to relieve pain or other symptoms; it is not curative used in this way. Because of this, beneficial results must be weighed against side effects of these potent medications. As more is learned about various drugs and combinations of drugs, chemotherapeutic agents hopefully will become more valuable as cures for cancer.

Combinations of drugs have an additive effect because different drugs attack the cancer cell in different ways and at different stages of development.

Common drugs used for chemotherapy include:

Methotrexate	Doxorubicin
5-Fluorouracil	Vincristine
Cyclophosphamide	Vinblastine
Chlorambacil	Hydroxyurea
Dactinomycin	Cis-platinum
Bleomycin	Hormones

New agents are being tested all the time. Each acts in a different way—in the way they affect cancer cells and normal cells. These drugs are used with strict care and supervision by your doctor, especially to monitor side effects or complications. Common side effects include:

• Nausea and vomiting. Giving the drug at night or in combination with medications for nausea may help.

• Hair loss. This may be a problem. Your hair will return, but use of a wig during treatment can be helpful.

• Decrease in production of blood cells (bone-marrow depression). This must be watched closely and can be monitored by regular blood counts. Decrease in certain blood cells can seriously affect your immunity and your ability to fight infections.

• Other less common side effects include loss of appetite, fatigue and damage to kidneys or liver.

Chemotherapy can be administered to you orally or intravenously, or it can be administered directly into the cancer area.

Cancer chemotherapy is an area of future and present hope. New agents are constantly being developed, evaluated and improved, providing longer and better survival rates to patients with cancer.

RADIATION

Everyone is constantly exposed to various forms of radiation. Many biologic processes rely on radiation, such as sunlight, to provide heat, light and energy for cell photosynthesis. In general, most forms of radiation are not harmful in ordinary amounts.

However, certain types of high-energy (ionizing) radiation can be useful tools in medical treatment. These high-energy sources of radiation injure living material. Their use in cancer treatment relies on the ability of these energy sources to cause injury to cancer cells—injury from which normal cells can recover. Any radiation, whether for diagnostic tests, therapeutic treatments or accidental radiation exposure, can be harmful to your body. Because of this, any exposure to X-ray, even dental X-ray, should be minimized.

Radiation from radium and cesium elements is used for treatment of human cancers. Radiation from X-ray machines has also been used for several decades in treating cancers. Roentgen rays (X-rays) were first discovered in 1896 by Roentgen in Germany.

How does radiation work? To oversimplify, high-energy electrons are produced by the X-ray machine and directed toward the target area. These electrons interact with the cancer cells and damage the protein and other vital parts of the cell nucleus, hopefully causing its death.

This selective destruction (some cells are more vulnerable to X-ray than others) of tissue forms the basis of treatment with radiation. Some cancers are not affected by radiation; they are radiation-resistent. Others are killed (radiation-sensitive) easily.

Radiation is measured in units called *rads*. The number of rads is controlled by the radiologist or radiation specialist. Different parts of the body and different cancers may be sensitive to different doses of radiation.

Radiation can be given by several methods.

• It can be given by X-ray machines (similar to X-ray machine for chest X-ray).

• Special instruments can be loaded with radioactive elements, such as cesium or radium, and placed inside the area to be treated and left for a period of time. This is called *intra-cavitary radiation*.

• Needles containing radium or cesium can be placed directly in the tumor.

• Solutions containing radioactive elements may be used when a surface area, such as inside your abdomen, must be treated.

All these treatments are calculated very precisely by a specialist in radiation treatment called a *radiation oncologist*.

Some of the high cure rates of female cancers are attributable to easy accessibility of female organs, such as the cervix and uterus. Because of this accessibility, high doses of radiation can be given to the cancerous tissues without exposing nearby normal tissues.

Side effects of radiation occur because normal tissues are exposed to radiation. Every effort is made to radiate *only* cancerous tissues, with as little exposure as possible to normal tissues.

Your bowel is particularly sensitive to radiation, so care must be taken not to damage the bowel. This is accomplished by exact placement of the least-effective amount of radiation. Your bladder is also very close to your pelvic organs, and it can be damaged by radiation. Diarrhea, intestinal obstruction, urinary frequency and urgency, plus rare fistulae (false passages into bowel or bladder), are serious complications. They can occur when your pelvic organs are radiated. Some of these problems may not appear until several months after treatment.

In certain cancers, such as cancer of the cervix, radiation may be the primary method of treatment. It may be more effective than surgery. For other cancers, such as cancer of the uterus, radiation may be used along with surgery—either before or after—or chemotherapy.

Cancer of the Breast

DEFINITION OF CANCER OF THE BREAST

Cancer of the breast is a condition in which your breast contains a malignant growth. If left untreated, the growth continues to grow and cause your death. "Cancer" is a term that describes many different diseases that share these same characteristics.

ABBREVIATIONS AND OTHER NAMES

Surgical removal of the breast is called *mastectomy* or *simple mastectomy*. When surrounding lymph glands, underlying muscles, fatty tissue and a wide area of skin are also removed, the operation is called *radical mastectomy*.

For many years, radical mastectomy has been the operation of choice in the treatment of cancer of the breast when cancer had not spread beyond immediate lymph nodes. However, in recent years the use of radical mastectomy has been questioned, especially when a simple lumpectomy (removal of the breast lump) or a simple mastectomy (removal of the breast without underlying muscles), followed by radiation therapy, may provide the same rate of cure.

PARTS OF BODY INVOLVED

In certain situations, cancer of the breast spreads during premenopausal years. Some doctors believe that removal of both ovaries may help halt estrogen production, which seems to retard growth of the breast cancer in some women. This is especially true if your cancer is sensitive to estrogen

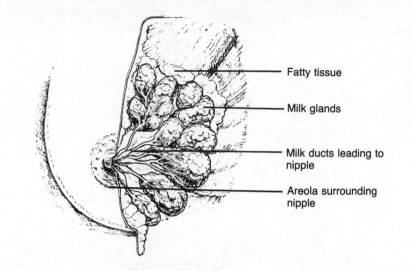

Fatty tissue

Milk glands

Milk ducts leading to nipple

Areola surrounding nipple

Structure of normal breast.

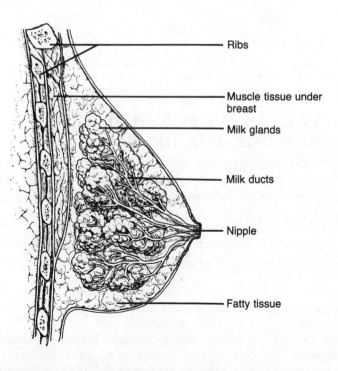

Ribs

Muscle tissue under breast

Milk glands

Milk ducts

Nipple

Fatty tissue

Side view of normal breast structure.

(produced by your ovaries) and the cancer has not spread. See illustration below. There is no uniform agreement on this subject, and it will require further study. So each case must be considered individually.

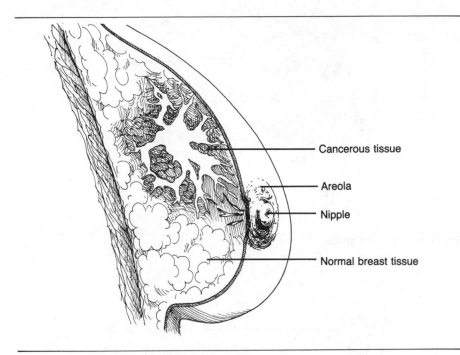

Cancer of the breast is beginning to spread.

COMMON REASONS FOR SURGERY FOR CANCER OF THE BREAST

Although some surgeons prefer radical mastectomy over lumpectomy and radiation treatments, their numbers are diminishing. Women are better informed today and want to be part of the treatment and surgery decision-making process.

It is difficult to argue with statistics. Chances for survival seem to be as good when you have a simple lumpectomy, followed by radiation therapy, as when radical mastectomy is performed. In time, radical mastectomy may be relegated to history.

Radiation therapy and X-ray treatments are used interchangeably. Technically speaking, radiation therapy can refer to treatment with radium, but when radium is used, it is named specifically.

Endocrine therapy (treatment with hormones) is also important in treatment of breast cancer. Its success depends on receptors (proteins) that are found in a few special cancers. These receptors are called *estrogen receptors*.

If you have a choice between a simple, safe procedure, such as lumpectomy plus radiation, and a grossly deforming radical mastectomy, with equal chance of recovery in either method, which would you choose? Your situation must be evaluated individually, but you have a choice. Discuss it thoroughly with your doctor *before* any surgery.

HOW COMMON IS SURGERY FOR CANCER OF THE BREAST?

Breast cancer is the most common type of female cancer. More than 1 out of 13 women (some statisticians claim 1 in 11), or about 7%, develop breast cancer at some time. Breast cancer is also the leading cause of cancer death in women, accounting for about 20%. Breast cancer is the leading cause of death from *all* causes in women 40 to 44 years old. Every 15 minutes, a woman dies of breast cancer in the United States.

All these women don't need a radical mastectomy, although that might have been the case several years ago. In the future, we may see more women having only a lumpectomy or simple mastectomy followed by radiation therapy to treat cancer of the breast. Because of the relatively recent change in treatment to simple lumpectomy, it's difficult to know exactly what percentage of women with cancer of the breast are still subjected to a radical mastectomy instead of lumpectomy or simple mastectomy.

FUNCTIONS INVOLVED IN SURGERY FOR CANCER OF THE BREAST

Every breast is composed of milk glands and fatty tissue in varying proportions. Breast tissue remains inactive from birth until adolescence. During adolescence, estrogen causes a growth of the ducts, and progesterone causes your breast glands to grow and develop. Insulin, cortisol, thyroxine, growth hormone and prolactin are hormones that also cause development of your breasts.

During pregnancy, increasing amounts of estrogen, progesterone and human placental lactogen produce active growth of your breast tissue. Amniotic fluid contains 100 times as much of the hormone prolactin (stimulates milk production and breast growth) as the baby's blood or your blood early in pregnancy. This is the reason your breasts become larger during pregnancy.

It's believed that fibrocystic disease of the breast is caused by too much estrogen without the countereffect of progestin — both are female hormones. Studies reveal there is 2 to 4 times as much cancer of the breast with fibrocystic disease, yet cancer does not develop in the cysts themselves.

A breast containing cancer is still capable of producing usable milk. There has been no evidence a nursing baby has ever "caught" cancer from its mother.

HOW SURGERY FOR CANCER OF THE BREAST IS PERFORMED

RADICAL MASTECTOMY

Radical mastectomy is a lengthy, difficult, deforming operation in which your breast, the surrounding lymph glands, underlying muscles and a wide area of skin are removed. In many cases, your arm on the surgery side remains swollen indefinitely after radical mastectomy because lymphatic drainage in the arm system is impaired.

Surgery for a radical mastectomy begins with an incision in your skin around the breast. See illustration below. All the breast tissue and overlying skin are removed. After this, the muscles under the breast are identified and removed. Surgery includes removal of lymph nodes from the middle of the chest out to the nodes under your arm. The surgery is carried all the way down to the ribs; even some of the thin muscle layers covering the ribs are removed. See illustration on opposite page.

It is obvious why this operation is so disfiguring. The muscle and fat layers are important components of your body contour, along with your breast.

SIMPLE MASTECTOMY

In a simple mastectomy, only your breast is removed. No attempt is made to remove your lymph glands or to operate on the muscle under your breast.

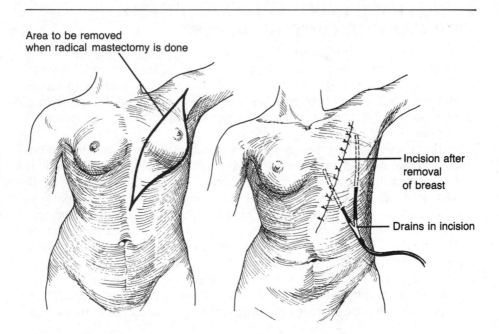

Area to be removed when radical mastectomy is done

Incision after removal of breast

Drains in incision

Radical mastectomy. This shows approximate amount of breast tissue and surrounding skin that is removed and incision after surgery is completed.

Because less skin is removed, it is easier to insert a prosthesis (silicone gel-filled envelope). This is sometimes done at the same time the breast is removed. Your entire breast is removed instead of the lump because the tumor is large or has spread within your breast.

A simple mastectomy is performed through an incision in your skin, but no skin is removed. Once the skin is opened, the underlying breast tissue is removed down to, but not including, the muscle layers below, as in a radical mastectomy. After the breast tissue is removed, attempts at cosmetic restoration of your breast include placement of the prosthesis.

In a newer technique, a pedicle of fat is transplanted from your abdomen and is brought up under the skin to the breast area to form a "breast." Discuss this with your surgeon before surgery. This type of surgery is similar to surgery for breast augmentation. See page 262.

LUMPECTOMY

In a lumpectomy, only the cancerous breast lump is removed. This operation is feasible when the cancer is small and confined to the lump. Lumpectomy is not disfiguring and requires no plastic reconstruction of the breast. It is followed by radiation therapy.

Performing a lumpectomy is similar to a biopsy except the entire lump is removed. The skin is opened over the lump, and the lump is identified and cut out in one piece. Bleeding is stopped, and the skin is closed over the area.

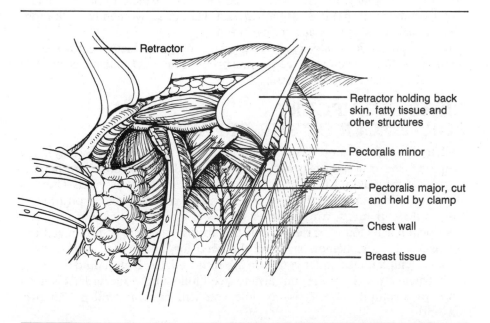

Retractor

Retractor holding back skin, fatty tissue and other structures

Pectoralis minor

Pectoralis major, cut and held by clamp

Chest wall

Breast tissue

When a radical mastectomy is performed, your breast, underlying pectoral muscles, lymph nodes under your arm and additional skin and fatty tissue are removed down to the chest wall.

If cancer spreads to other organs besides your breast, there may be no reason for any surgery to be performed. Chemotherapy or radiation therapy are administered to relieve symptoms, and rarely, a cure.

PROPHYLACTIC MASTECTOMY

Some women become so obsessed with fear of cancer of the breast they want their breast removed to avoid the *possibility* of cancer. This is called *prophylactic mastectomy,* and it is not a logical reason for having a mastectomy.

It's possible if you have severe fibrocystic disease that causes agonizing pain or if you must undergo repeated biopsies and cyst aspirations, you might be a candidate for this type of surgery. Consult your doctor about having a mastectomy to relieve pain and emotional upset. Because the lumps in fibrocystic disease are cysts, they should first be aspirated, which is a relatively painless procedure. If your lump disappears, your problem is solved. Actual biopsy is necessary *only* when a lump is still present after fluid has been removed or if the fluid is bloody or otherwise suspicious of malignancy.

Certain types of fibrocystic disease are accompanied by increased risk of breast cancer, but this increased risk is *not* sufficient to warrant mastectomy in the absence of the *diagnosis* of cancer. One survey showed 11,000 prophylactic subcutaneous mastectomies (removal of the breast leaving the skin and nipple) were performed in 1981.

This operation is not without complications, such as infection, hemorrhage, loss of the nipple due to anesthesia, risk of anesthesia and risk of hardening around the implant. Prophylactic subcutaneous mastectomy is mentioned only to emphasize that it is rarely justified. Half of all women have "lumpy" breasts, and most lumps are *not* cancerous.

If a prophylactic mastectomy is suggested by your doctor, get a second opinion. Go to a breast-cancer center or a breast-cancer specialist. See page 88 for a list of breast-cancer centers.

RISKS OF SURGERY
FOR CANCER OF THE BREAST

There is little, if any, risk if only a lump is removed (lumpectomy). If a simple mastectomy is performed, there is a small risk of infection, hemorrhage and sensitivity to the anesthetic if local anesthesia is used. There is always a risk with general anesthesia, such as vomiting and aspiration of vomit into your lungs, cardiac arrest or sensitivity to medications or gas.

Radical mastectomy carries with it the additional risks of prolonged anesthesia, infection, hemorrhage and the need for, and risk of, transfusion. Because lymph nodes under your arm are removed, the lymph fluid drainage is obstructed, which causes your arm to swell following surgery. This is *not* a temporary complication. It is possible you will have a swollen arm permanently.

The pectoral muscles that underlie and support your breast are also removed. A radical mastectomy is deforming and adds to the trauma of losing your breast. A large area of the skin surrounding your breast is removed so the remaining skin must be drawn taut to close the wound. As a result, the blood supply may be compromised enough to cause poor, delayed or incomplete healing, even sloughing (death and loss of skin). The risk of blood clots forming and being carried to other vital areas is considerably greater with a radical mastectomy than with a lumpectomy or simple mastectomy.

It is difficult to implant a breast prosthesis (silicone gel-filled envelope) after a radical mastectomy to give you a normal breast contour because of the amount of skin that is removed. If your doctor suggests a radical mastectomy, get a second opinion.

ADVANTAGES OF SURGERY FOR CANCER OF THE BREAST

Surgery is the treatment of choice in breast cancer and is used in addition to chemotherapy or radiation. It offers the best chance for cure when followed by radiation. The question arises as to what kind of surgery you need.

It is also important to have surgical removal of cancer of the breast as early as possible. The rate of cure is directly proportional to the containment of the cancer. The earlier cancer is discovered and removed, the greater your chance of a cure.

DISADVANTAGES OF SURGERY FOR CANCER OF THE BREAST

RADICAL MASTECTOMY

A radical mastectomy has many disadvantages and risks, as we've already discussed. Hopefully we have convinced you to get a second opinion if your doctor suggests a radical mastectomy to you.

There is a great deal of disfigurement involved with radical mastectomy, in which a wide resection of skin, breast tissue, muscles and lymph glands are removed. Your arm will probably be swollen after surgery and may remain swollen. It will be difficult, if not impossible, to insert an implant or correct the deformity left by a radical breast amputation.

SIMPLE MASTECTOMY AND LUMPECTOMY

A simple mastectomy leaves you without a breast, but many doctors now insert a breast implant at the same time as surgery so there won't be any deformity. This is one of the best treatment plans. It may be followed by X-ray treatments or chemotherapy, depending on what your doctor finds.

A lumpectomy causes practically no deformity and entails little, if any, risk.

WHO OPERATES?

It's important to have a specialist perform your surgery who has treated many cases of breast cancer. In most instances, this is a general surgeon.

Together, you will decide whether you should have a lumpectomy or a simple mastectomy and whether you should have a prosthesis implanted at the same time. He will also arrange for radiation treatment.

DIAGNOSTIC TESTS BEFORE, DURING AND AFTER SURGERY FOR CANCER OF THE BREAST

In addition to urinalysis and complete blood count, your doctor will order a chest X-ray to rule out spread of cancer to your lungs. He may order other X-rays of bones, kidneys, liver and other organs to check for spread.

WHERE IS SURGERY PERFORMED?

Radical mastectomy is always performed in the hospital. It's better to have a lumpectomy performed in the hospital because the cancer may have spread beyond its capsule. If it has invaded surrounding tissue, your doctor may decide to perform a simple mastectomy rather than a lumpectomy.

The exception to this rule is aspiration (withdrawal of fluid) of a breast cyst. This simple procedure can be done safely in your doctor's office. Fluid removed from the cyst is sent to the lab for examination. If a mass remains in your breast after aspiration, the tumor is biopsied or completely removed.

HOSPITALIZATION AND DURATION

Radical mastectomy requires 2 to 3 hours in the operating room and 1 week in the hospital. Simple mastectomy is often a matter of an hour in the operating room and 2 or 3 days in the hospital. Lumpectomy is an outpatient procedure, which means you can be in and out of the hospital the same day.

RADICAL MASTECTOMY

Radical mastectomy is further complicated by drains and the possibility of skin slough along your incision. Pain is greater than with a simple mastectomy because dissection is greater and muscles have been removed.

Your arm will have to be supported for several days after a radical mastectomy, and you won't be able to move it. Anesthesia lasts longer, so you'll be slower to recover from it. You're more likely to have nausea following surgery, and it may take longer for you to regain your appetite. Intravenous fluids are continued longer, and you may have to have a transfusion.

You will be encouraged to get out of bed the day after surgery, but you may not feel like moving very far because of pain in your arm and chest. Plan on at least 1 week before you are fully ambulatory.

SIMPLE MASTECTOMY

A simple mastectomy is also painful, and this is part of the reason for your stay in the hospital. You will be offered pain-relieving drugs as you need them.

Your intestinal tract is not involved in the surgery, so you should be able to eat whatever you want by the day after surgery. You will probably sleep most of the day of surgery.

You can get up, but use your arms as little as possible. Pain may restrict you — the main reason for caution is so you won't cause hemorrhage in your incision. Within a few days, you'll be able to move your arms without too much discomfort.

Dressings are tight enough to control and prevent bleeding in your incision yet loose enough to permit good circulation. You may have some slight draining from the incision for a few hours, but this probably won't happen after the first day.

LUMPECTOMY

There is little, if any, pain following a lumpectomy. Over-the-counter analgesics should be sufficient to relieve discomfort. An icepack may help if you need it, but if you have more pain than aspirin or acetaminophen will relieve, check with your doctor for complications.

ANESTHESIA

A simple or radical mastectomy requires general anesthesia and subjects you to premedication with a sedative and a drug to decrease the flow of your saliva. The drug, called *scopolamine,* dries up secretions throughout your body and decreases the risk of aspirating secretions into your lungs.

A general anesthetic is never given without intravenous fluids running, in case you must be given emergency medication. An I.V. is a safeguard in the event of drug sensitivity, cardiac arrest or any other complication that requires immediate intravenous medication.

You will remain drowsy for some time after awakening from a general anesthetic, and you may have some nausea or vomiting. You may wake enough to be helped out of bed the same day of your surgery but will definitely be ambulatory beginning the day after surgery.

Following radical breast surgery, you'll probably remain asleep the entire day because of the prolonged anesthesia time. The longer you are under anesthesia, the longer it takes your bladder and bowel to begin to function. When it takes you longer to begin to take fluids by mouth, you require intravenous fluids for a longer time. However, you will be fully awake from your anesthesia the morning following surgery, although you may be drowsy from pain relievers.

A lumpectomy is performed under local anesthesia. It carries with it only a slight risk of sensitivity to the local anesthetic.

PROBABLE OUTCOME OF SURGERY FOR CANCER OF THE BREAST

RADICAL MASTECTOMY

Side effects are numerous in a radical mastectomy. One of the most difficult to deal with is the psychological effect of losing your breast and a feeling you are "no longer feminine."

Before agreeing to a radical mastectomy, discuss the possibility of swelling of your arm post-operatively. Ask your doctor how he has handled this problem in the past.

Urgency of treatment exists, but this urgency must give way to allow you time to ponder, discuss and review each fact, including the type of surgery and the need for radiation treatment. This knowledge can give you peace of mind and the assurance you're pursuing the best possible plan of therapy for you. The outcome of surgery for breast cancer depends on the type of cancer you have and the extent of spread before surgery.

SIMPLE MASTECTOMY AND LUMPECTOMY

Simple mastectomy and lumpectomy carry smaller risks than those for radical mastectomy. They remove the cancer for diagnosis and treatment and are followed by X-ray and chemotherapy. Lumpectomy and simple mastectomy should be well-tolerated without the added problems of risks and disfigurement of a radical mastectomy.

A woman may feel unfeminine after her breast is removed, and this is the reason many doctors try, with a simple mastectomy, to implant an artificial breast as part of the operation. Not every case permits immediate implantation, but techniques are steadily improving and it's becoming more common.

Discuss the matter of a prosthesis with your surgeon to see if it's possible in your case, and listen to his reasons. Don't be afraid to ask all your questions *before* surgery. Ask if the prosthesis can be implanted immediately when the breast is removed.

POST-OPERATIVE CARE

RADICAL MASTECTOMY

Radical mastectomy is a major operation and demands prolonged rehabilitative therapy to restore maximum use of your arm. Swelling of your arm may or may not be helped by treatment.

With radical mastectomy, you will have considerable discomfort when you go home after 5 to 7 days, so your doctor will give you pain relievers to take at home. He will dress your incision daily while you are in the hospital and will probably want to see you in his office several times a week to check you.

Your doctor may take some stitches out in a week, then remove the rest a few at a time over a period of 7 to 10 days.

The skin has been stripped of much of its blood supply during surgery, so your doctor will watch your incision for any evidence of separation or sloughing. He will also check it for redness, swelling, infection and drainage. He can usually tell within a month if your incision will heal without further problems.

SIMPLE MASTECTOMY

Simple mastectomy is performed in the hospital and requires a 2- or 3-day stay. Pressure dressings and follow up to prevent hemorrhage and infection are supervised by your doctor and hospital personnel.

Movement of your arm may be painful for a few weeks. Rehabilitation exercises are recommended as soon as soreness permits. Your doctor will give you pain relievers to take at home. Pressure dressings may be left in place for a week or more. Stitches are removed in 7 to 14 days.

You may have a permanently implanted breast prosthesis if you required removal of a breast. If you don't have an implanted prosthesis, an external appliance can be worn under your clothes and is undetectable by any ordinary observer.

LUMPECTOMY
Lumpectomy requires only a pressure dressing to prevent hemorrhage. Pain is minimal and easily controlled by over-the-counter medication, such as aspirin or acetaminophen. Your doctor may give you some medicine to take home, but this is not usually necessary. He will allow you to remove the dressing in 1 or 2 days and also allow you to bathe or shower. Stitches are removed in about 1 week.

DIET
There is no special diet to follow after any of these three procedures. It's important to know that obesity may hinder rehabilitation if you must have a breast removed.

MISCONCEPTIONS ABOUT SURGERY FOR CANCER OF THE BREAST

A diagnosis of cancer of the breast means I'm going to die.
If your cancer has not spread, the cure rate of cancer of the breast is about 86%. Diagnosis of this type of cancer doesn't mean you must have a disfiguring operation. It's more likely you'll have a lumpectomy, followed by radiation.

Cancer of the breast means an end to my femininity.
This is untrue. Many women have had a breast removed, and it has not meant an end to their femininity. You may be surprised to discover how many of your friends or acquaintances have had cancer of the breast. Many are alive and well and functioning as well as before surgery.

I don't have any place to go for information about breast cancer.
If you want information about breast cancer, there are many places to find it. Popular women's magazines often carry articles about breast cancer; you might contact some of the researchers mentioned in articles to find out more. Many universities conduct cancer screenings. Call the local branch of the American Cancer Society to find out if there are any in your area. Or contact your local county medical society to obtain information regarding the breast center nearest you.

There are breast centers in many cities. A breast center offers:
- immediate care
- information about your condition
- mammography and other screening tests
- good follow up of your condition
- team approach with an oncologist, radiologist and surgeon

Below is a list of some breast-cancer centers to call for more information:

Dana-Farber Cancer Institute
Breast Evaluation Center
Boston, Massachusetts
(617) 732-3666

Fort Sanders
Comprehensive Breast Center
Knoxville, Tennessee
(615) 971-1624

The Breast Center
Van Nuys, California
(818) 787-9911

The Breast Care Center
San Diego, California
(619) 287-8837

Memorial Breast Center
Memorial Medical Center
Long Beach, California
(213) 595-2211

Children's Hospital of San
Francisco—Breast Health Center
San Francisco, California
(415) 387-8700, ext. 5336

Genesis Women's
Diagnostic Center
Atlanta, Georgia
(404) 853-0200

Ochsner Breast Screening Clinic
New Orleans, Louisiana
(504) 838-4021

Mease Breast Health Center
Dunedin, Florida
(813) 734-6391

Cancer Prevention Center
Crump Cancer Center
Houston, Texas
(713) 791-7950

ALTERNATIVES TO SURGERY
FOR CANCER OF THE BREAST

Breast cancer *does* have alternative methods of treatment! If this book serves no other purpose than to inform you that you *do* have alternatives to radical mastectomy, it will have served its purpose.

Discuss your diagnosis with your doctor. Let him know your feelings about treatment. Let him know you are informed and are aware lumpectomy and simple mastectomy (when needed), followed by radiation, give the same cure rates as radical mastectomy.

CALL YOUR DOCTOR IF . . .

1. You have hemorrhage or drainage from your incision.
2. There is redness, swelling or extreme soreness around your incision.
3. You have chills or fever.
4. You have more pain than you think you should have.
5. You just don't feel as good as you should.

QUESTIONS TO ASK YOUR DOCTOR

How extensive is my cancer? How far has it spread?
Your doctor should be able and willing to provide you with this information. You want to know what your condition is and be as well-informed as possible about your cancer. You can't make plans for the future without knowing what your medical outlook is.

Is it a fast-growing cancer?
Ask your doctor to be as specific as possible.

Which is better in my case — a lumpectomy or simple mastectomy? Why?
This is a question to ask your doctor *before* surgery and a subject you should discuss in detail with him.

Is this a cancer that should respond to radiation or chemotherapy treatment?
This depends on the type of cancer. Your doctor may use one treatment or a combination of treatments.

Do you intend to implant a breast prosthesis at the same time my breast is removed?
Your doctor may have special reasons for these decisions, but discuss them. You'll be a better patient if you know what's going on and why.

How long will I be in the hospital? How soon will I be able to return to work?
These answers may vary with each doctor and with your individual cancer, but they will help you adjust to the situation. The average stay after a simple mastectomy is about 5 days. After a radical mastectomy, the average stay is about 1 week.

Will you refer me to a physical therapist to help restore complete use of my arm, if necessary?
This will be necessary only after radical mastectomy.

Cancer of the Cervix

DEFINITION OF CANCER OF THE CERVIX

The cervix is the part of the uterus that protrudes into your vagina. Cancer of the cervix is a disease in which the cells covering your cervix undergo a change.

Your doctor can see your cervix with his instruments when he does a vaginal exam. The cervix is the part of your vagina you can reach with your finger. If you've used an intrauterine device, you feel for the string protruding from your cervix to make certain the IUD is in place.

The cause of cancer of the cervix is unknown, but it seems to be related to damage and injuries sustained by the cervix. Cancer of the cervix is virtually unknown among celibates, and it is uncommon in childless women. By contrast, it's common in women who engage in sex at any early age and those who have had multiple partners. There has been some evidence that may link it with herpes-2 virus and the human papilloma virus, but this is still being researched. There is even more evidence that it is linked to sexually transmitted warts (condylomata).

ABBREVIATIONS AND OTHER NAMES

There are no other names for cancer of the cervix except for the medical name carcinoma of the cervix. Other conditions mentioned are carcinoma-in-situ (localized) or microinvasive disease (beginning to spread). Although the cervix is part of the uterus, when cancer of the uterus is mentioned, it's assumed it is a cancer of the body of the uterus, also called *endometrial cancer*. See page 121 for more information on cancer of the uterus.

PARTS OF BODY INVOLVED

Unless there is spread to other organs, cancer of the cervix is limited to the cervix. See illustration below. If the cancer spreads to surrounding lymph glands, then your uterus, bones, liver, lungs and brain become targets for spread. There is a small area near the opening of the cervix where two different kinds of tissue meet — tissue lining the canal of the cervix, which is glandular in nature, and tissue covering the outside of the cervix, which is a flat, covering-type of tissue.

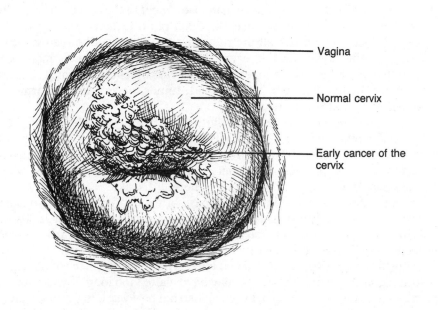

Early cancer of the cervix.

At the junction of the two tissues is the place where cancer of the cervix begins. This is an area of constant turnover of cells, with rapid change. Growth of the cell lining makes the possibility of malignant change more likely. It is from this junction that your Pap smear is taken because a smear picks up discarded cells of the cervix that show early changes that could eventually (5 to 10 years later) develop into cancer of the cervix.

COMMON REASONS FOR SURGERY OF CANCER OF THE CERVIX

One of the monumental milestones of medicine was the discovery that cancer of the cervix could be diagnosed *before* it developed into cancer. It took Dr. George Papanicolaou 25 years to convince the medical profession that smears of cells taken from the cervix and vagina could demonstrate early changes that would predict the eventual development of cancer. Dr. Papanicolaou first developed this technique in the 1920s, but it was not accepted by the medical profession until about 1945. Today, a Pap smear is a common and vital part of every pelvic examination.

Cancer of the cervix is usually a slow-growing cancer that takes an average of 5 to 10 years to change from a localized (cancer-in-situ) to an invasive stage. But no one can predict how slow or fast a cancer will grow. This slow growth provides you with adequate time to diagnose cancer of the cervix so almost no woman needs to die of this disease. But don't put off exams and regular Pap smears. Cancers *can* break all the rules and can grow and spread rapidly.

Cancer begins just inside the cervix; this area can be accurately monitored by Pap smears. If there are changes in your smears that indicate early cancer is developing, further tests, which may include minor surgery, are performed to diagnose and treat the early changes.

Cancer of the cervix may be due to a virus or other factors. Herpes has been suspected, but not definitely identified, as one culprit. Cancer of the cervix is more common in women who begin sexual activity at an early age, women who have multiple sex partners and women of limited economic means. Many doctors consider this type of cancer a venereal disease.

Cancer of the cervix used to be a disease of women in their 40s, but Pap smears have gradually reduced this age of discovery to women in their 20s and 30s. In fact, cancer of the cervix is occasionally diagnosed in its earliest stages in teenagers. This is due to earlier sexual activity among teens.

Unfortunately, if you wait until you have symptoms of cancer of the cervix before consulting your doctor, you may have waited too long. If you have any painless spotting or bleeding between menstrual periods, even a thin, watery, blood-tinged vaginal discharge, or bleeding after intercourse, report it to your doctor immediately.

Late symptoms are pain in legs, groin, bladder, bowel or back. These are often signs of spread of the cancer.

You can detect cancer of the cervix long before you have any of the above symptoms by having a regular Pap smear. When properly obtained and expertly examined under the microscope, a Pap smear will detect any changes in your cervix early enough to avoid the tragedies of cancer.

DES (DIETHYLSTILBESTROL) AND ITS PROBLEMS

It seems appropriate to mention diethylstilbestrol (DES) and the children of women who were given DES during pregnancy. DES is a non-steroidal synthetic estrogen given to some women to keep them from having a miscarriage.

In the 1940s and '50s, it was common practice to prescribe DES for a pregnant woman who threatened to miscarry or who habitually miscarried.

When the offspring, especially female, of DES-treated women were followed into their teens, severe changes in the teenagers' vaginal mucous membranes were discovered. Since then, these changes have been shown to be due to DES.

A study done in 1970 uncovered eight cases of cancer of the vagina in women between the ages of 15 and 22. This was a higher number than recorded in all previous medical literature. It was found the mothers of the young women with vaginal cancer had been treated during the first trimester of the relevant pregnancy with DES.

Since 1970, other cases of cancer of the vagina have been discovered in children of DES-treated women. The youngest patient with these changes was 7, and the oldest was 29. The development of cancer seemed to be unrelated to the size of the dose of DES that was given. All that was important was the fact DES *had* been given. The incidence of cancer of the vagina in female children of DES-treated mothers is about 0.14 to 1.4 per 1,000. About 90% of the cases occur in girls 14 years of age or younger.

A benign condition called *vaginal adenosis* (a benign cellular change of the cervix) is extremely common in DES offspring and is always present in those girls who have clear-cell cancer of the vagina. Although vaginal adenosis can be found anywhere within the vagina, it is most often found in the upper part of the vagina surrounding the cervix. Vaginal adenosis is superficial and can often be treated locally. At least 60% of all women treated with DES during early pregnancy have female offspring in whom vaginal adenosis can be diagnosed.

In general, all daughters of DES-exposed mothers should have a gynecologic exam every 6 to 12 months beginning at age 14 or at the onset of menstrual periods. Colposcopic exams at regular intervals are recommended. See page 102 for more information on colposcopy. The purpose of this regular examination is to detect the development of cancer of the vagina at its earliest stages. At present, there is no treatment for vaginal adenosis. Except for a little increase in vaginal discharge, there are no other symptoms.

In male offspring of DES-treated mothers, about 30% have developed some abnormalities of the reproductive tract.

There is no satisfactory treatment for vaginal adenosis (other than regular exams, vaginal adenosis requires no specific treatment) or clear-cell cancer of the vagina. Surgery and radiation are used, but recurrence is common. Chemotherapy has been disappointing.

TREATMENT OF CANCER OF THE CERVIX

Treatment of cancer of the cervix is not always surgical; treatment is extremely simple if your cancer is detected early. Detection and treatment of cervical cancer proceeds somewhat as follows.

Cancer Smears — Pap smears are obtained on a regular basis as soon as you begin to have intercourse. If you have two consecutive negative smears, the

American Cancer Society recommends you have a regular cancer smear every 3 years, until age 60. High-risk patients need yearly or more-frequent exams. If all your smears have been negative to age 60, you require no further smears. Most doctors recommend Pap smears be done more frequently.

Classification of Cancer Smears — Cancer smears are classified in degrees of change. The term *dysplasia* is used to describe abnormal changes in cells of the cervix. The term *carcinoma-in-situ* is used for a lesion that has passed from the stage of dysplasia (benign) to neoplasia (cancerous).

This classification uses the term *cervical intraepithelial neoplasia* or *CIN*, which means abnormal, precancerous cells in the cervix. All lesions have the potential to progress to cancer. Classification and a short description of management are shown below.

CIN I	Mild dysplasia.
	Colposcopy with biopsy for diagnosis.
	Treated with cryosurgery (freezing) or laser.
CIN II	Moderate dysplasia.
	Colposcopy with biopsy for diagnosis.
	Treated with cryosurgery or laser.
CIN III	Severe dysplasia.
	Colposcopy and biopsy for diagnosis. Must be closely examined because CIN III is close to carcinoma-in-situ.
	Treated with cone biopsy, cryosurgery, laser or hysterectomy, if childbearing is completed.
Overt	Carcinoma-in-situ.
Cancer	Cone biopsy used to evaluate extent of the disease.
	Treatment will be a hysterectomy or radiation, depending on the extent of the disease.

Punch Biopsy of Cervix — A biopsy can be by punch or conization. Many doctors now have colposcopes, or access to them, so when a smear is abnormal, your doctor will take a look at your cervix with a colposcope. This is an instrument like a telescope that magnifies the tissue that lines your vagina and cervix. After staining of your cervix with a 3% acetic-acid solution, your doctor can tell *where* the abnormal tissue is on your cervix so he knows exactly where to take the punch biopsy.

Conization of Cervix — Conization is the removal of a cone of tissue from your cervix when your cancer has not spread. See illustrations on opposite page. The cone of tissue is sent to the lab for examination. In the laboratory, a pathologist can tell how much, if any, spread of the cancer has occurred.

In some instances there has been no spread of cancer, and the conization effects a cure by removing all the cancer. If there has been only microscopic (minimal) invasion of less than 3 millimeters in depth through the basement membrane of the cervix, then a hysterectomy is performed. Often a simple hysterectomy is sufficient treatment. In other cases, total abdominal hysterectomy, plus removal of adjacent lymph nodes, is performed if the cancer

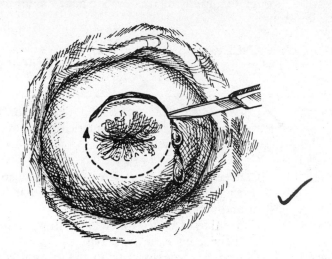

Cone of tissue is removed from cervix with a scalpel to remove chronic area of inflammation that does not heal.

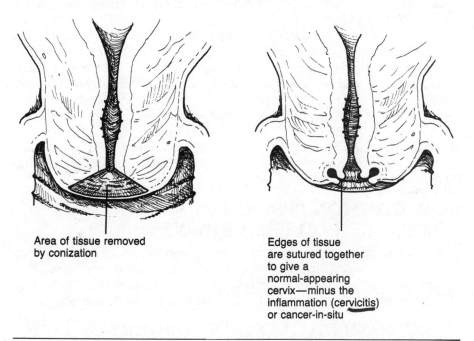

Area of tissue removed by conization

Edges of tissue are sutured together to give a normal-appearing cervix—minus the inflammation (cervicitis) or cancer-in-situ

Area of tissue removed by conization. Edges of tissue are stitched together to give a normal-appearing cervix.

has spread through to underlying tissues. See page 218 for more information on hysterectomy.

STAGES OF CANCER

Cancer of the cervix is also classified clinically in stages. Stages are listed below.

Stage 0 ✓	Cancer-in-situ has not begun to spread. It has not broken through the basement membrane of the layer of tissue that covers the cervix.
Stage I	Cancer is limited to the cervix.
Stage II	Cancer has spread to the vagina but not to the lower third. It has spread outward to tissues that lie alongside of and support the cervix.
Stage III	Cancer has extended to the lower third of the vagina or to the side walls of the pelvis.
Stage IV	Cancer has spread outside the genital tract (pelvic organs), such as to the bladder, rectum, liver, brain or bones.

✓ Stage 0 is treated by conization of your cervix, especially if you still want more children. If you're older or do not wish more children, you may be offered a hysterectomy.

Stage I and II are occasionally treated with a radical hysterectomy (also called a *Wertheim hysterectomy)* in which the uterus and pelvic lymph nodes are removed. But it has been shown that survival statistics in cases in which the cancer has spread beyond its earliest stages are better if radium and X-ray therapy are used. This is where staging is important. To generalize, Stage I and Stage IIA (early Stage II) are treated with surgery. Stages above this (more-extensive disease) are treated with radiation.

Large cancer centers occasionally remove all pelvic organs plus bladder and rectum (called *pelvic exenteration)* in some Stage II, III and IV cancers of the cervix.

HOW COMMON IS SURGERY FOR CANCER OF THE CERVIX?

Cancer of the cervix is detected in its earliest stages by means of Pap smears, so conization and hysterectomy are fairly common. Before Pap smears, most cancers were discovered late, usually after the patient had already developed symptoms, and it was too late for surgical treatment.

FUNCTIONS INVOLVED IN SURGERY FOR CANCER OF THE CERVIX

If cancer of the cervix is detected early, only the diseased part of your cervix is removed by conization. This leaves all pelvic organs intact so you can still have menstrual periods and pregnancies. There should be no hormone changes because your ovaries still function normally.

If your cancer has spread, interference with other body functions and physiology depends on *where* the cancer has spread to and how extensively. Treated or untreated, cancer of your cervix can spread to almost any organ in your body and interfere with its function.

Early symptoms of cancer of the cervix are a thin, watery, blood-tinged vaginal discharge that may not even be noticed. You may bleed after intercourse or after douching. You also may notice occasional episodes of heavier bleeding between menstrual periods.

As your cancer grows, you have heavier, longer menstrual periods and more bleeding between periods. Bleeding may become continuous.

Late symptoms may include pain in the side of your abdomen or legs, secondary to involvement of your ureters, pelvic wall or sciatic nerves. You may have painful urination, blood in your urine, rectal bleeding or even inability to have bowel movements if your bowel is involved severely. All these symptoms worsen, with eventual swelling of your extremities and massive hemorrhage as involvement of your organs becomes overwhelming.

HOW SURGERY FOR CANCER OF THE CERVIX IS PERFORMED

PUNCH BIOPSY

Punch biopsy is done with special hollow forceps that actually cut out a round piece of tissue when the forceps are closed over a suspicious area. This suspicious area is revealed by staining with iodine and more definitely determined by examination with a colposcope.

Tissue that is removed is sent to the laboratory for staining and examination under the microscope. This examination determines if the tissue biopsied is cancerous and if cancer has invaded the tissue layers underlying your cancer.

CRYOSURGERY

Cryosurgery can be used for treatment of cervicitis, CIN lesions and some cases of dysplasia and carcinoma-in-situ (CIS). Carcinoma is a medical term for cancer. The procedure is most often used with colposcopy when the abnormal area on the cervix can be seen well.

Cryosurgery is performed in your doctor's office without anesthesia. A very cold probe (from gases, such as nitrous oxide or carbon dioxide) is placed on the cervix to cover the abnormal area. Tissue is frozen for 3 to 5 minutes, allowed to "thaw" for a few minutes, then frozen again.

Cryosurgery works by freezing and killing the abnormal tissues. The cervix then heals with normal tissue. It's important to check for "cure" of the problem with a Pap smear every 3 months for 1 year.

The main disadvantage of this treatment is that no tissue is removed and sent to the lab to look for more severe disease that might have been missed in the preliminary evaluation.

LASER

Use of the laser is becoming more common in almost all fields of medicine. Laser surgery is described in more detail in the section on endometriosis. See page 211. Its use with cervical cancer is becoming more common.

Laser surgery can be performed in the office or outpatient surgery area. A laser beam is directed at abnormal areas of tissue and vaporizes the tissue. The primary advantage of laser treatment is that abnormal tissue can be destroyed very precisely without damage to adjacent normal tissue.

CONIZATION

In conization, or cone biopsy, a cone of tissue is cut out with a knife or laser. It is called *cold-knife conization,* in contrast to removal with a hot cautery loop. The cone of tissue encompasses the opening of the cervix, the area in which cancer of the cervix originates. Bleeding vessels are cauterized to stop bleeding.

The cervix has no sensation of pain except when stretched, so conization requires no anesthesia. But if stretching and manipulation of the vagina are necessary to do the surgery, anesthesia is required. Your doctor usually does a D&C at the same time, unless you're pregnant, to be certain there is no cancer in the endometrium. For the D&C part of the operation, you will require anesthesia.

If you're pregnant, your doctor will perform a shallow, coin-shaped, flat biopsy of your cervix instead of a conization. This is a very specialized technique requiring special equipment and skills. The procedure is still called a cone biopsy, but it may be cut a little differently.

HYSTERECTOMY

If your cancer is invasive or microinvasive (less than 3 millimeters of penetration), radical hysterectomy may be performed. Your uterus, tubes, ovaries (ovaries are removed if you are over 45, otherwise they are left in), pelvic lymph nodes and a cuff of vaginal tissue from the upper part of your vagina are removed.

When removing this extra cuff of vaginal tissue, your doctor must be very careful not to injure your bladder or rectum, which are very close to your vagina. Adjacent extra tissue is removed to avoid the spread of the cancer.

Dissection of your pelvic lymph nodes is a long, difficult, tedious procedure, and great care must be taken to avoid injury to pelvic blood vessels, bladder, rectum and ureters. This dissection may cause adhesions.

PELVIC EXENTERATION

Pelvic exenteration is an "ultraradical" surgery for the treatment of advanced or recurrent pelvic cancer. It is not for every patient because of the radical nature of the surgery, but for some it is the only choice available. Although it has been used for several types of pelvic malignancies, its greatest use is for recurrent or advanced cervical cancer.

Exenteration involves removal of the uterus, tubes, ovaries and adjacent organs, including the bladder and bowel. If the bowel and bladder are removed, new structures must be "constructed." Surgery for exenteration may require more than 8 hours, with a mortality rate of about 5%. For some women with advanced disease, this is all that can be done.

RISKS OF SURGERY
FOR CANCER OF THE CERVIX

Treatment of cancer of the cervix is specialized. Unless your doctor is experienced in treating this type of cancer, ask for consultation with, and possible referral to, someone who treats many of these cases, such as a gynecology-oncologist.

There is little or no risk in punch biopsy of your cervix. Cryosurgery also carries few risks. Laser surgery is new, technical and expensive, and most doctors don't have laser facilities. Most laser treatment is performed in medical centers. However, it's an exciting new area of medicine.

Conization may remove many connective fibers and interfere with support from the fibers, resulting in an "incompetent cervix." Hemorrhage is always a possibility with conization of the cervix. Bleeding may be severe enough to require admission to the outpatient department or even to the hospital to replace blood and to control surgically any bleeding.

Hysterectomy carries with it the usual risks of major surgery and general anesthesia, such as drug sensitivity, post-operative blood clots, pneumonia, shock, hemorrhage, infection and bowel obstruction. If a radical hysterectomy is performed, risks are even greater because of extensive additional dissection of lymph nodes and longer anesthesia time. There is also the risk of injury to your ureters and bowel with subsequent development of false openings from these organs and drainage of urine or feces.

As we've already discussed, risks and complications of pelvic exenteration are great, but for some women this is the only option.

ADVANTAGES OF SURGERY
FOR CANCER OF THE CERVIX

Treatment for cervical cancer may be surgical, with radiation, chemotherapy or a combination of all of these. Surgery is most often applied to earlier stages. Surgery for cancer-in-situ is by conization or simple hysterectomy and should have few complications. Surgery gets rid of the cancer by removing the site.

Radical hysterectomy surgery encompasses many risks, as we have stated. It may not be a great advantage because radium and X-ray therapy are also very successful, but surgery may carry less risk.

Surgery is an advantage if your cancer is extremely early because your childbearing ability can be preserved if surgery is conservative. The ovaries may or may not need to be removed as part of the surgical procedure.

Surgery may also carry the advantage of not exposing your ovaries to radiation that could damage their function. This is important to your continued production of hormones.

DISADVANTAGES OF SURGERY FOR CANCER OF THE CERVIX

Radiation therapy by insertion of radium into the cervical canal, alongside your cervix, followed by (or occasionally preceded by) X-ray treatments may be preferred over surgery when the cancer has spread to organs that are close, such as the bladder or bowel. The radium treats the cancer where it is — in your cervical canal and in the most common area of spread — alongside the cervix. Surgery removes the uterus and cervix, but it can't always reach lymph nodes as thoroughly as radiation therapy.

But the side effects of radiation treatment, such as loss of ovarian function, must be taken into consideration as to which therapy is best for you.

WHO OPERATES?

Only specialists perform these surgeries. Sometimes even gynecological specialists don't treat enough cancer to be proficient at it and will refer you to an oncologist, a doctor who specializes in the treatment of cancer. If you discuss your surgery or radiation treatment with your doctor, he'll probably suggest consultation with and referral to a gynecology-oncologist.

DIAGNOSTIC TESTS BEFORE, DURING AND AFTER SURGERY FOR CANCER OF THE CERVIX

PAP SMEAR

Whenever cancer of the cervix is discussed, it begins with a Pap smear. The Pap test has been acclaimed by the American Cancer Society as the most significant advance in cancer detection in our time.

At least three cancer specimens are taken for a Pap smear. Specimens are taken from:

1. The vaginal pool of cells and secretions found just behind your cervix.
2. Inside your cervix to obtain cells from your cervical canal.
3. Tissue on the inner surface of the cervical opening.

These specimens are smeared on a slide and dropped into a special solution or sprayed with a solution that keeps them from drying before they reach the lab. In the laboratory, smears are specially stained and examined by someone who is trained to detect any changes in the cells from the cervix. In this way abnormalities are identified early — before they become cancer —and can be treated.

PAP-SMEAR DIAGNOSIS

The Pap test is *not* a diagnostic tool; it is a screening test. Before cancer of the cervix can definitely be diagnosed, a biopsy of your cervix must be taken.

It must be performed carefully and accurately, or it will yield many false-negative results (a Pap smear that is read as negative but really is positive—an abnormality is present).

A Pap test is designed to screen only for cancer of the *cervix*. By chance, cancer cells from your endometrium, tubes or ovaries may be discovered in a Pap smear. But additional tests are necessary to confirm the diagnosis in cancer of these organs.

If you are sexually active, you should begin having regular Pap smears at age 18. A repeat smear should be done in 1 year. If both smears are normal, you should have a repeat smear at intervals of every 3 years until age 35 and at 5-year intervals until 60. Many doctors still recommend a yearly exam, including a Pap smear, with a complete exam and a blood-pressure check.

The problem with this type of program is a Pap smear screens only for cancer of the cervix. The advantage of an annual Pap smear is that it brings you to your doctor once a year for an examination, which may reveal other health problems.

In the course of taking yearly Pap smears, we have uncovered cancer of other organs and diseases, such as diabetes, hypertension, gallbladder disease, hemorrhoids and hernias.

These discoveries happen only when a gynecologist performs a physical examination — not just a pelvic examination. In many cases, your OB-GYN doctor may be the only doctor you see regularly.

PRE-INVASIVE CANCER OF THE CERVIX (SUSPICIOUS PAP SMEAR)

Pap smears are merely screening tests. Even if a Pap test is strongly suggestive of cancer of the cervix, the diagnosis must be confirmed by tissue examination. When your smear is suspicious or suggestive of cancer, it may be called *precancerous*. The next step is a biopsy of the cervix, along with colposcopic examination.

With the use of colposcopy, the cervix can be examined carefully and biopsies taken of abnormal areas. A solution of 3% acetic acid is applied to help delineate abnormal areas. Iodine also may be used (the Schiller test). Normal cervical tissue is readily stained; suspicious areas do not take the stain and are then biopsied.

Punch biopsies are obtained from non-stained areas. If punch biopsies don't confirm the diagnosis, a conization of your cervix may be done. This confirms the diagnosis and may provide the treatment because it removes all suspicious tissue.

Some smears and some biopsies show changes that are not yet cancerous. But experience has demonstrated these eventually may develop into a definite cancer.

CARCINOMA-IN-SITU

The earliest stage of definite cancer of the cervix is called *carcinoma-in-situ*, which means the cancer has not broken through the basement lining of the mucous membrane — it has not begun to spread. At this stage, cancer of the cervix should yield at least a 90%-cure rate. At this stage, hopefully your cancer of the cervix has been diagnosed by means of cancer smears.

CRYOSURGERY

Freezing tissue is used to treat inflammation of the cervix and early changes of the cervix in which cells show abnormality but not actual cancer. This applies to CIN I and II and sometimes CIN III. It is not advocated when cancer has been definitely diagnosed.

Cryosurgery is performed about 1 week after cessation of your last menstrual period. This avoids treating you when you are pregnant and allows for healing before the next menstrual cycle.

LASER

Laser is an acronym for "light amplification by stimulated emission of radiation." The laser produces a coherent light, which is a parallel beam of uniform wavelength that can be focused by a lens into a small area.

Laser surgery takes more time and causes more pain than cryosurgery, but healing is much faster. Laser surgery is not available in all areas of the United States, but its use is growing. Laser equipment is expensive and should only be used by those specially trained in this special procedure.

CONIZATION

Cancer-in-situ can be cured by conization. This is the method of choice if you desire further pregnancies. If you desire no further pregnancies, a hysterectomy is the treatment method of choice.

Schiller's staining helps mark the area that needs to be removed from your cervix. This also helps determine the depth of the cone of tissue to be removed. A cone of tissue is then removed using a scalpel. Conization can also be done with the laser.

When skillfully performed, conization is an excellent procedure for removing the site of cancer-in-situ of the cervix. Occasionally bleeding occurs following surgery, but this can be controlled.

If you desire further pregnancies, other methods of treatment, such as punch biopsy, cryosurgery or laser surgery, are preferred because conization occasionally impairs cervical function. A "coned" cervix may interfere with fertility or the ability to carry a pregnancy to full term.

If cancer-in-situ is diagnosed during pregnancy, the pregnancy may be allowed to progress to full term. After vaginal delivery, further evaluation with Pap smears and conization could be undertaken, depending on the situation.

COLPOSCOPY

Meticulous study and diagnosis of early cancer of the cervix is also done by colposcopy. Tissues are examined through the vagina by means of a colposcope. The colposcope allows magnified examination of the cervix and vagina, and allows the abnormal areas to be biopsied for diagnosis. The cervical canal is also scraped to look for abnormal cells. This procedure is called *ECC* or *endocervical curettage.*

Colposcopy may be performed in your doctor's office. It requires 15 to 20 minutes and is usually no more uncomfortable than a regular pelvic exam.

The principal value of colposcopy is that it may avoid the necessity of a cervical conization, which might risk miscarriage in a pregnant woman. Colposcopy can zero in on the exact area to be biopsied and enable your doctor to obtain a punch biopsy without disturbing your pregnancy. It can also locate the most suspicious area on the cervix for biopsy and examination of the tissue for cancer.

REASONS FOR TESTS

All these tests play a role in the diagnosis and treatment of cancer of the cervix. Most of them are also used in collaboration with your doctor's pelvic examination. Sometimes your doctor can tell by his examination if there is thickening alongside your cervix, which might indicate your cancer has spread outward toward your pelvic wall. In advanced cases of cervical cancer, your doctor may even be able to feel thickening or cancer nodules in your rectum, indicating spread of the cancer.

WHERE IS SURGERY FOR CANCER OF THE CERVIX PERFORMED?

Pap smear, punch biopsy, cryosurgery and laser surgery are performed in your doctor's office. Some doctors prefer to do conization and D&C in the hospital or in outpatient surgery.

Hysterectomy, insertion of radium and X-ray therapy are performed in the hospital.

HOSPITALIZATION AND DURATION

Hysterectomy involves being admitted to the hospital the night before, or the morning of, surgery. You will have urinalysis, complete blood count, type and crossmatch of blood for surgery. If he anticipates difficult surgery, your doctor may have you donate a pint of your blood 1 to 4 weeks before surgery in case you need a transfusion. Then you can receive your own blood during surgery. This is called *autotransfusion.*

Chest X-ray, intravenous pyelogram (X-ray of your urinary system to see if it is involved by cancer), barium enema to check your lower bowel, cystoscopy (examination of your urinary bladder by scope) and even rectosigmoidoscopy (using a special scope to look into the rectum and lower bowel) may be done before surgery to make certain these organs are not involved.

You may be offered a sleeping pill the night before surgery to ensure your rest. An enema is sometimes given to clear your bowel to cut down on post-operative gas.

Early on the morning of surgery, you'll be given an injection containing a drug to dry secretions to prevent aspiration of secretions into your lungs. The shot also contains a pain reliever that decreases the amount of anesthetic you will require. Because of this injection, you may not remember going to the operating room.

Intravenous fluids are started, and it is through this tubing you receive pentothal or brevital in the operating room to put you to sleep. You will not be aware of going to sleep.

After you're asleep, a tube is inserted into your trachea to assure an open airway throughout surgery. It is through this tube that your gas anesthetic is administered. You may also be given a muscle relaxant to relax abdominal muscles and make it easier for your doctor to visualize and operate on them.

Surgery takes about 1-1/2 hours for a simple hysterectomy but may require several hours longer if a radical hysterectomy is performed. Most of that time will be spent in locating and removing cancer-involved lymph nodes.

After surgery, you are taken to the recovery room to awaken from your anesthesia. In recovery, you're carefully monitored for any bleeding from your incision or from the vagina. Your blood pressure, pulse and respiration are closely watched.

After about an hour in recovery, you are returned to your hospital room where you will be drowsy, if not asleep, for the remainder of the day.

Plan on 5 to 7 days hospitalization after your hysterectomy. During this time, you will be up and about, begin to eat and possibly move your bowels on your own. Your bladder should be working well by the time you go home.

Some doctors leave stitches in longer than others. Yours may be removed before you go home. Injections are given for pain relief as you need them, but you may not require any after the first post-operative day. Your doctor may give you pain pills to take home with you to take as you need them.

If your ovaries have been removed, your doctor will probably give you estrogen tablets. They will prevent surgical menopause (hot flashes, nervousness, insomnia) that ordinarily follows removal of your ovaries.

ANESTHESIA

The cervix contains few nerve endings, so it can be cut, sewed and cauterized with minimal pain. But it is painful to stretch the cervix. Cauterization, punch biopsies, cryosurgery and laser surgery can be performed without anesthesia. If a D&C is performed along with these surgeries, anesthesia is necessary. This is usually I.V. pentothal or brevital. For a hysterectomy, general anesthesia is used.

When radium is inserted, the cervix is stretched to accommodate the pencil-sized rubber tube containing the two capsules of radium that are inserted into the cervix. For this procedure, anesthesia is required.

Two other radium-filled applicators are inserted into the upper vagina on either side of your cervix. Packing is inserted to hold these in place. Intravenous or gas anesthesia is used when radium is inserted. The radium will be left in place for several hours or as long as a day or two. No anesthesia is necessary when the radium is removed.

PROBABLE OUTCOME OF SURGERY FOR CANCER OF THE CERVIX

Treatment is extremely successful for cancer of the cervix. It takes an average of 5 to 10 years before this type of cancer begins to spread. It is considered by many doctors to be a preventable disease—no woman should die of cancer of the cervix if it is detected early.

If cancer of the cervix has begun to spread, the outcome is less favorable in direct proportion to the extent of its spread. Average 5-year-cure rates for cancer of the cervix in subgroups is shown below. Statistics are based on 2,000 patients treated at the M.D. Anderson Hospital and Tumor Institute in Texas.

Stage I	91.5%	Stage IIIA	45%
Stage IIA	83.5%	Stage IIIB	36%
Stage IIB	66.5%	Stage IV	14%

POST-OPERATIVE CARE

PUNCH BIOPSY

There is rarely any bleeding following punch biopsy. These are shallow specimens, so bleeding is easily controlled by pressure or cautery. A watery, blood-tinged discharge is present for 1 to 2 weeks. You may want to douche if the discharge becomes foul smelling.

CRYOSURGERY

Hemorrhage is uncommon following cryosurgery. If it does occur, it is late, when the remaining dead tissue is sloughed away. Discharge is likely to continue for a month. It may be blood-tinged and may become foul smelling.

LASER THERAPY

Discharge is light, and bleeding is light. Discharge is less foul smelling because less tissue is destroyed.

CONIZATION

Hemorrhage is common, due to large blood vessels that are cut or during the healing process. Discharge may be heavy, bloody and foul smelling. Douches must be taken with care so the douche tip does not cause additional bleeding. If hemorrhage occurs, it usually can be controlled by cautery. If this doesn't stop it, a couple of stitches will stop the bleeding.

HYSTERECTOMY

There is always a chance of bleeding and infection following hysterectomy, but it is uncommon. You will be permitted to continue exercises begun in the hospital, which include walking, climbing stairs and increasing activity such as household chores. Don't lift more than 10 pounds to begin with. You can gradually increase to normal amounts after about 6 weeks.

After a month, sexual activity can return to normal. Undertake sports gradually, especially golf, tennis and jogging. Swimming is good for you, and it is easier on your body than other sports because of buoyancy in the water.

DIET

There is no special diet following surgery for cancer of the cervix. As with any major surgery, you must avoid overeating while you are inactive, or you will gain more weight than you want.

If you've had a pelvic exenteration (removal of bladder and lower bowel), you will have special training in control of these functions, and a diet will be prescribed to fit your special needs. Your recovery will take longer and may require many weeks.

MISCONCEPTIONS ABOUT SURGERY FOR CANCER OF THE CERVIX

Cancer of the cervix is incurable.
Many cancers are curable, and cancer of the cervix has one of the highest cure rates. Just because you have cancer doesn't mean you're going to die.

Having cancer means I'll have to have extensive surgery.
A conization may cure you, or a simple hysterectomy may cure you. Even a radical hysterectomy can be performed with great skill and few complications today. Pelvic exenteration is uncommon, and it is unlikely you will ever need one.

If I receive radiation treatments, it means my cancer is incurable (inoperable).
This is untrue in cancer of the cervix. Radiation treatments are often more effective than surgery in cancer of the cervix when the cancer is beyond the earliest stage. Chemotherapy is rarely used in treatment of cancer of the cervix.

ALTERNATIVES TO SURGERY FOR CANCER OF THE CERVIX

Cautery is not used for treatment of cancer of the cervix, even in its earliest stages. Cryosurgery is used by some doctors for treatment of cancer-in-situ, but conization is better because it is more exact, and cure rates are higher. Radium and X-ray are the best combination treatment for cancer of the cervix when it has begun to spread.

CALL YOUR DOCTOR IF . . .

1. You have fever or chills.
2. You have redness, swelling or irritation of your abdominal incision.
3. You have bleeding heavier than a menstrual period.
4. You have a foul-smelling, profuse discharge, heavier than what your doctor has told you to expect.

QUESTIONS TO ASK YOUR DOCTOR

Explain what kind of cancer I have, how extensive it is and what I should expect in the way of treatment.

You can better understand the clinical stages of cancer if your doctor explains them to you. You will be able to understand and accept the treatment for your particular stage of disease.

Explain what effect this treatment will have on my body, my menstrual periods, my chances for pregnancy and menopausal symptoms.

Write down any questions that enter your mind. Write down your doctor's answers, and be certain you understand as much as possible about your condition.

What about activity, exercise, sports, lifting, going back to work? How soon? What limitations?

Your doctor can give you some guidelines, although you may have to wait and see how your surgery turns out and how you feel.

What did you find at surgery? Had the cancer progressed farther than you anticipated? What does this mean?

It's better if you know exactly what you have and what can be done for you.

Cancer of the Ovary

DEFINITION OF CANCER OF THE OVARY

Cancer of the ovary is not one disease — it is a common term for many different diseases of the ovary. Some of them are very different from the others. Ovarian cancer is a term for cells of the ovary that have changed their biology so they no longer follow the rules that normal cells adhere to. See the explanation of cancer-cell growth on pages 71 and 72.

A cancer cell becomes independent of its parent cell and changes its structure and pattern-of-growth characteristics. It then transmits these changes to successive generations of cancer cells. As far as we know, cancer cells eventually kill you if they are not treated and eradicated.

Extensive research has failed to uncover any specific causes for cancer of the ovary. The incidence is greater in older women, women who have had no children and Caucasian women.

ABBREVIATIONS AND OTHER NAMES

Cyst, tumor, mass, lump, thickness, growth, lesion—any of these terms could refer to cancer of the ovary. But they could also refer to benign or non-cancerous growths. So if you say you have a tumor or a growth on your ovary, it could mean almost anything and not necessarily cancer. If your doctor says you have a growth on your ovary, ask him to be specific and tell you if he thinks you have cancer. Ask how you and he can be sure.

PARTS OF BODY INVOLVED

When it begins, cancer of the ovary may be limited to your ovary, see illustration below, but it can involve almost any part of your body if it spreads. Ovarian cancer typically spreads to surface areas inside your abdomen. These areas include adjacent areas in the abdomen—the intestines and the omentum.

LYMPH NODES

You may have wondered why cancers spread to lymph nodes. Your body has a separate system of circulation, in addition to the bloodstream, that carries special lymph fluid. This fluid pools in glands called *lymph nodes.*

One of the primary functions of lymph fluid is to carry white blood cells to fight infection wherever it occurs in the body. That is why you have "swollen glands" with a sore throat.

Your body treats cancer as though it were an infection (an enemy of your body) and sends white blood cells to fight the cancer cells. This is why cancer spreads by way of the lymph channels to your lymph glands, which then become swollen. When you have cancer, the first place your doctor looks for spread is in the surrounding lymph glands.

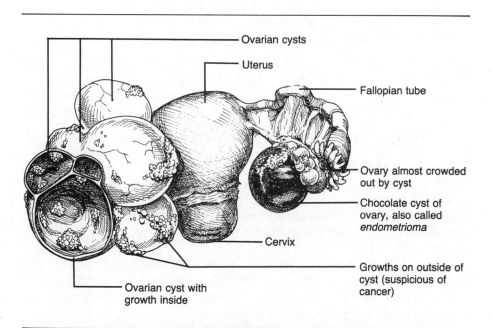

Composite shows endometrial cyst (chocolate cyst) on one side and many cysts on the other side, with growths on the inside and outside of the cyst.

COMMON REASONS FOR SURGERY FOR CANCER OF THE OVARY

Cancer of the ovaries is called a *silent cancer* because there are no symptoms — until it has progressed far enough to compress other organs, invade and involve organs, interfere with their function or become large enough to cause your abdomen to enlarge. This is another reason to have a yearly pelvic exam. Many cancers of the ovary have been detected early because they were found on routine pelvic examination.

Some doctors or other medical personnel recommend a Pap smear (for cancer of the cervix) only once every 3 years or even less frequently. We recommend this smear on an annual basis because it takes you to your doctor yearly for a pelvic exam, at which time he can also check for ovarian cancer as he performs other routine tests.

You probably see your OB-GYN fairly regularly during childbearing years, but a yearly examination is even more important *after* you have had your family, certainly after age 35. When a pelvic exam reveals an ovarian mass or growth, it must be investigated to see if it is cancerous. The way to be certain about an ovarian cancer is to *look* at it. The most common reason for surgery involving the ovaries is to determine if an ovarian growth is cancerous and to remove it.

HOW COMMON IS SURGERY FOR CANCER OF THE OVARY?

Cancer of the ovary is becoming more common and is now the fourth leading cause of cancer death in American women. Cancer of the cervix is declining as a cause of death because of the Pap smear, but cancer of the ovary has doubled, from 3.2 to 8.9 per 100,000, in the period from 1930 to 1968.

FUNCTIONS INVOLVED IN SURGERY FOR CANCER OF THE OVARY

It's surprising that cancer can exist in your ovary and not interfere with your ovarian function. Yet, until cancer is far advanced, it causes *no* symptoms of any kind. Menstrual periods continue as usual (these are controlled by ovarian hormones), even though part of your ovary may have been invaded by cancer.

It would aid early diagnosis if you had some signs or symptoms to warn you that you might have ovarian cancer. With the exception of masculinizing or feminizing tumors (see explanation on next page), there are no typical symptoms of ovarian cancer, especially early symptoms.

Perhaps because your ovaries are in close proximity to your bowel, and because of the nature of spread (surface spread) of the cancer, cancer of your ovaries may produce lower abdominal pain or pressure and vague digestive disturbances (indigestion, belching, gas). But these are usually *late* signs of the disease. Vaginal bleeding occurs if you have an estrogen-producing ovarian cancer that causes the uterus to bleed. Only about 15% of all women with ovarian tumors have vaginal bleeding.

Masculinizing tumors may cause growth of hair on your face and body, deepening of your voice and enlargement of your clitoris. Unfortunately, most of these symptoms occur only when your tumor has advanced beyond the early stages.

Feminizing cancers may cause heavier menstrual flow or bleeding between periods.

One tumor of the ovary is a *dermoid,* which characteristically contains teeth, hair and other tissues. If a dermoid becomes malignant, it is called a *teratoma.* It is often diagnosed by X-ray when a tooth can be seen on the X-ray. See illustration below.

When a pelvic mass is discovered on routine pelvic exam, it might be due to many things. These include gas or stool in your bowel, infected pockets of your bowel (diverticulitis), cancer in the lower part of your bowel, a fibroid

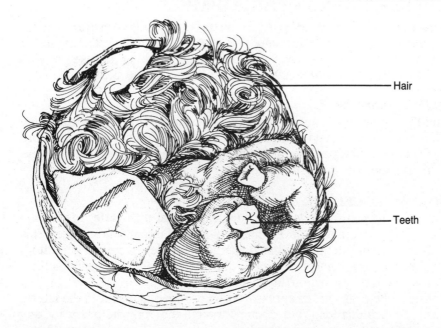

Dermoid cyst is a benign cyst that has various tissues in it. It can become cancerous and is then called *teratomas.*

tumor of your uterus, a "pelvic kidney" (one that can be felt because it is lower than normal), an enlarged Fallopian tube or any number of other masses. In any event, a mass in your pelvis that is 2-1/2 inches or larger that persists through two menstrual cycles should be examined by laparoscopy, especially when thought to be ovarian. For more information on laparoscopy, see page 237. If you are post-menopausal, any ovarian mass that can be felt on exam must be considered to be ovarian cancer until proven otherwise by surgery.

Although most benign ovarian tumors are smooth-walled, cystic, freely movable and less than 3 inches in diameter, there is no way to be certain of malignancy without further studies, such as laparoscopy, ultrasound and X-ray. X-ray may uncover teeth in a dermoid ovarian tumor, but other tumors also show calcium deposits, so ultrasound and laparoscopy are necessary.

Examination of the urinary system may show displacement (by the mass) of the tube from the kidneys to the bladder. Bowel X-ray may reveal involvement of your large or small intestine. Tests on bladder and bowel are carried out when the tumor is believed to be extensive and may have spread to your small or large intestine or bladder.

Examination of the large intestine just above your rectum, called *sigmoid-scopy,* and rectal examination can evaluate or discover 80% of cancers of the lower left bowel. This exam should be done *before* major surgery is performed for an ovarian mass, to be sure the mass isn't in your lower bowel or rectum.

HOW SURGERY FOR CANCER OF THE OVARY IS PERFORMED

Surgery for ovarian cancer is performed through a *midline incision.* This is made, instead of the bikini incision, because your doctor must examine all parts of your abdomen and pelvis to determine the extent of the disease. This type of exam cannot be done adequately through a bikini incision.

MIDLINE INCISION

A midline incision is somewhat easier to perform than the pubic hairline incision, and it is faster, especially for large tumors. A midline incision is more likely to break open if you have a coughing episode or if you put undue stress on your incision post-operatively.

SURGICAL PROCEDURE

After entering your abdomen, your doctor looks at the ovaries to evaluate the extent of your tumor, to determine what kind of tumor it is and see if it is malignant. Although definite diagnosis cannot be made, except in a laboratory under a microscope, in most cases your doctor can recognize a benign follicle cyst or a dermoid cyst by looking at it.

A piece of the ovary or the entire ovary is removed and sent to the lab for microscopic examination. Your doctor inspects the opposite ovary for any evidence of the same tumor and checks your other pelvic organs and abdominal organs for evidence of tumor or other abnormalities.

Whether or not your doctor removes part or all of your ovary or any other pelvic organ depends on the type of tumor, the extent of its spread, your age and your desire for more children. From a survival standpoint, the ideal treatment of ovarian cancer is removal of your uterus, along with Fallopian tubes and ovaries. If you are past menopause, this presents no problem. If you're younger and want to preserve your childbearing ability and ovarian hormone function, it's essential that a firm diagnosis of ovarian cancer be established *before* such radical treatment is undertaken.

Common practice is to send ovarian-tumor tissue to the lab for a frozen biopsy while you're still on the operating table. A frozen biopsy is not as accurate as a paraffin-prepared biopsy, but that test requires waiting a few days for the report. Waiting a few days may be worth it to be sure organs are not removed unnecessarily, especially in younger women.

If your ovarian tumor has wartlike growths on its surface or inside its cystic mass, it's more likely to be cancerous. Adhesions to other organs, growth of the tumor in the abdominal cavity or blood-filled areas in your ovary are also suspicious of cancer. Your doctor will examine both ovaries carefully because spread from one ovary to the other is common. A biopsy is always done if there is any question.

At the time of surgery, the extent of possible spread of cancer is evaluated by removal of the lymph nodes. This is one of the primary areas of spread by many cancers because cancer cells collect in nodes.

Another method of evaluation is to obtain pelvic or abdominal washings. Fluid from your abdominal cavity is examined to see if there are cancer cells in it. This is done immediately, while your abdomen is still open. A third way to evaluate your situation is to biopsy other structures that appear to be involved by cancer, such as your diaphragm, liver and omentum (the protective apron of the abdomen). Your surgeon will also check the inside of your abdominal cavity for evidence of spread of the cancer.

If the cancer seems to be localized in one ovary and you want to preserve your childbearing ability, only the involved ovary will be removed. However, you must realize the risk you take. The only way to know for sure is to remove any possible source of cancer — in this case, both ovaries. Usually all your female organs are removed — uterus, tubes and both ovaries — to reduce the risk of spread, but this depends on the type of cancer you have and your particular situation.

If there's any evidence of spread to your lymph glands or other organs, or if the particular cancer has a high rate of spread, X-ray treatment maybe more effective than treatment with anti-cancer drugs. There is evidence both methods give greater relief of symptoms and prolong life longer than either method used alone. X-ray treatment and chemotherapy (and their combination) are still being evaluated to determine the best treatment method for various types of ovarian cancers.

You have about a 25% chance of developing baldness if you are treated with chemotherapy, but this is usually temporary. Other side effects of chemotherapy and radiation vary according to the agents used. The most common side effects are nausea, vomiting, diarrhea and weakness.

Even if your cancer has already spread, surgical attempts to remove as much of the tumor as possible may be made to reduce the number of surviving tumor cells.

A gradual reduction of tumor mass through surgery, X-ray and chemotherapy, one following the other, occasionally reduces the number of surviving tumor cells to the point where your own defenses may overcome the remaining tumor.

RISKS OF SURGERY
FOR CANCER OF THE OVARY

Risks of surgery for cancer of the ovary depend on how much surgery must be performed. If your cancer has not spread, and if surgery consists of removing an ovary or removing all the pelvic organs, the risk is no greater than an ordinary hysterectomy.

There is always the risk of post-operative bowel obstruction in any abdominal surgery. There is also the risk of hemorrhage and the risk from general anesthesia. But modern surgery is safe, and complications are rare.

If your cancer has begun to spread, there is the risk of damage to blood vessels, to the ureters (tubes from kidneys to bladder) and the risk of bowel obstruction if the intestines are involved.

Occasionally ovarian cancer spreads to adjacent organs, such as the bowel. When this occurs, extensive surgery may *not* be undertaken because chemotherapy and X-ray treatment may be more effective, or surgery may not be possible because of the extent of the disease. In some cases, if the cancer is widely spread, your abdomen is closed, and you will be treated with chemotherapy and X-ray treatment.

ADVANTAGES OF SURGERY
FOR CANCER OF THE OVARY

A diagnosis first must be established so your doctor will know the course of action for the best treatment. Diagnosis may include history, careful physical exam, ultrasound and X-ray studies, as previously mentioned. Laparoscopy may be used to see your tumor and take a biopsy, but many doctors believe laparoscopy should not be used because an adequate biopsy may not be taken. Laparotomy, which is major surgery, is performed only after all the tests are completed, such as D&C if there is vaginal bleeding.

In the final analysis, surgery is almost always the ultimate treatment for ovarian cancer. It permits your doctor to confirm the diagnosis and remove the cancer, if it can be removed, or evaluate the extent of it for treatment with chemotherapy or X-ray treatment.

DISADVANTAGES OF SURGERY FOR CANCER OF THE OVARY

The only disadvantage to surgery is if your cancer has spread so much that it is inoperable. Other organs are so involved that the cancer cannot be removed or the other organs would require removal. This would be more serious to your overall outlook. If there is spread to other organs, chemotherapy and X-ray treatments are the only methods to treat your cancer. Surgery might be considered unnecessary, except it helps determine the extent of your cancer and the fact it must be treated in some other way.

WHO OPERATES?

In general, an obstetrician-gynecologist or possibly an oncologist will operate on you because he has trained and specialized in this type of surgery. However, some general surgeons perform this surgery and are competent to care for you. Your surgery may be extensive and involve bowel surgery, so a gynecologist may join with a general surgeon in performing the surgery.

DIAGNOSTIC TESTS BEFORE, DURING AND AFTER SURGERY FOR CANCER OF THE OVARY

The only way to discover an ovarian tumor early is to find it during a pelvic exam. One strong argument in favor of having regular annual physical exams is to uncover unsuspected ovarian tumors *early*. It can be discovered "early" if your doctor feels an enlarged ovary (on routine exam for Pap smear) or by ultrasound if done for another reason.

Any ovary as large as 2-1/2 inches in diameter (about the size of a tennis ball) should be observed through two menstrual cycles. Or it may be treated with hormones to make certain it does not contain a simple ovarian cyst. This does not apply to a woman who is post-menopausal — cancer must be ruled out, so this means surgery. About 95% of all simple cysts under 2-1/2 inches are benign; they cure themselves by spontaneous rupture or spontaneous resolution. Many cysts break while your doctor is examining them — this is a simple cure with no ill effects.

Simple cysts often come and go, rupturing spontaneously and spilling their contents into your peritoneal cavity with no adverse symptoms. If enlargement of the mass persists, laparoscopy may determine the type of tumor in your ovary and whether it needs to be explored and removed by major surgery.

STAGING OF CANCER OF THE OVARY

As with most cancers, cancer of the ovary is classified according to how far it has spread. This is called *clinical staging*.

Stage I	Growth limited to ovaries. There are subgroups A, B and C, according to whether cancer is found in one or both ovaries and whether there are cancer cells in the fluid found in the peritoneal cavity.
Stage II	Growth in the ovaries extends to other pelvic organs (tubes and uterus).
Stage III	Growth in ovaries extends to other organs in the pelvis (bowel, omentum) and to lymph nodes in the peritoneal cavity but outside the pelvis.
Stage IV	Growth in ovaries with distant spread, such as liver and lungs.

It is surprising how large an ovarian tumor can become without causing any symptoms. On routine pelvic examination, many doctors discover ovarian cysts that have reached massive proportions. You may be surprised to learn there is something wrong with you because you had no unusual symptoms. You may have noticed only an increasing abdominal girth or that clothes were too small.

Any pelvic mass in the post-menopausal period demands immediate investigation by surgery to determine if removal is necessary. Some doctors feel an ovarian mass cannot be adequately evaluated by laparoscopy in the post-menopausal period, and laparotomy must be performed. Perhaps their cautious attitude is prompted by the high incidence of ovarian cancer in women after menopause.

The best diagnostic test for ovarian cancer is an accurate pelvic examination. Your doctor may even want to examine you under anesthesia to be certain of his findings.

Besides the pelvic exam, as mentioned, laparoscopy, ultrasound and X-ray may be helpful in establishing a definite diagnosis of a pelvic mass. Complete blood count and urinalysis are routine. Special blood chemistries are performed prior to surgery if your doctor feels they are necessary. A barium enema and an intravenous pyelogram are ordered by your doctor before surgery if he suspects bowel or urinary-tract involvement by the cancer.

WHERE IS SURGERY PERFORMED?

This is major surgery and will be performed only in the operating room of a hospital. This is definitely *not* outpatient surgery.

HOSPITALIZATION AND DURATION

Much depends on what your doctor found on laparoscopy, ultrasound, X-ray and bowel and bladder studies to see if the cancer has spread. Ideally, as much of the cancer (hopefully all of it) will be removed with surgery, followed by chemotherapy.

If you are having surgery, you will be admitted the day before surgery for urinalysis, complete blood count, blood-chemistry studies and blood type and crossmatching for possible transfusion. You may have already donated your own blood for autotransfusion.

You will have nothing to eat after midnight to keep your stomach empty. Early on the morning of surgery you will receive an injection of sedative-tranquilizer and a drug to dry your secretions for general anesthesia.

An I.V. with an extra-large needle is started, in case blood must be given. Blood requires a larger needle than I.V. fluids. It is through this continuous I.V. that nearly all your medications will be given during surgery, including one to put you to sleep before switching to a mask for gas anesthesia.

Your doctor will make a midline incision so your abdomen can be examined. Adhesions and large ovarian tumors require a longer incision.

After extending your incision into your abdominal cavity, the doctor will thoroughly examine your ovaries, tubes, uterus and the rest of your abdominal cavity and organs. He will look for any evidence of spread of the cancer.

Sometimes your doctor can tell what kind of cancer you have just by looking at it. But he always depends on laboratory analysis for ultimate treatment.

Surgery can involve the removal of only one ovary or include hysterectomy and removal of both tubes and both ovaries. Discuss with your doctor the possibilities before surgery. He should have authorization from you to do whatever is necessary and whatever will give you the best results.

After the surgery is finished and your incision is closed, you will be taken to the recovery room where you will awaken. When your vital signs—pulse, blood pressure and respiration—are stable, you will be taken to the intensive-care unit (if extensive surgery was performed) or to your hospital room.

Unless spread of your cancer necessitates additional surgery, your operation takes 1 to 3 hours in the operating room. You'll be in the recovery room about an hour, then taken to your hospital bed. Plan on 3 to 7 days in the hospital, although this could vary according to your doctor and the extent of your surgery.

You'll be out of bed the day after surgery to go to the bathroom. The following day you may be walking up and down the hall with help; you'll be completely ambulatory by the time you go home.

You may have a problem emptying your bladder if surgery was extensive. Otherwise bowel and bladder function will be normal. Gas pains are common but short-lived (24 hours). Enemas are used sparingly because most patients seem to go to the bathroom on their own, if given time.

You may feel you're being rushed as nurses and attendants hustle you out of bed, but this is your best safeguard against phlebitis. You will be given pain-relieving shots and pills as you need them.

ANESTHESIA

You will be asleep from the medication given through your I.V. needle so you won't know when the mask is placed on your face. You won't be aware that a tube is placed in your trachea during anesthesia to ensure an adequate airway. The tube will be removed before you awaken enough to be aware of its presence. You will be watched constantly, in case you vomit, so you don't suck vomit into your lungs.

You will probably be given a general anesthetic. If you prefer epidural or spinal anesthesia, discuss this with your anesthesiologist when he visits you the night before surgery. Because of improved methods of anesthesia, you will have little nausea, vomiting or gas pains following surgery.

PROBABLE OUTCOME OF SURGERY FOR CANCER OF THE OVARY

Fewer than 30% of all ovarian cancers have not spread when they are diagnosed. This is tragic because when cancer has not spread beyond the ovaries, a 5-year survival rate of almost 75% can be expected, while only a 12% 5-year survival rate is possible when cancer has spread. One out of every 100 women in the United States, between 30 and 45, will eventually die from ovarian cancer.

One survey showed that less than 50% of the internists in Massachusetts performed routine pelvic exams. Often vague abdominal complaints are treated with antacids without a thought that the problem could be ovarian cancer. Every doctor should perform a pelvic exam as part of a complete physical exam.

Ovarian cancers vary. Some are highly malignant; others grow very slowly. Some cancers, such as dysgerminomas, a rare cancer similar to cancer of testicle in male, respond well to X-ray treatments. Others do not. Surgery is effective for some cancers. Have confidence in your doctor and his judgment. He will probably seek consultation with a cancer specialist or a tumor clinic, and together they will individualize your treatment. Follow their advice.

Surgery for your ovarian cancer is not the real problem. The outcome depends on the extent and type of your ovarian cancer. Surgery may be the first step, followed by X-ray treatment or chemotherapy. Or it could represent the entire treatment.

POST-OPERATIVE CARE

When you're discharged from the hospital, you'll be walking around, able to go to the bathroom and able to look after yourself. It's not unusual to have a "let-down" feeling after you return home and find you're weaker than you thought.

Be easy on yourself, but don't stay in bed — the danger of blood clots forming in your legs is greater. But don't feel you need to clean your house or entertain visitors.

You should get stronger each day, although you'll have good and bad days. Stairs won't hurt you nor will driving your car. Start gradually with things like sweeping the floor or running the vacuum cleaner.

Sports can wait until after you go back to your doctor for your checkup in 1 month. Then see how you feel. You may not want to stretch or strain abdominal muscles for a while.

DIET

You won't have a special diet following surgery for ovarian cancer. There is a tendency to eat more as you feel better, so be careful of gaining weight during the time you are relatively inactive.

MISCONCEPTIONS ABOUT SURGERY FOR CANCER OF THE OVARY

Cancer is incurable.
This is untrue. Outcome depends on the type of cancer and how extensive it is. Many cancers are curable; yours may be one of these.

Pelvic surgery will make me old, wrinkled and sexless.
None of these fears are based in fact. Many women fear removal of their ovaries for various reasons. In certain cancers of the ovary, your ovaries will not have to be removed (at least not both of them).

My ovaries will have to be removed, and I'll go through menopause now.
With rare exceptions, both ovaries will have to be removed, and this would normally put you through a surgical menopause. However you will probably be able to take estrogen to prevent any menopausal symptoms.

CALL YOUR DOCTOR IF . . .

1. You have chills or fever.
2. You have any redness, tenderness, swelling or discharge around or from your incision.
3. You have any separation of your incision.
4. You don't feel as good as you think you should.

QUESTIONS TO ASK YOUR DOCTOR

What about consultation with another physician?
If surgery is recommended, don't be afraid to request a second opinion. You should have the right to choose the consultant, if you wish.

What kind of tumor do I have? Is it malignant? Has it spread? How extensively?

"Cancer" is a collective term used to describe many different tumors. Find out all you can about your ovarian tumor so you will know what to expect.

Were you able to remove the entire tumor mass? Did you find any of the lymph glands involved with cancer? Any other organs?

It's important to know if your cancer has spread to your lymph nodes and if your doctor feels he was able to remove all of your cancer. If it has spread to other organs, then you'll probably need chemotherapy or X-ray treatment. Your discussion clears the air and lets you know what to expect. In this enlightened age, you want to know, and have the *right* to know, all about your cancer.

Do I need any further treatment? X-ray therapy? Chemotherapy?

You want to know what kind of treatment you may receive and how effective it should be in your particular case.

Is this type of cancer inherited? What about my daughters? Are they likely to get it?

This is probably unlikely, although some families do have a greater tendency to develop cancers.

If my ovaries are removed at surgery, what about menopause? Will I still experience it?

If your ovaries are removed, you'll have menopausal symptoms, but they can be relieved by taking estrogen.

Will I be taking hormones? For how long? Will hormones affect the cancer or make it recur?

If you have few or no menopausal symptoms — hot flashes, nervousness, insomnia — you may not require hormones. Hormones should have no effect on some cancers but may have dramatic effects on others. There are a few cancers that may be related to female sex hormones, such as some breast cancers or cancer of the uterus, and you would not be given hormones if you had one of these cancers. Many advantages are now known about hormones and your current and future well-being. The decision to prescribe hormones depends on your individual case and will require continued discussion with your doctor. After surgery, don't "disappear," thinking you are cured. Continue to consult with your doctor on regular visits to get the best care possible for you.

Cancer of the Uterus

DEFINITION OF CANCER OF THE UTERUS

Cancer of the uterus is really cancer of the *lining* of the uterus. It is a very common type of cancer in female organs. Cancer of the uterus can occur in the cervix (neck) or in the corpus (body) of the uterus. Common usage has divided the two cancers — *cancer of the uterus* refers to cancer of the endometrium (lining of the cavity of the uterus), *not* cancer of the cervix. This section deals with cancer of the lining of the uterus (the endometrium). Cancer of the cervix is covered in the section that begins on page 90.

ABBREVIATIONS AND OTHER NAMES

Cancer of the endometrium is also called cancer of the womb. The surgical treatment of endometrial cancer is hysterectomy and removal of tubes and ovaries, sometimes called a complete hysterectomy or total hysterectomy with bilateral salpingo-oophorectomy. If cancer has spread, surgery can include removal of lymph nodes.

PARTS OF BODY INVOLVED

The first area of spread is deeper within the uterus. Additional spread is to the lymph glands of the pelvis, to the peritoneal cavity, both tubes and ovaries and to adjacent organs, such as the bowel or bladder. See illustration on page 122.

Cancer cells can spill out the ends of the Fallopian tubes into the peritoneal cavity. There they implant themselves on almost any abdominal organ. When

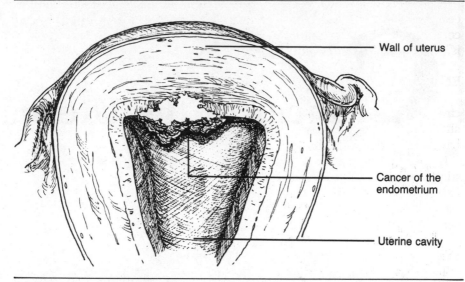

Wall of uterus

Cancer of the endometrium

Uterine cavity

Cancer of the endometrium is cancer of the lining of the uterine cavity. It is commonly called *cancer of the uterus.*

cancer cells invade the bloodstream, they can be carried throughout the body. They seem to seek organs that have the best blood supply, such as liver, lungs and brain.

COMMON REASONS FOR SURGERY FOR CANCER OF THE UTERUS

The most common signs of endometrial cancer are bleeding after menopause or prolonged, heavy menstrual bleeding during periods and intermenstrual spotting. The average age for cancer of the uterus is 61; about 20% of all women who bleed after menopause will have endometrial cancer.

When uterine cancer occurs in young women, they are often massively overweight. Most of these women do not ovulate, possibly because of their obesity. If you are overweight and have any change in your menstrual periods, check with your doctor.

Biopsy of the endometrium can detect many uterine cancers, but a complete D&C is more accurate. Only 1/3 to 1/2 of all women with cancer of the endometrium have an abnormal Pap smear on routine screening. This means you need more than a Pap smear to determine the cause of abnormal uterine bleeding.

The best way to determine what causes abnormal bleeding is to perform a *fractional D&C.* A specimen is obtained by scraping the canal of your cervix, and a second specimen is obtained by scraping the cavity of the uterus. This shows where the cancer is located. A Pap smear is valuable and must not be overlooked, but D&C is absolutely essential.

Just as Pap smears have been able to diagnose premalignant changes in the cervix, D&C and office biopsies have helped us diagnose a premalignant condition of the endometrium called *endometrial hyperplasia.* This condition is not malignant, but because it often leads to cancer, we discuss it below.

ENDOMETRIAL HYPERPLASIA

Endometrial hyperplasia is an overgrowth of the lining of your uterine cavity. Instead of a normal menstrual cycle in which the lining builds up and sheds, your lining continues to thicken. Progressive changes in this endometrium may lead to cancer. See illustration below.

Endometrial hyperplasia is believed to be due to continuous or excessive stimulation by estrogen without the normal opposing effect of progestin. *Estrogen* causes a growth and thickening of your endometrium. *Progestin* causes the glands in the thickened lining to grow and produce a nutritious, perfect environment to receive a fertilized egg and begin a pregnancy.

SYMPTOMS OF ENDOMETRIAL HYPERPLASIA

Typical symptoms of endometrial hyperplasia are irregular, prolonged or occasionally profuse episodes of uterine bleeding, sometimes accompanied by

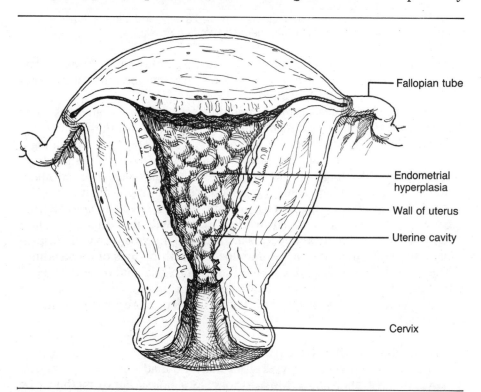

Fallopian tube

Endometrial hyperplasia

Wall of uterus

Uterine cavity

Cervix

Endometrial hyperplasia is an overgrowth of the lining of the uterus. When it becomes thick, it tends to bleed.

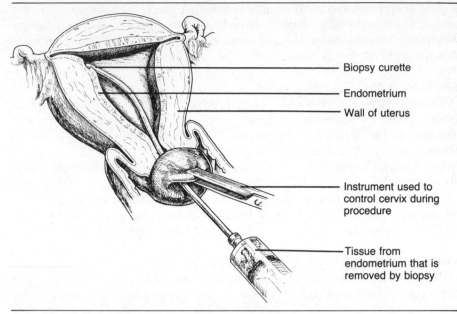

Biopsy curette

Endometrium

Wall of uterus

Instrument used to
control cervix during
procedure

Tissue from
endometrium that is
removed by biopsy

With an endometrial biopsy, tissue can be removed easily, and often painlessly, from the endometrium to determine if the endometrium is normal.

uterine cramps. Some believe cramping is due to painful contractions as your uterus attempts to expel the blood clots. The most common cause of endometrial hyperplasia is lack of ovulation.

Endometrial hyperplasia is most commonly seen in young women just after puberty or in women around menopause (ages 40 to 60). At these times, you are more likely to have bleeding without giving off an egg (anovulatory). Bleeding from endometrial hyperplasia is anovulatory, so it is not *menstrual* bleeding. This bleeding permits clots to form. Menstrual blood normally contains an anticoagulant that keeps blood from clotting. This may be Nature's way of permitting the blood to escape more easily from your uterus.

No eggs are released from your ovaries, so you will not become pregnant when you have endometrial hyperplasia. Bleeding may be heavy, light, prolonged, in the form of spotting or interspersed with periods of no bleeding.

There are different kinds of endometrial hyperplasia, and the incidence of cancerous change is higher in some types than others. Progression from hyperplasia to cancer is usually slow; it may take 5 or more years to make the transition.

DIAGNOSING ENDOMETRIAL HYPERPLASIA

Diagnosis of endometrial hyperplasia may be made by an endometrial biopsy. See illustration above. Most doctors feel a more accurate method is by D&C. The diagnosis is rare during childbearing years. When it occurs at this time, it often occurs along with polycystic ovaries (ovaries riddled with benign cysts) and menstrual cycles in which no egg has been released from the ovary.

TREATMENT OF ENDOMETRIAL HYPERPLASIA

When symptoms are severe enough to suggest endometrial hyperplasia, D&C *must* be done to rule out endometrial cancer. Removing the thickened uterine lining by D&C often cures your endometrial hyperplasia, which means the D&C is diagnostic and therapeutic. Treatment varies somewhat according to age.

Teenage Years — After confirming diagnosis by endometrial biopsy or D&C, treatment consists of 6 months of artificial cycles produced by estrogen and progestin given monthly in cycles, with artificial hormones producing menstrual cycles. If repeat biopsy still shows you have hyperplasia, progestin (progesterone hormone) is given orally each day for 10 days. After this you will have an artificial menstrual period, and bleeding may be heavier than usual.

Some doctors call this procedure a *medical D&C.* No surgery is involved, but the same effect is achieved. The lining of your uterus is completely shed, as though it had been scraped by D&C.

This same treatment program can be repeated until regular menstrual periods occur on their own or until you are ready for childbearing. At that time you can be given fertility medication to stimulate ovulation if you don't ovulate on your own. Endometrial hyperplasia in teenage years rarely converts to cancer.

Childbearing Years — Estrogen-progestin artificial cycles for 3 months are followed by endometrial biopsy to be certain you have established a benign pattern in your uterine lining. Artificial cycles can be stimulated until you desire a pregnancy, at which time you can take fertility drugs to stimulate ovulation if you do not ovulate. Endometrial hyperplasia during your childbearing years can, and occasionally does, become cancerous.

Menopausal Years — The average age of menopause is around 50, but it can vary. If everything else is normal, you can take progestin on a cyclical basis for 7 to 10 days at the end of each month to produce artificial cycles for treatment of endometrial hyperplasia. It is believed the progestin is helpful because it opposes or counterbalances the action of your estrogen, decreasing the development of endometrial hyperplasia.

If you have other reasons requiring hysterectomy, such as a fallen bladder, a dropped uterus, a hernia of your rectum into the vagina or severe, persistent bleeding due to hyperplasia, hysterectomy is the cure for these conditions and your hyperplasia. If your D&C shows the tissue has a glandular appearance, called *adenomatous hyperplasia,* which is often linked with cancer of the endometrium, hysterectomy may be recommended. It depends on your age and general health. Hyperplasia around the menopause is *more likely* to develop into cancer.

Post-Menopausal Years—Unless there are medical reasons why you should *not* have surgery, a hysterectomy is the best way to treat endometrial hyperplasia if you are post-menopausal. The chance of cancer of the endometrium is too great to leave your uterus as a source of trouble.

HOW COMMON IS SURGERY
FOR CANCER OF THE UTERUS?

The American Cancer Society estimates that about 40,000 women developed cancer of the uterus in 1984. Endometrial cancer is twice as common as cancers of the ovary and cervix, and it is increasing in frequency each year. In spite of the increase in the number of women developing uterine cancer, fewer are dying of it. Medical treatment is improving, and women are seeking help earlier for abnormal bleeding.

After diagnosis of uterine cancer is made, treatment should begin immediately. Exact methods of treatment are controversial, but treatment should begin by staging your cancer or classifying it as to how far it has progressed.

Below is a chart showing the various stages of cancer of the uterus.

Stage I	Cancer is limited to the body of the uterus.
Stage II	Cancer is limited to the body and cervix of the uterus.
Stage III	Cancer extends outside the body of the uterus but is still confined to the pelvis.
Stage VI	Cancer involves bladder or rectum or has extended outside the pelvis.

If you have Stage I endometrial cancer, you will probably have a total abdominal hysterectomy, along with removal of tubes and ovaries. There is still some debate about giving X-ray treatments, progestins and chemotherapy after surgery.

Patients with Stage II cancer of the uterus first may be given X-ray treatment, then have radium inserted into the uterus. This is followed by hysterectomy and bilateral removal of ovaries and tubes about 6 weeks later.

If you have Stage III or IV cancer of the uterus, your case will probably consist of a combination of X-ray, radium and surgical removal of your pelvic organs, followed by hormonal treatment (progestins) or chemotherapy.

RECURRENCES

If the cancer recurs in the top of your vagina, it can be treated with surgery and X-ray treatment. If the cancer recurs in other areas, you will be given chemotherapy and progestins.

Usually about 1/3 of all women with recurrence respond to progestins (the cancer decreases in size). About 1/3 of those who do not respond to progestins find relief with chemotherapy.

FUNCTIONS INVOLVED IN SURGERY
FOR CANCER OF THE UTERUS

If spread of the cancer has not occurred, only the uterus is involved. If spread occurs, any of your pelvic organs or abdominal organs may be involved. Distant spread is first to liver, lungs and brain, with bones and other organs ultimately becoming involved.

HOW SURGERY FOR CANCER
OF THE UTERUS IS PERFORMED

Surgery begins with a fractional D&C. A fractional D&C differs from an ordinary D&C because the cervical canal is first scraped by curette as specimen No. 1. Your uterine cavity is then scraped as specimen No. 2. The purpose of a fractional D&C is to determine if your cervix is also involved, along with your endometrial cavity.

If a hysterectomy must be performed, hospitalization will be required, and preparations are more involved.

In your room, you may be given two drugs by injection on the morning of surgery. One drug is to dry up your secretions to prevent aspiration of saliva during anesthesia. The other is to make you drowsy and decrease the amount of gas anesthesia that is necessary.

Intravenous fluids are started, and it is through this in-dwelling I.V. needle that you usually are given enough barbiturate to put you to sleep. A breathing tube is then inserted into your trachea to maintain an airway and to administer your gas anesthetic. Sometimes a drug is given that further relaxes your muscles around the incision so your doctor can see better. A catheter is placed in your bladder and may or may not be left in place during surgery.

After cleansing your abdomen and placing sterile drapes over the cleaned area, your doctor is ready to make an incision in your abdomen. This incision can be a midline incision from your navel to your pubic bone or a bikini (pfannenstiel) incision within the pubic hairline. Surgery performed for cancer is often done with a midline incision to allow removal of all the cancer and for evaluation of other pelvic and abdominal organs.

After making the incision, your doctor inspects all your abdominal organs to search for any evidence of extension of cancer. Cancer may appear as a white, thickened growth in or on any organ or on the lining of your abdominal cavity. Your doctor also feels for any thickening or enlargement of your lymph nodes.

There are two main sources of blood supply to your pelvic organs — the ovarian and uterine arteries and veins. These are carefully dissected free on either side of your uterus and ovaries and doubly clamped. A cut is made between the clamps, and sutures are placed around them.

An incision is made into your vagina; this incision is carried around the cervix, amputating your uterus from the vagina. Extreme care is taken to avoid injury to your bladder, ureters or bowel.

If cancer is limited to the uterine cavity, this may be all the surgery you require. If lymph nodes are involved, these must be located and removed.

Your gallbladder is examined for stones, but these are not removed, even if they are found. The advantage of checking the gallbladder is in *knowing* you have stones in case you have gallbladder attacks in the future. The stones are not removed because the gallbladder is located high in the abdomen. It is difficult to reach, and this might prolong anesthesia time and increase the risk of your surgery.

Your doctor will check your kidneys for size, feel your liver and spleen and check your small and large bowel for any evidence of spread of your cancer.

When the procedure is completed, your incision is closed in layers. After this, your doctor may insert a tiny tube into your bladder to be left in place until you are able to empty your bladder without difficulty.

RISKS OF SURGERY
FOR CANCER OF THE UTERUS

Risk is the same as for ordinary hysterectomy if cancer is only Stage I. If lymph nodes must be dissected and removed because cancer has spread beyond the body of the uterus, there is risk of injury to your pelvic blood vessels causing hemorrhage, injury to your ureters and increased risk of bowel obstruction. The risk of recurrence increases with the extent of spread.

ADVANTAGES OF SURGERY
FOR CANCER OF THE UTERUS

One of the advantages of surgery for cancer of the uterus is that you are rid of the organ where the cancer originated. The problem is you can't be absolutely certain your cancer has not spread to some of your lymph nodes. If your cancer is confined to the uterus, then surgery is certainly the best treatment, and further therapy is unnecessary.

The necessity of radiation therapy *before* surgery varies, depending on the extent of disease and the particular cancer. Some doctors insert radium in the uterus and give you X-ray treatments before removing your uterus. Others feel this is frequently unnecessary and may compromise other organs. Each group has its own statistics to prove it is right.

Surgery is necessary in cancer of the uterus. The question is when, how much and what kind of additional treatment should be given.

DISADVANTAGES OF SURGERY
FOR CANCER OF THE UTERUS

Surgery for cancer of the uterus subjects you to the usual risks of major surgery: anesthesia, sensitivity to drugs and possibility of bowel obstruction following surgery. Perhaps the greatest disadvantage of surgery is that you can't be certain all the cancer has been removed. If it has spread to your lymph nodes, you can search for involved nodes, but it is almost impossible to be sure all cancer-containing nodes have been removed.

In addition to determining the stage of your cancer, doctors try to evaluate the cancer according to its appearance under the microscope (fast or slow growing), degree of invasion, even the depth of your uterine cavity. All these factors help evaluate your tumor and the possibility of cure, but Nature brings in other factors that are difficult to evaluate.

Your doctor and his consultants will weigh these variables as carefully as possible, then decide on surgery, chemotherapy, radiation or hormone therapy, and in what combination. In this way, most disadvantages of surgery will be eliminated.

WHO OPERATES?

Obstetrician-gynecologists perform this surgery, although some general surgeons are also trained in female surgery. Your surgery could be extensive, involving dissection of lymph nodes and possibly even bowel resection, so gynecological specialists often operate with general surgeons when you require surgery for cancer of the uterus. A gynecologist who specializes in female cancer may be consulted; he may perform your surgery, depending on its severity.

DIAGNOSTIC TESTS BEFORE, DURING AND AFTER SURGERY FOR CANCER OF THE UTERUS

In addition to a Pap smear, you should also have a fractional D&C to help establish the extent of your cancer and to determine if the canal of your cervix is also involved.

Consultation with other doctors, sometimes called a *tumor board,* will help determine the stage of the cancer, evaluate the extent of it and submit a consensus on the treatment.

Urinalysis, complete blood count, type and crossmatch for transfusion are standard tests before major surgery. There probably will be insufficient time to withdraw your own blood to keep for autotransfusion because you would need a few weeks to build your blood up again before surgery can be done.

WHERE IS SURGERY PERFORMED?

This major surgery could be extensive, so it is always performed in the operating room of a hospital. It definitely is *not* outpatient surgery.

HOSPITALIZATION AND DURATION

You will be admitted to the hospital the day before surgery. You will already have had a fractional D&C and smear. Besides urinalysis and complete blood count, your blood will have been typed, crossmatched and some will be held ready in case it is needed.

You may be offered a sedative the night before surgery to ensure a good rest. If any bowel surgery is anticipated, because of spread, you will be given a cleansing enema and antibiotics to free your bowel of infection.

Your anesthesiologist will visit the night before surgery to discuss possible drug sensitivities, heart or lung disease and the type of anesthetic you will have.

Surgery requires 2 to 4 or more hours, depending on the extent of spread of the disease.

You will be asleep and "waking up" most of the day, after spending perhaps 1 hour in recovery. When you return to your room, you are checked carefully until you are completely awake. Your incision is checked for evidence of bleeding, and your blood pressure and pulse are monitored to make certain they are normal.

The day following surgery you will be helped up to the bathroom and encouraged to walk around your room with assistance. You may not feel like walking, and it will be painful, but ambulation helps prevent blood clots from forming in your pelvic veins. These clots could be carried to other parts of your body, such as lungs and brain, where they could cause serious problems.

You'll be given intravenous fluid until you can take sufficient fluid by mouth. After you are able to pass gas by rectum, your intestinal tract is usually able to handle a liquid diet, followed by soft foods, gradually increasing to a full diet.

Your hospital stay lasts 5 to 7 days, depending on the extent of your surgery. You will be given pain-relieving drugs while you're in the hospital, but aspirin and acetaminophen are usually sufficient when you go home. Stitches or staples may be removed in the hospital, or your doctor may have you come to his office in a week to have them removed.

ANESTHESIA

Although some doctors use spinal anesthesia, most anesthesiologists prefer general anesthesia, and most patients want to be asleep during their surgery.

PROBABLE OUTCOME OF SURGERY FOR CANCER OF THE UTERUS

Outcome of the surgery should be excellent because this surgery is so highly developed today. The total outcome of your cancer depends on the extent and type of cancer you have.

Don't expect your surgery and recovery to be like anyone else's. Everyone responds differently. Allow yourself about a month to regain your strength and several months to return completely to normal following this major surgery.

POST-OPERATIVE CARE

There is no special post-operative care for uterine cancer. You can expect some vaginal drainage for 1 or 2 weeks, but this should gradually taper off. After a week, you may use an internal tampon to take care of the discharge.

Tub baths may be allowed after 1 week or after stitches are removed. Defer douching until 1 month. Intercourse can be resumed after 1 month. Although gentleness is recommended until you see how you feel, you should have no pain with intercourse.

Normal discomfort keeps you from stretching your abdomen very much, but you can gradually resume moderate exercising. Begin by walking each day, including more distance to suit your tolerance. If you become too fatigued, slow down. Don't be afraid to bend over to pick things up. Sweeping and vacuuming won't harm your incision. Avoid heavy lifting for 4 to 8 weeks, depending on how rapidly you heal. Sports may have to wait 2 months, after which you may slowly resume golf, tennis, horseback riding and other activities. Swimming is easier and is permissible almost any time after the first month.

DIET

The most important advice regarding diet is to avoid overeating. After recovering your appetite, you may be tempted to overeat. Don't! Overeating and inactivity have caused many women to gain weight after surgery. Having surgery will *not* cause you to gain weight.

MISCONCEPTIONS ABOUT SURGERY FOR CANCER OF THE UTERUS

Surgery is *not* always the best, or only, treatment and may be combined with radiation, chemotherapy and hormone treatment. In very early cases, your cancer is limited to a small, superficial area of your uterus, so usually surgery alone is the treatment of choice.

Many cancers are cured; the rate of cure in cancer of the uterus is high, perhaps because it is discovered early. It is impossible to give rates of cure because so many factors enter into the prognosis, such as your age, general health and the extent of the progression of the disease.

Although cancer of the uterus is increasing, the number of deaths from this disease is decreasing.

ALTERNATIVES TO SURGERY FOR CANCER OF THE UTERUS

Alternatives to surgery include radiation, chemotherapy and hormone treatment. But these, *without* surgery, are reserved only for relief of symptoms in advanced cases. Surgery *is* the method of choice for treatment of cancer of your uterus, but it is combined with other methods of treatment. These methods are *not* substitutes for surgery.

CALL YOUR DOCTOR IF . . .

1. You have chills or fever.
2. You have redness, soreness or swelling of your incision.
3. You have drainage — pus, fluid or blood — from your incision.
4. You have any bulging of your incision.
5. You don't feel as well as you think you should following your surgery.

QUESTIONS TO ASK YOUR DOCTOR

What kind of cancer do I have? How extensive is it? Has it spread? To what organs? Is it fast-growing?

These are intelligent questions that you have a right to have answered. Ask your doctor to explain these things to you in terms you can understand.

What do you feel are my chances for a cure?

Your doctor can only give you figures based on averages. But no one is average because each cancer and each patient is different. He can give you his opinion.

Do I need any further treatment, such as radiation, chemotherapy or hormone treatment?

You'll want to know how long this will take, if it will make you sick and how much good he expects it to accomplish.

How soon will I be able to return to work, resume exercise, sports, sex?

Your doctor has his own program of rehabilitation. Follow his advice.

Cancer in Pregnancy

DEFINITION OF CANCER IN PREGNANCY

Cancer is a malignant growth of any kind that will eventually kill you if it is not treated and destroyed. Unfortunately cancer has no respect for pregnancy and can occur during pregnancy. In fact, there is a cancer that is caused by pregnancy — *cancer of the placenta.*

Cancer in anyone brings with it many problems, but cancer during pregnancy presents an entirely new set of circumstances because the presence of the fetus must be considered. Should your pregnancy be terminated? Are you close enough to delivery that your baby could be saved if treatment were deferred for a few weeks or a few months? Will your fetus be harmed more by the malignancy or by the therapy necessary to treat your cancer? What about your life versus the life of your baby?

These questions would be easier to answer if cancer were one disease instead of many and if all cancers ran the same course and responded equally well to various methods of treatment. But each case is individual, and you will receive the best care possible.

Optimum treatment occurs when you are given the benefit of a team of specialists that include your physician, a radiologist, an oncologist (cancer specialist), an obstetrician (if your own physician is not qualified in this field) and yourself and your husband.

ABBREVIATIONS AND OTHER NAMES

Almost any cancer can occur during pregnancy, but there are two conditions that may become cancerous; one is a cancer (choriocarcinoma) and the other is a growth (hydatidiform mole). Both are tumors of the placenta. They are discussed in detail on pages 138 and 139.

PARTS OF BODY INVOLVED

Cancers that occur during pregnancy can involve any organ of your body. But tumors of your placenta primarily involve your uterus, unless cancer spreads to your liver, lungs, brain, vagina or other organs.

COMMON REASONS FOR SURGERY FOR CANCER IN PREGNANCY

Although you are pregnant and concerned with the welfare of the baby you are carrying, your primary concern and the concern of your doctor is for your health and survival. Your life must be preserved to take care of any children you have, to have more children and to survive as an individual.

If you are just beginning a pregnancy, it may have to be ignored to start treatment of your cancer without delay. As you approach full term you, your doctor and consultants may confer as to the risk of delaying treatment until you can give birth to a baby that will survive.

Other than consideration for the length of your pregnancy and survival of your baby, treatment of your cancer will proceed as usual.

In this section, we discuss cancers of your pelvic organs that occur during pregnancy and cancer of your afterbirth, cancers that are *due to your pregnancy.* Pregnancy is divided into three trimesters — first trimester is 1 to 12 weeks, second trimester is 13 to 24 weeks and third trimester is from 25 weeks until full term.

WARNING SIGNS OF CANCER

The warning signs of cancer, which also apply during pregnancy, include:
- change in bowel or bladder habits.
- a sore that doesn't heal.
- unusual bleeding or discharge.
- thickening of lump in breast or elsewhere.
- indigestion or difficulty in swallowing.
- obvious change in wart or mole.
- nagging cough or hoarseness.

Together, these signs spell *caution.* It will be up to you to notice most of these warning signs and symptoms and seek help for them. Tell your doctor if you have any of these signs, and he will take it from there.

Cancer during pregnancy is discovered the same way as when you are not pregnant. In fact, pregnancy may help diagnose a cancer because it brings you to your doctor. A Pap smear and physical exam, including a pelvic exam and breast exam, are performed when you first visit your doctor after your diagnosis of pregnancy.

When you are examined, cancer of the cervix may be identified by Pap smear. Breast cancer, ovarian cancer and other cancers may be identified by examination. Cancers of the placenta (involving the pregnancy) are identified by bleeding from the vagina or by abnormal growth (often too fast) of the pregnancy.

If cancer of any kind is suspected, biopsies or other methods of diagnosis should not be delayed. When dealing with any cancer, early diagnosis is the key to giving you the best chance of a cure.

CANCER OF THE VULVA

Cancer of the vulva (external female organs) during pregnancy is extremely rare, with less than 50 total cases reported in medical history. Most of the patients were between 25 and 35 years old. If cancer of the vulva has not begun to spread, treatment can be delayed until after the delivery of your baby.

If it has penetrated into deeper tissues, and vulvar cancer is diagnosed during the first or second trimester of your pregnancy, your vulva is removed surgically (after the 14th week of pregnancy) along with the lymph nodes of your groin. Pregnancy is allowed to continue to full term.

When cancer of the vulva is diagnosed during the third trimester, your vulva is removed immediately, but dissection of your groin lymph nodes is delayed until after delivery. If you conceive after this treatment, you will probably deliver subsequent pregnancies by Cesarean operation, but this depends on the extent of your surgery and the state of the disease.

The outcome of cancer of the vulva is not influenced by pregnancy.

CANCER OF THE VAGINA

The vagina is an extremely rare site of cancer during pregnancy, but it seems to be slightly more common now because of cancers of the vagina in the daughters of mothers treated with DES (diethylstilbestrol — a synthetic female hormone). There are also other types of cancer of the vagina that are not influenced by pregnancy. Treatment is generally by radical surgery (removing lymph nodes, upper vagina, uterus, tubes and ovaries) if your cancer is early and limited. Radiation therapy is reserved for more-advanced cases, but cancer of the vagina during pregnancy is very rare.

CANCER OF THE CERVIX

Even experts do not agree concerning cancer of the cervix in pregnancy. Some claim cancer of the cervix prevents pregnancy; others claim pregnancy prevents cancer of the cervix. Some believe cancer of the cervix is slowed by pregnancy, while others believe pregnancy accelerates the growth of cancer of the cervix. *None* of these claims has been substantiated.

At this time, most doctors and researchers agree that there are no changes in the cervix during pregnancy that make you more susceptible to cancer of the cervix.

Controversy exists as to whether youth is an advantage or disadvantage in cancer of the cervix in pregnancy. Some doctors favor radiation treatment. Others lean toward primary radical surgery removing the uterus (called a *radical hysterectomy)*, with lymph-node dissection, as soon as possible. It is difficult to settle these disputes because cancer of the cervix during pregnancy is rare — perhaps 1 in 2,500 pregnancies.

In one sense, pregnancy protects younger women against advanced or incurable cancer of the cervix because it brings them to a physician frequently, where a Pap smear is taken and the condition diagnosed early. Pregnancy does not seem to have an adverse effect on the outcome of the cancer. Cesarean operation may be selected for delivery because of the possibility of hemorrhage or infection if the cancer lesion is large.

If cancer is preinvasive, treatment can wait until after delivery. If invasion has begun, and the cancer is in Stage I or early IIA (see page 96 for stages of cancer), and you are in your first or early second trimester of pregnancy, radical surgery is performed immediately. Radical surgery includes a hysterectomy, which terminates the pregnancy, lymph-node dissection and removal of adjacent tissue but preservation of the ovaries.

If cancer has advanced beyond these stages, radiation therapy is used after removal of the fetus by abortion or Cesarean section is performed, depending on the number of weeks gestation.

CANCER OF THE ENDOMETRIUM

This cancer is also called *uterine cancer.* During pregnancy, it is rare. In fact, the few cases that were discovered were found incidentally when a D&C was performed to treat miscarriage.

It is possible cancer interferes with the normal growth and development of the pregnancy, resulting in miscarriage.

Treatment of cancer of the endometrium when it exists coincidentally with pregnancy consists of a total hysterectomy along with removal of Fallopian tubes and ovaries. This usually means termination of the pregnancy, with removal of the uterus. Radiation treatment is used by most doctors. Some physicians favor only surgery in the treatment of cancer of the endometrium, especially if it is in its early stages.

The outlook is generally good for cancer of the endometrium because the disease is usually discovered early.

CANCER OF THE FALLOPIAN TUBE

The average age for cancer of the Fallopian tube is between 50 and 55. This type of cancer is very rare. For this reason, its presence in pregnancy is extremely remote. It occurs most often in only one tube. Diagnosis is almost impossible *during* pregnancy and is usually discovered accidentally when post-partum tubal ligation for sterilization is done immediately after delivery.

Treatment consists of total abdominal hysterectomy, bilateral salpingo-oophorectomy (removal of both tubes and ovaries) and radiation therapy, depending on the findings at surgery.

CANCER OF THE OVARY

Ovarian tumors are uncommon in pregnancy, but they do occur. Not only are they difficult to diagnose, because they are obscured by the enlarged uterus especially later in pregnancy, but they can cause various complications. Ovarian tumors may become twisted on the blood vessels or ovarian ligaments, shutting off their blood supply and causing acute pain that requires emergency surgery.

Ovarian tumors may become impacted behind a pregnant uterus, causing pain as your uterus enlarges. Ovarian tumors also may obstruct labor if they become lodged in the birth canal ahead of the baby in the pelvis.

Ovarian cysts, whether cancerous or benign, may rupture, bleed, become infected or twist on their pedicle. If the cysts are malignant, they are a great hazard because they may not be diagnosed until after delivery, perhaps not until your first post-partum checkup.

When diagnosed, treatment of ovarian cancer during pregnancy depends on the type of cancer, how aggressively it grows, how large it is, if both ovaries are involved and how far along you are in your pregnancy. Your doctor will confer with a cancer specialist to weigh these two factors. Pregnancy does not adversely affect ovarian cancer.

Cancer of the ovary must be placed in a category according to the extent of your cancer before intelligent treatment can begin. Early Stage I cancers of the ovary during pregnancy may be treated conservatively with a hysterectomy and removal of tubes and ovaries. For more information on the stages of ovarian cancer, see page 116.

Radiation therapy depends on the type of cancer, your doctor's method of treatment and the duration of your pregnancy. Anything beyond early Stage I should receive the full treatment of complete surgery plus radiation therapy or chemotherapy. If you are near term, treatment of your ovarian cancer may be delayed until after delivery. If the pregnancy is less than 6 months, treatment may have to take priority over the baby to save your life.

OTHER PELVIC CANCERS

Cancer of the bladder or colon and rectum are other pelvic cancers. In general, treatment of any cancer is carried out in spite of pregnancy, except in the last trimester of pregnancy. Controversy exists over treatment when your baby is beyond 20 weeks gestation.

Some doctors wait until 2 weeks after performing a Cesarean to undertake treatment. Others proceed with surgical resection of the cancer in spite of your pregnancy, usually with no resulting interference with your uterus or its contents. But each situation is different, and treatment will be individualized.

TUMORS OF THE PLACENTA (AFTERBIRTH)

There are two tumors of the placenta called *trophoblastic tumors:*

• *Hydatidiform mole,* which is benign but may become cancerous. It starts out as a benign mole but may become cancerous.

• *Choriocarcinoma,* which is cancerous from the beginning.

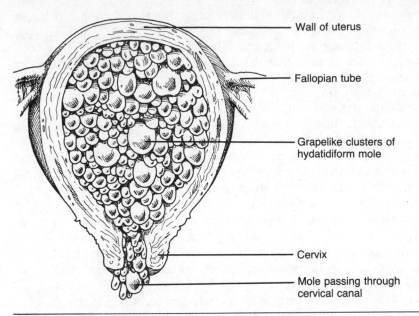

Wall of uterus

Fallopian tube

Grapelike clusters of
hydatidiform mole

Cervix

Mole passing through
cervical canal

Hydatidiform mole is a tumor of the placenta in which cells swell with fluid and have the appearance of skinned grapes.

Both of these tumors are serious and must be monitored very closely to make certain all the cancer has been removed. Monitoring is done principally by blood tests similar to pregnancy tests. A specific hormone or chemical is produced in pregnancy (whether in a normal pregnancy, a mole or choriocarcinoma) called *human chorionic gonadotropin (HCG).* This is the hormone that is tested for in a pregnancy test. The presence of enough hormone in your blood gives a positive pregnancy test.

A mole and choriocarcinoma also make HCG, usually in large amounts. The success of treatment or recurrence of disease can be monitored by measuring the amount of HCG in your blood. The pregnancy test (HCG level) is negative and remains negative if all your mole or choriocarcinoma are removed.

HYDATIDIFORM MOLE

This tumor looks like a bunch of skinned grapes because the cells of the afterbirth become bloated with fluid. See illustration above. Hydatidiform moles occur once in about 1,200 pregnancies in the United States. It may cause bleeding during pregnancy and may co-exist with the pregnancy or exist in the absence of a fetus. For some unknown reason, moles are 5 times as common in Asia and parts of Africa as they are in the United States.

A mole may grow rapidly. This rapid enlargement of your uterus during pregnancy may be the first clue something is wrong. Other symptoms include vaginal bleeding, excessive nausea and vomiting, and elevated blood pressure in *early* pregnancy. Occasionally some of these grapelike moles pass through the vagina, along with your bleeding. Ultrasound shows a snowflake pattern. Nausea and vomiting are often more severe than with a normal pregnancy. A mole is also more common in women over 45 years of age who become pregnant. It is seen infrequently in teenagers.

Treatment consists of immediate suction curettage, followed by regular pregnancy tests. The placenta produces the hormone HCG that gives a positive pregnancy test, and this is a tumor of the placenta, so it also produces a positive pregnancy test. These blood pregnancy tests or hormone (HCG) levels must remain negative for at least 1 year before you can be considered cured and ready for another pregnancy, if you desire one.

After you have a D&C for a molar pregnancy, blood pregnancy tests will be done at 1-to-2 week intervals until they are normal. This will indicate a "cure" or remission and should occur in about 8 out of 10 patients. The HCG test will then be done bimonthly for a year. During this time, reliable birth control is essential so you don't confuse a pregnancy with the recurrence of the disease.

A positive pregnancy test (or blood HCG level) is evidence there is still molar tissue present that may have spread from the uterus or become malignant. The tumor may have spread to other organs. Chest X-ray, liver, brain and general CAT (computer tomography tests) scans, along with general blood chemistry tests, may also be used to show spread. If they are positive, as much tissue is removed surgically as possible, which may include hysterectomy if no further pregnancies are desired. This is followed by chemotherapy. Fortunately chemotherapy is effective in the treatment of invasive hydatidiform mole.

CHORIOCARCINOMA OR GESTATIONAL TROPHOBLASTIC NEOPLASIA

About 2 to 5% of hydatidiform moles convert to choriocarcinoma, cancer of the placenta. It is now commonly called *gestational trophoblastic neoplasia*. This type of cancer has also been known to develop following normal pregnancy, ectopic (tubal) pregnancy or abortion. The cancerous change can occur immediately or several months after pregnancy. Sometimes the choriocarcinoma has already spread to the liver, lungs or brain by the time it is diagnosed.

There are no typical symptoms, although the pregnancy test remains positive after delivery when choriocarcinoma is present. Nausea and vomiting may be worse than with a normal pregnancy because of higher hormone levels. The problem is that your doctor has no reason to run a pregnancy test after delivery when there are no symptoms to provoke such investigation. Usually the first sign of trouble is persistent bleeding from the uterus, a cough or bloody sputum from lung invasion.

Treatment depends on whether the choriocarcinoma is confined to your uterus or whether it has already spread to your lungs, brain, liver or vagina. Newer chemotherapy techniques have been remarkably effective in treating this type of cancer. Chemotherapy is combined with surgery if cancer is limited to your uterus. Follow up consists of regular pregnancy tests, which must remain negative for at least 1 year to indicate cure.

HOW COMMON IS CANCER IN PREGNANCY?

According to a 1968 study of 700 cases, reported in the *American Journal of Obstetrics and Gynecology,* the most common cancers in pregnancy were breast tumors, leukemia and lymphomas as a group, melanomas, cancers of female organs and bone tumors, in that order. Fortunately, cancer in pregnancy is uncommon, perhaps because cancer is less common during the childbearing years.

FUNCTIONS INVOLVED IN SURGERY FOR CANCER IN PREGNANCY

Cancers of any part of your body can occur during pregnancy, and almost any bodily function can be affected. For many years it was believed cancers in general were adversely affected by pregnancy, possibly because of the increased blood supply to organs during pregnancy. This could be true, but no one has proved it applies to average cancers.

Leukemia does not interfere with your pregnancy unless you are required to take chemotherapy to treat it. The same conditions would apply with Hodgkin's Disease (cancer of lymph glands).

Melanomas are skin cancers found in pigmented moles. They grow and spread rapidly. They must be treated immediately, regardless of your pregnancy.

HOW SURGERY FOR CANCER IN PREGNANCY IS PERFORMED

The only difference in surgery for cancer in pregnancy is when cancer occurs near delivery time. When cancer is detected early in pregnancy, if possible it is best to wait until your pregnancy is at least 14 weeks along before performing surgery (if you are not going to terminate the pregnancy). This decreases exposure of the fetus to medication used for anesthesia during critical developmental stages of the baby. It may be possible for treatment to be deferred until after delivery so your baby can survive.

Some cancers are best treated by chemotherapy, some by X-ray treatment, others by surgery. Most are successfully treated by a combination of these methods. Certain drugs used in treating cancer are more harmful than others to you and your baby. All anti-cancer drugs are *potentially* harmful to a fetus and may cause abortion or deformities. X-rays are also capable of causing abortions or fetal deformities.

Surgery itself can cause miscarriages. In some cases of cancer in pregnancy, the best treatment is complete removal of both tubes, both ovaries and your uterus, thus meaning the loss of the pregnancy. Nowhere is the judgment of your doctor tested more than in trying to treat cancer in pregnancy, especially cancer of your female organs.

You have a voice in treating your cancer when it occurs during pregnancy. Whether to abort your pregnancy or try to carry it to full term and take the chance that the cancer treatment will not harm the baby are difficult decisions to make. Many factors must be considered, such as the nature of and location of your cancer, how many children you have, how difficult it has been for you to conceive, your present age and the opportunity you might have for more pregnancies. Every situation is different and will require all the knowledge your doctor and consultants have.

Religious convictions and medical ethics also play an important role when destruction or possible deformation of a living fetus are contemplated. You must also consider the possible effect on the next generation if the sex organs of your fetus receive X-rays or cell-poisoning anti-cancer drugs. If you contemplate life-saving surgery that produces a miscarriage and perhaps permanent sterility, you must understand all the ramifications so you can cope with your decision.

CHEMOTHERAPY DURING PREGNANCY

All drugs used in chemotherapy have the potential to cause fetal abnormalities and can result in abortion, fetal death, malformations and growth retardation. The dangers to your fetus must be weighed against the possible detrimental effect on your own survival of withholding these life-saving agents from you.

During your first trimester of pregnancy, certain cancer-killing drugs almost invariably cause abortion or an abnormal fetus. If drugs are administered to you during your first trimester and you do not abort, you should have a therapeutic abortion.

RADIATION THERAPY DURING PREGNANCY

The greatest problem facing you and your doctor when radiation therapy must be administered during pregnancy is the effect on the fetus. What dose of X-ray is safe, and when is it safe?

We know rapidly multiplying cells are more sensitive to radiation than normal cells. Fetal cells multiply rapidly. This same principal of radiosensitivity in rapidly growing cells makes cancer cells more sensitive and vulnerable to X-ray radiation.

In general there are three significant periods of fetal development as far as radiation effect is concerned.

Before Implantation—Radiation at this time has an all-or-none effect. It either destroys the egg or has no effect at all, as far as is known.

When Organs Are Forming—This is usually before 40-days gestation, especially from days 18 to 38. Small doses of 10 to 40 rads can cause maldevelopment of the brain, eye damage, growth retardation, foot damage and other deformities. Even 4 rads and less are thought to cause some fetal damage.

Development After 40 Days — Larger doses of X-ray are required to produce malformations at this stage, but doses over 50 rads can cause mental retardation and brain damage.

A barium enema (X-ray study of your lower bowel) results in about 6 rads exposure to the gonads (ovaries or testicles) of the fetus. A chest X-ray results in exposure of 300 millirads per plate. Your chest is X-rayed, but your abdomen, including the baby, is shielded. There is evidence exposure of as little as 3 to 5 rads may cause an increase in benign and malignant tumors in your child *after birth.*

It's better not to expose a pregnant woman to chemotherapy or radiation. But if you have a malignant tumor, it may have to be treated in spite of your pregnancy with whatever method gives the greatest chance for survival.

HODGKIN'S DISEASE

Hodgkin's Disease is a painless, progressive, sometimes fatal enlargement of the lymph nodes, spleen and general lymphoid tissues. It often begins in the neck and spreads through the body. One of the triumphs of modern medical treatment over cancer is the fact that most cases of Hodgkin's Disease can now be treated, controlled and perhaps cured. Remission rates up to 90% have been obtained.

Hodgkin's commonly affects young people and may be found in pregnancy. Approximately 1 in 6,000 deliveries is affected by the discovery of Hodgkin's Disease. Hodgkin's must be treated with radiation or chemotherapy; it is fortunate many women have the disease above the diaphragm, making it possible to shield their pregnant uterus from the rays by covering their abdomen with a lead shield.

Radiation to the abdomen and chemotherapy are postponed until after delivery and are never administered during the first and second trimesters. Pregnancy has no adverse effect on Hodgkin's Disease.

Staging of Hodgkin's Disease, according to extent of spread, makes treatment more scientific and exact. Rapid improvements are being made in the treatment of this disease, and they point toward a complete cure in the future.

LEUKEMIA IN PREGNANCY

The average age of a patient with leukemia in pregnancy is 28; these patients usually deliver their babies about 1 month early. Characteristic of leukemia in pregnancy is a rate of about 10 to 15% post-partum hemorrhage. Leukemia seems to be unaffected by pregnancy, except that vigorous treatment of the disease with chemotherapy and radiation is limited to protect your baby.

Babies of leukemic mothers are as normal as those born of unaffected mothers. Chemotherapy is not administered during the pregnancy, and radiation therapy is not given to the uterine area.

The type of leukemia and aggressiveness of the disease, combined with the period of gestation, determine the course of therapy. Your desire in regards to continuing your pregnancy are important when the disease is diagnosed early in pregnancy. Your doctor will discuss alternatives with you. Treatment may cause you to abort.

Later in your pregnancy, the question of carrying the baby until you can deliver him *before* treatment begins becomes a possibility. Discuss these alternatives with your doctor.

MELANOMA IN PREGNANCY

One of the typical symptoms of pregnancy is an increased pigmentation of certain tissues, notably around your nipples and in a strip from your navel to your pubic hairline. It is not known how this ties in with malignant melanoma, which is cancer in a pigmented mole, but pregnancy seems to activate and worsen a melanoma. Spread from a melanoma to adjoining lymph nodes is more rapid during pregnancy. There are conflicting reports, but most doctors feel pregnancy has an adverse affect on maligant melanomas.

If you develop a melanoma during pregnancy, it will have to be removed surgically, even though you are pregnant.

BREAST CANCER DURING PREGNANCY

Cancer of the breast is a rare complication in pregnancy, probably because cancer of the breast is uncommon in women under age 35. Unfortunately pregnancy does have an adverse effect on breast cancer, dropping the overall survival rate from 50 to 20% in those who are pregnant, making cancer in pregnancy a more-serious complication. Pregnant patients have a much higher incidence of spread to their lymph nodes at the time of discovery.

If there is no spread to the lymph nodes at the time of diagnosis of cancer of the breast during pregnancy, the outlook is about the same as in a non-pregnant woman (70 to 80% survival). Of all patients with breast cancer, 1 to 2% are pregnant at the time of diagnosis.

Contrary to popular belief, pregnancy does *not* usually hasten the spread of cancer of your breast, even though spread has often already occurred when diagnosed. Abortion of your pregnancy will not improve the course of the disease. Some doctors recommend termination of pregnancy during the first trimester, even though there is no evidence this improves the survival rates, so chemotherapy, radiation or combination treatments can be used to give the maximum chance of survival.

The debate over the type of treatment — radical mastectomy versus lumpectomy — continues, even though survival rates are about the same. It is agreed that if cancer of the breast is diagnosed during the second or third trimester, pregnancy is usually not terminated. The problem becomes considerably more complex during the last two trimesters because you want your baby to be normal, yet you know you need treatment. You may have mixed feelings.

There are certain instances in which positive estrogen-binding (the tumor is fed by estrogen) is demonstrated. For example, any source of estrogen, such as from pregnancy or the ovaries, must be eliminated because estrogen feeds the cancer and makes it grow. In these cases, your pregnancy might be terminated and your ovaries removed to improve the chance for remission of the disease. This is controversial and must be individualized for each woman.

Most surgeons recommend that you not nurse on the remaining breast because of increasing the blood supply and spread of the cancer if it should begin in that breast. The cause of breast cancer is unknown; some believe it might be a virus that could be passed through breast-feeding. They recommend you don't breast-feed.

Chemotherapy is often beneficial in cases of recurrent breast cancer and as a follow-up (to check for the return of the cancer) after radiation therapy, when cancer was found in the lymph nodes at the time of initial surgery.

HOW SURGERY FOR CANCER IN PREGNANCY IS PERFORMED

In some cancers of the ovary, only the involved ovary must be removed, and your pregnancy can continue without ill effects. There is a small possibility that any surgery might cause you to miscarry.

It is safe to say your cancer, wherever it is and regardless of its type or extent, will have to be treated to save your life. If it means major surgery, it means major *abdominal* surgery or removal of a breast in breast cancer. If it means taking all of your pelvic organs, including your baby, it may have to be done to save your life. You are an important consideration. Any variations in this attitude that are made to obtain a live, normal baby must be weighed against considerations of you as the mother and your health and survival.

RISKS OF SURGERY FOR CANCER IN PREGNANCY

All your tissues have a greater blood supply during pregnancy. For this reason, there may be more bleeding during surgery than when you are not pregnant.

The risk of miscarriage due to surgery is greater in earlier pregnancy and is also affected by how extensive surgery is. Anesthesia poses minimal risk as long as your body receives plenty of oxygen for you and your baby. Anesthesia is constantly monitored to ensure plenty of oxygen in your blood and, consequently, in your baby's blood.

The risk of the surgery itself depends on the extent of surgery and whether the surgery involves pelvic organs. Shock, hemorrhage, infection and post-operative bowel obstruction can occur with any surgery, including during pregnancy.

ADVANTAGES OF SURGERY FOR CANCER IN PREGNANCY

Surgery does not carry the danger of deformity to your baby that chemotherapy or radiation therapy do. It seems to be an all-or-nothing situation, in which surgery causes you to lose your baby or there are no ill effects. You are fortunate if you have a cancer that can be removed by surgery and won't require chemotherapy or radiation therapy.

Surgery is usually a one-time treatment. Chemotherapy and radiation therapy require many treatments and close follow up with blood tests.

You cannot always choose whether or not to have surgery. Your cancer must be diagnosed, so it can be determined which type of treatment will give you the best chance for cure.

DISADVANTAGES OF SURGERY FOR CANCER IN PREGNANCY

Surgery carries the risk of anesthesia, with its danger of aspiration pneumonia (most often due to sucking vomit or stomach acids into your lungs), decreased oxygen to your baby, post-operative nausea and vomiting, and sensitivity to drugs used for medication or to the anesthetic agents.

WHO OPERATES?

Cancer during pregnancy is uncommon. But if you do have it, it's important you have a doctor who is a cancer specialist and has sufficient experience to treat you. A doctor who treats many cancers and has wide experience will usually be welcomed as a consultant by your doctor. Your obstetrician may be relieved to have a cancer specialist give expert help. You have the right to request consultation if your doctor does not suggest it.

DIAGNOSTIC TESTS BEFORE, DURING AND AFTER SURGERY FOR CANCER IN PREGNANCY

After your cancer has been diagnosed, your doctor will seek consultation with a cancer specialist, unless he offers this kind of treatment himself. Ultrasound tests can often tell much about tumors before surgery.

If a positive Pap smear showing abnormal cells is obtained on your first prenatal visit, your doctor will biopsy your cervix with the use of colposcopy. During pregnancy, he may take a flat biopsy, rather than a cone biopsy, but this depends on the severity of the cancer. It will cause less bleeding and hopefully not interfere with the ability of your cervix to contain your pregnancy to full term.

It is important not to do anything that will interrupt the pregnancy. At the same time, possible cancers cannot be ignored and must be evaluated properly, even if it means taking a biopsy.

Before major surgery for cancer during pregnancy, your doctor will order a urinalysis, a complete blood count and possibly a type and crossmatch for possible transfusion.

A chest X-ray will be necessary if there is a possibility of spread of your cancer to your lungs. If cancer has spread to your lungs, surgery will probably be replaced by chemotherapy or X-ray treatment.

WHERE IS SURGERY PERFORMED?

Minor surgery is performed in your doctor's office or in an outpatient surgical department. Pregnancy does not alter the fact that the cancer must be treated, regardless of the method.

If your pregnancy is far enough advanced, and if your surgery is major, your doctor will probably monitor your baby's heart rate during surgery. Through the use of such monitoring, every effort will be made to see that your baby (through your system) receives adequate oxygen at all times.

HOSPITALIZATION AND DURATION

Your doctor will probably want to admit you to a hospital rather than perform surgery in an outpatient facility. In this way, you can have bed rest and total care before and after surgery.

Your stay in the operating room, the recovery room and in the hospital will depend on the extent of your surgery, rather than the fact you are pregnant. If you are having problems during pregnancy, such as threatened miscarriage, threatened premature labor, elevated blood pressure or other problems, your stay in the hospital might be prolonged.

Intravenous fluid, medications for pain relief and general nursing care will be essentially the same as if you were not pregnant. Your doctor will take every precaution to prescribe medication that will not harm your unborn baby.

There is an increased risk of phlebitis in your legs because of your pregnancy. This is due in part to the increased pressure on your pelvic veins and because of a small increase in coagulation of your blood during pregnancy. For this reason, you'll be helped out of bed as early as possible and perhaps more often than if you were not pregnant.

You should be completely ambulatory when you go home; you must be careful to remain ambulatory after you get home because of the danger of phlebitis. Your recovery depends on the type and extent of surgery you have and how well you heal.

ANESTHESIA

General anesthesia is usually the anesthesia of choice for pregnancy-related surgery, perhaps because the anesthesiologist feels he has better control of your oxygen intake. Sometimes there is a fall in your blood pressure with spinal anesthesia that can cause decreased oxygen flow to your baby.

If general anesthesia is used, your abdomen is prepared, shaved, cleansed and draped, ready for your doctor to make his incision *before* anesthesia is started. This procedure cuts down on the amount of anesthetic your baby receives. When you are anesthetized, your baby is also anesthetized because whatever is in your system passes through the umbilical cord to your baby.

By contrast, if you have a spinal or an epidural anesthetic, you are first given the anesthetic, *then* prepared and draped for surgery. When possible, spinal or epidural anesthesia may be used to cut down on medications given to you and exposure to your baby.

PROBABLE OUTCOME OF SURGERY FOR CANCER IN PREGNANCY

The outcome of the surgery depends on the type of cancer you have and the extent of its spread. The combination of cancer and pregnancy creates a very emotional situation because decisions made must take into consideration not only you, but your unborn child.

POST-OPERATIVE CARE

Post-operative care may have to be altered due to your pregnancy if you threaten to miscarry (spotting blood or cramps) or if you are close enough to term that surgery could put you into labor.

Special precautions are then necessary, such as additional bed rest and sedation to stop cramps or threatened labor. You must wait to see if the threat of miscarriage or labor passes.

DIET

Unless your surgery causes prolonged intestinal upset requiring intravenous feedings, the fact you are pregnant should not require any special diet. Your doctor will check your blood to see if you need to take iron and vitamins post-operatively.

MISCONCEPTIONS ABOUT SURGERY FOR CANCER IN PREGNANCY

Surgery during pregnancy is much more dangerous than at any other time.
Surgery during pregnancy, whether for cancer or otherwise, is about the same as if you were not pregnant. You withstand anesthesia and the trauma of surgery just as well as if you were not pregnant. Modern surgery and anesthesia are so exact and sophisticated that they pose little threat to your pregnancy. The fetus will be a major consideration in all parts of your treatment, including safeguarding it.

Cancer means I'm going to die.
Cancer does not mean you will die. Many cancers, including those that occur during pregnancy, can be cured. One of the great advances in the last few decades has been in the treatment of cancer that begins in placental tissue. This formerly lethal disease is now cured in most women.

ALTERNATIVES TO SURGERY FOR CANCER IN PREGNANCY

In some instances, chemotherapy or X-ray are better than surgery for the treatment of cancer that develops during pregnancy. Sometimes a combination of two or all three of these treatment methods give you the best chance for cure.

If you develop cancer during pregnancy, your doctor will request consultation or refer you to a doctor who treats cancer. The result will be the best method(s) to save your life.

CALL YOUR DOCTOR IF . . .

1. You have any of the warning signs of cancer.
2. You have chills or fever.
3. You have soreness, redness, discharge or bleeding from your incision.
4. You feel you are not progressing as you think you should.

QUESTIONS TO ASK YOUR DOCTOR

What kind of cancer do I have? Has it spread? How far? What are my chances for cure?

You have a right to know and will be a more cooperative patient if you know these things.

What lies in my future? One month from now? Six months? A year? Five years?

Your doctor often cannot predict these things, but he can give you averages so you can make plans. If the outlook is excellent, you want to know it.

What about my pregnancy? Will I have more difficulty later on? Is there a chance that I will not be able to carry it to full term?

You don't want to get your hopes up if the outlook is not good. It is better for you and your doctor not to play games with each other. Most people want to *know* what to expect and what is being done for them in their treatment.

What about future pregnancies? How soon? Should I expect any difficulty with other pregnancies?

There is usually no hold-over effect, except with hydatidiform mole and choriocarcinoma. You will have to have negative pregnancy tests for at least 1 year before you can consider yourself cured. You may even want to wait longer than this before you begin another pregnancy.

Will I need chemotherapy? How long it will take, how many treatments, what are the side effects?

Every cancer is different; the response to therapy is different in every patient. For this reason, standard answers cannot be given. But discuss *your* cancer with *your* doctor. He can answer the above questions for you.

Cesarean Operation

DEFINITION OF CESAREAN OPERATION

Cesarean operation means delivery of your baby through an abdominal incision rather than through your vagina. It is called Cesarean operation because Caesar is alleged to have been born this way.

ABBREVIATIONS AND OTHER NAMES

It is also called a Cesarean-section or C-section. Occasionally it is referred to as "delivery per abdominal route."

PARTS OF BODY INVOLVED

Having a Cesarean operation involves your abdominal wall and the wall of your uterus. Both must be cut to enter the uterus to remove your baby. This operation also indirectly involves your bladder. The bladder must be carefully separated from the lower segment of your uterus because the cut in your uterus is made directly underneath your bladder.

The lining of your uterus—the endometrium—is cut, and it must heal following surgery. It is from this lining that your menstrual flow originates.

COMMON REASONS FOR CESAREAN OPERATION

PREVIOUS CESAREAN

The most common reason for performing a Cesarean operation is a previous C-section. There is danger of rupture of your previous incision through the wall of your uterus when it's subjected to the strain of labor contractions. The added pressure from the abdominal wall as you strain to expel your baby may also cause rupture.

If the reason for your first C-section is likely to recur, such as a normal-sized baby that doesn't fit through your birth canal, you may talk with your doctor about a planned or repeat C-section. Repeat C-section is the most common reason for a Cesarean at this time.

The risk of rupture is usually minimal if the incision was made in the non-contractile area of your uterus and if there was no infection or other complication with a previous Cesarean section. *(Non-contractile* means the area of the uterus not involved in uterine contractions during labor; it is not subjected to as much stress or strain.) See illustration below. The reason for your first Cesarean section greatly influences whether or not subsequent pregnancies must be delivered by C-section.

Many women may now deliver vaginally, without C-section, after a previous Cesarean. A Cesarean is *not* automatically performed because you had a previous C-section. There are well-defined indications and contraindications.

If for some reason a *classical incision* was made through the contractile part of your uterine wall, you are *never* subjected to labor. This type of incision

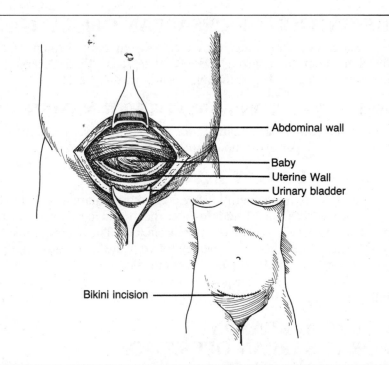

Abdominal wall

Baby
Uterine Wall
Urinary bladder

Bikini incision

Incision in non-contractile portion of uterus. An incision of this type is less likely to rupture in subsequent pregnancies and vaginal deliveries.

increases the risk of rupture of the uterus during labor. All subsequent pregnancies must be delivered by Cesarean operation.

FETAL DISTRESS

Another, less common, reason for a C-section is if the baby is "in trouble." This is called *fetal distress.* Many pregnancies are monitored throughout labor, and the fetal heartbeat is continuously recorded. If the heartbeat slows too much or if any other monitor changes indicate fetal distress, the fetus is even more carefully monitored.

Your baby may be monitored by use of "scalp pH." This is a blood test done on the baby while you are in labor. A small cut is made on the baby's scalp, and blood is collected with a long tube. A test is performed on the blood that indicates whether the baby is in trouble or stressed and not getting enough oxygen. This test may be repeated several times during labor.

If giving you oxygen or other measures, such as changing your position, doesn't relieve the distress, immediate delivery must be considered. Sometimes the pressure of the fetus on your aorta or vena cava may cause your blood pressure to fall, which can put the fetus in distress. Turning you on your side relieves this pressure and may relieve the fetal distress.

If your cervix is fully dilated and your distressed baby is ready, immediate delivery through your vagina may be accomplished. If delivery through your vagina is not immediately possible, a C-section becomes urgent.

UMBILICAL-CORD COMPRESSION

Sometimes fetal distress is caused by compression of the umbilical cord between the baby's head and your pelvic wall. See illustration on page 152.

Sometimes the cord has slipped down (prolapsed) next to the part of your baby that is coming first and can be seen or felt in your vagina. A prolapsed cord can occur in any delivery, but it is more likely to occur in a breech or transverse presentation. It is also more common if there is an excess of amniotic fluid because the cord may be flushed out with the gush of fluid when your waters break.

If the baby's cord prolapses and becomes compressed, the oxygen and nutrition supply are shut off, and death of the unborn infant will occur. An emergency C-section can overcome this hazard in a breech or other abnormal presentation.

Continuous fetal monitoring helps recognize this condition early, but in labor the possibility of a prolapsed cord in a breech presentation still threatens the life of the baby.

If your cervix is fully dilated and the presenting part is low enough so safe delivery can be accomplished immediately through your vagina, the problem can be solved, even if forceps must be used. But your cervix may not be fully dilated or the presenting part may be too high or too large for safe, immediate vaginal delivery. The doctor then must keep his hand in your vagina to prevent pressure on the prolapsed cord until a C-section can be done.

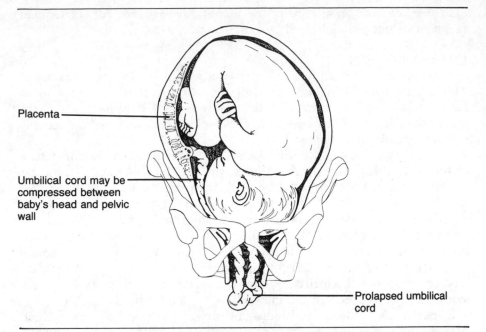

Placenta

Umbilical cord may be compressed between baby's head and pelvic wall

Prolapsed umbilical cord

Prolapsed umbilical cord shows oxygen is shut off when the cord is compressed between baby's head and the pelvic wall. Cesarean operation may save the baby.

KNOT IN CORD

Occasionally fetal distress is due to a knot in the umbilical cord that is pulled taut as your baby descends in the birth canal. Or the cord may be wrapped around the baby's neck so his descent gradually shuts off circulation through the blood vessels of the cord. The umbilical cord is the baby's lifeline. Immediate delivery by C-section may be necessary.

BREECH PRESENTATION

When the baby comes feet first or buttocks first, it is called a *breech presentation.* See illustration on opposite page. Many obstetricians believe a breech baby should be delivered by C-section, especially if it's your first baby. The head doesn't have time to narrow quickly enough to pass through the birth canal without danger of injury.

The buttocks and rest of the lower body may pass through the birth canal fairly easily, but the baby's more rigid head may have difficulty molding to pass through the birth canal in a breech delivery. Brain hemorrhage could occur in the process. A C-section avoids possible serious injury.

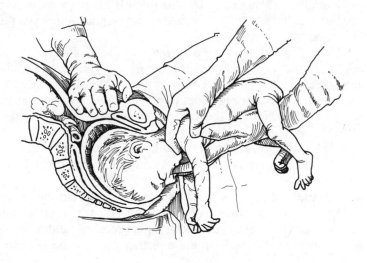

Delivery of after-coming head in breech delivery.

PREMATURE BREECH

In a premature breech, the same conditions exist — plus an additional hazard. With a full-term birth (280 days), the diameter and circumference of your baby's head and his shoulders are about the same. A premature baby's head is larger than its shoulders. This discrepancy increases proportionately with the number of weeks your pregnancy is premature. After full term, the circumference of the baby's shoulders becomes larger than the circumference of your baby's head.

The hazards of breech delivery can be multiplied in a premature baby. This is not a factor in a baby born before it is mature or developed enough to survive, but after 24 to 26 weeks, a premature breech presents a serious problem if delivered through your vagina. A premature infant has a head much larger than his shoulders. Because the body of a breech baby delivers before his head, it is often difficult to deliver the larger head through the birth canal.

PREMATURE SEPARATION OF PLACENTA

Sometimes the afterbirth separates during labor. If separation is sufficient, it endangers the life of your baby by shutting off his oxygen and nutrition supply. See illustration below. Unless immediate vaginal delivery is possible, delivery must be by Cesarean.

Bleeding from separation of the placenta may be obvious when blood is released through your vagina, or the bleeding may be concealed and detected only through fetal distress. If bleeding is massive, yet concealed in your uterus, it may be detected through your own symptoms, such as shock. If this condition is diagnosed before the baby is damaged, he can be delivered immediately by C-section and avoid impairment or death.

Diagnosis is made with ultrasound combined with your doctor's clinical judgment. Sometimes there is external bleeding; at other times bleeding is completely concealed.

With this condition, the uterus becomes stony hard and extremely tender to the touch, depending on the amount of separation of your placenta. The baby's heart rate speeds up at first, then slows and becomes fainter until death occurs. A fetal monitor will pick up these changes in your baby's condition.

PLACENTA PREVIA

The afterbirth may come ahead of the baby; this is called *placenta previa.*

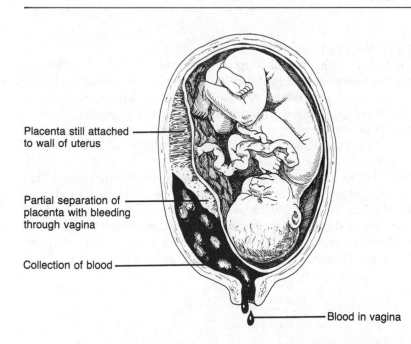

Placenta still attached to wall of uterus

Partial separation of placenta with bleeding through vagina

Collection of blood

Blood in vagina

Premature separation of placenta. Separation is partial, and bleeding is obvious through vagina.

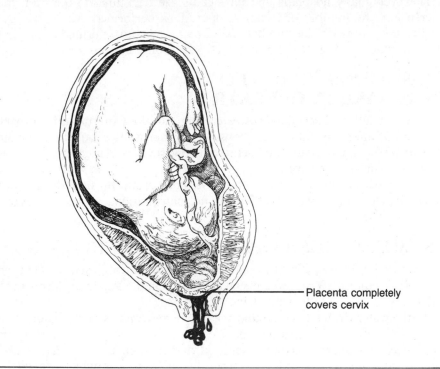

Placenta completely covers cervix

Complete placenta previa in which placenta covers cervix completely. Any further dilatation of the cervix produces more hemorrhage.

This condition is accompanied by hemorrhage, depending on the amount of placenta that overlies your dilating cervix.

If you develop painless bleeding (more than the few drops that might come from your dilating cervix or from exams by your doctor), especially before labor begins, you must suspect placenta previa. See illustration above.

When your placenta becomes attached in the lower segment of your uterus, it is possible the enlarging placenta may encroach on your cervix. How low the placenta is implanted in your uterus may determine whether bleeding starts before labor begins or whether it occurs as your cervix begins to dilate.

If a large amount of placenta covers the cervical opening and results in excessive bleeding, your pregnancy must be terminated immediately by Cesarean. If bleeding is accompanied by rapid dilatation of your cervix, vaginal delivery may occur before a Cesarean can be done.

HOW COMMON IS CESAREAN OPERATION?

Twenty years ago the C-section rate was 2 to 4% of all deliveries. In 1985, it was almost 20%. Part of this increased rate is due to fetal monitoring and the abnormalities it detects.

However, many hospitals and physicians are beginning to question the increase in the number of Cesarean operations performed. Many are life-saving, but a questionable number of Cesareans may be performed because of an abnormal reading that is not understood or only temporary.

FUNCTIONS INVOLVED IN CESAREAN OPERATION

Even though a C-section involves cutting into your uterus, this surgery should not alter any future functions of the uterus. It should not change menstrual regularity, amount of menstrual flow, severity of menstrual cramps or your ability to conceive.

With modern techniques, a C-section does not measurably limit the number of pregnancies you may have if there are no complications, such as infections or severe hemorrhage.

HOW CESAREAN OPERATION IS PERFORMED

An incision is made first through your abdominal wall, then through the wall of your uterus. A second incision cuts through the amniotic sac containing the water surrounding the baby.

As the water drains from around the baby, your uterus immediately contracts and can make it difficult to remove your baby. When the amniotic sac is punctured, the baby is quickly removed and handed to an assistant who suctions out any mucus and water from the baby's throat, which allows the baby to take its first breath. The doctor then removes the placenta from your uterus while an injection of a drug causes the uterus to contract even more firmly to keep bleeding to a minimum.

The cut walls of the uterus are sewed together in layers. Your ovaries and tubes are carefully inspected to make certain they are normal. Then your uterus, tubes and ovaries are replaced in the abdominal cavity. Your abdominal wall is sewed together in layers, including your skin.

There are two methods of performing a Cesarean section — classical and low-cervical approach.

CLASSICAL CESAREAN

In a classical Cesarean, the incision into the uterus is made through the upper, muscular part of the uterus, which is involved in active contractions during labor. This incision is rarely used now, except in special circumstances such as a breech birth, because danger of uterine rupture in future pregnancies is greater with this type of incision. Even before labor begins, a previous scar in the uterus from this operation can thin to the point of rupture.

Once a Cesarean-section has been performed through a classical incision, all future pregnancies *must* be delivered by Cesarean operation. Each pregnancy must be carefully monitored for the possibility of rupture, even before labor begins.

LOW-CERVICAL CESAREAN

This is the most widely used type of incision for a C-section. The incision is made vertically or horizontally in your lower uterine segment, which contains very little contractile tissue. This area is not involved in contractions during labor, so it is not subjected to as much stress and strain. It is also partially protected from strain because it lies behind your pubic bone.

To reach this segment of your uterus, your bladder must be dissected away from the uterus. Dissection requires care, skill and more time on the part of the obstetrician to avoid injury to your bladder. Time is occasionally a factor in a fetal or maternal emergency.

Some doctors believe if a low-cervical C-section has been performed and if there were no post-operative complications, subsequent normal pregnancies can be delivered safely through the vagina. This assumes no other reasons for repeat C-section exist, such as large baby, a prolapsed cord, placenta previa or other condition. The old adage, "once a Cesarean, always a Cesarean" is not a hard-and-fast rule, and each situation must be considered separately. The final decision must be left up to the attending physician, after he has discussed the situation with you.

CESAREAN HYSTERECTOMY

There is the rare occasion when your uterus must also be removed during a Cesarean. For example, such problems as hemorrhage from your uterus that is uncontrollable by any other means, cancer of the cervix or severe infection of the uterus may necessitate removal of the uterus. But hysterectomy increases the risk of surgery because it almost doubles the amount of surgery. It would be undertaken only as a last resort. Either Cesarean or hysterectomy alone is a major operation, but the two operations together prolong anesthesia, and risks of hemorrhage, infection, shock and post-operative bowel obstruction are increased.

RISKS OF CESAREAN OPERATION

The trend toward more frequent C-sections is not necessarily negative. Many babies have been saved from trauma or death from difficult or prolonged labors. Some may have been spared the danger of brain hemorrhage due to a difficult forceps delivery. Some breech babies have also been spared the danger of brain hemorrhage, injury to arms or spinal-cord injury during delivery.

You and your doctor must balance the risks of a C-section against the risks of vaginal delivery. The mortality rate is 2 to 4 times greater for a mother who has a Cesarean as compared with a vaginal delivery. Mortality rates vary from hospital to hospital but average 20 to 70 deaths per 100,000 for Cesarean compared to 8 to 27 for vaginal delivery.

A C-section is still a major operation and carries the risk of anesthesia, whether general, epidural, spinal or local. It carries the risk of infection, hemorrhage, shock, blood clots, injury to other organs, such as the bladder or bowel, and abdominal adhesions and bowel obstruction. There may be abdominal adhesions immediately following a C-section, with the added risk of subsequent adhesions or bowel obstruction.

ADVANTAGES OF CESAREAN OPERATION

Some of these conditions are discussed earlier in this section. See common reasons for Cesarean operations, which begins on page 149. Other conditions are discussed below.

LARGE BABY — SMALL PELVIS

This is called *cephalo-pelvic disproportion* (CPD). With CPD, your baby's head cannot descend into your pelvis. Sometimes a large head converts to a brow presentation rather than a normal presentation. This further complicates the situation.

If there's a question about the ratio of the diameter of your baby's head to the diameter of your pelvis, the doctor will probably perform a C-section. The only way to determine this is to experience labor, called a *trial of labor* to see if the baby fits. See page 161 for more information. If your baby's head can pass through your pelvis, your labor will proceed, and the baby will deliver normally. If the head is too big for the pelvis, it will not descend through the birth canal and requires a C-section.

It is usually less hazardous to perform a C-section than to risk a difficult, possibly traumatic, forceps delivery. Paralysis or mental impairment of your baby can be avoided by a C-section when there is any question about CPD.

PREMATURE RUPTURE OF MEMBRANES

Rupture of your membranes before your labor starts is called *premature rupture of the membranes.* If your membranes rupture before the baby is mature, it is called *preterm rupture of the membranes.* If your membranes rupture, notify your doctor immediately, regardless of how advanced your pregnancy is.

If labor does not begin within 24 hours, there is increased danger of infection in your uterus, which can be dangerous for you and your baby. If your baby has reached the stage where it should survive outside the womb (it is mature), attempts are made to stimulate your labor.

If membranes rupture before your baby is mature, the risk of infection for you and your baby is weighed against delivery of a premature baby. Each situation must be considered individually. All factors are weighed, such as how premature the baby is, your risk of infection, how long your membranes have been broken and other factors.

Depending on the size and maturity of your baby, if labor does not begin within 24 hours and cannot be started with drugs, a C-section must be considered. Every case is different, and your doctor may feel safe waiting longer. But he may favor a C-section to deliver your baby and avoid possible infection.

MULTIPLE PREGNANCY

When there is more than one baby, especially more than two, it may be easier, quicker, less traumatic and safer to deliver them by C-section. When a second or third baby presents itself in a breech or transverse position, there is risk of a prolapsed umbilical cord and trauma to the baby if the doctor tries to correct the position or deliver a breech baby through the vagina.

An added risk is that a second or third baby may be larger than the first, which could mean difficulty with delivery. This is especially true if the larger second or third baby is breech.

When the uterus has been overstretched to accommodate a multiple pregnancy, it has more difficulty contracting and returning to normal. This increases the likelihood of post-partum hemorrhage, a condition that can be controlled or avoided during a C-section.

CANCER OF THE CERVIX

If a Pap smear taken on your first prenatal visit shows early, slow-growing cancer of the cervix, you may decide to continue your pregnancy. The doctor may decide to perform a Cesarean at full term to avoid the potential spread of cancer that trauma of labor, dilating of the cervix and vaginal delivery could cause.

HERPES

If you have an outbreak of genital herpes, or if there is evidence of the disease at labor or with the rupture of membranes, your baby is delivered by C-section. This avoids infecting the baby as he passes through your birth canal during labor and delivery and the subsequent serious problems that can occur. See illustration on page 160. If your membranes have been ruptured for several hours, giving time for the infection to proceed upward, then a "normal" vaginal delivery can occur.

OVER AGE 35

If you have your first baby after age 35, especially if you have had difficulty conceiving, a C-section may be considered. Your doctor might be more inclined toward C-section if there is any question as to prolonged labor or difficult delivery.

PREGNANCY-INDUCED HYPERTENSION

You may develop pre-eclampsia, also called *toxemia of pregnancy*, during pregnancy. Your symptoms could include high blood pressure, swelling, albumin in your urine and neurologic changes. A C-section may be required for the well-being of you and your baby. Each case must be decided on its own merits.

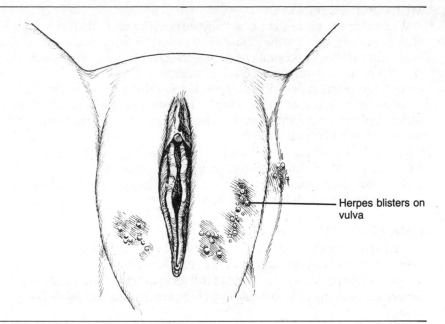

Herpes blisters on vulva

Diagnosis of herpes vaginalis is made by appearance of "cold-sore" blisters on vulva. This disease can be fatal to a newborn.

DISADVANTAGES OF CESAREAN OPERATION

MAJOR OPERATION

A Cesarean operation is a major operation, and it carries all the risks of major surgery — infection, bleeding, adhesions, shock, injury to other organs and hazards of anesthesia. These are complications of any major abdominal surgery, but you have the added concern of the health of your baby. The maternal mortality rate in C-sections is 2 to 4 times higher than it is for vaginal deliveries.

HOSPITAL STAY

Your hospital stay is longer — maybe 3 days to 1 week — as opposed to 2 to 3 days with vaginal delivery.

RECOVERY PERIOD

It may take a month before you can get around the way you want. It may require up to several months before you return to normal.

RISK OF RUPTURE OF UTERUS

There is always the risk of rupture of the old wound in your uterus with a subsequent pregnancy. This risk is reduced when a low-cervical incision is made. Sometimes a rupture in your uterus occurs even before labor begins. The risk of rupture of a previous incision is also greater if your wound became infected with a previous C-section. Rupture of your uterus threatens your baby's life and your own.

SELF-ESTEEM

Some women feel "less of a woman" because they have not experienced labor and delivery through the vagina. Some women feel they failed because they didn't labor and deliver in Nature's way. Don't feel you failed because you didn't deliver your baby vaginally. A happy mother and baby after delivery is the most important outcome.

ATELECTASIS

Atelectasis is a condition in which the baby's lungs fail to expand or inflate with air at birth. There is an increased risk of atelectasis for a baby delivered by Cesarean section. In a normal vaginal delivery, your baby's lungs are compressed, which helps expel amniotic fluid. The process of vaginal delivery also seems to stimulate your baby to breathe and get rid of secretions.

If general anesthesia is used, it may depress your baby's stimulus to breathe. In most hospitals, pediatricians or other trained personnel aspirate mucus from the baby's throat to help avoid atelectasis.

WHO OPERATES?

The type of doctor who performs a Cesarean varies, depending on the availability of specialists and the rules of the hospital. When available, board-certified obstetricians perform C-sections. When not available, general surgeons may perform C-sections. There are situations in which general practitioners are the only physicians available, and some have become expert in this type of surgery.

Your county medical society should be able to provide you with a list of doctors who are qualified to perform Cesarean operations.

DIAGNOSTIC TESTS BEFORE, DURING AND AFTER CESAREAN OPERATION

TEST OR TRIAL OF LABOR

If your doctor believes your baby might be too large to pass through your pelvis, he may give you a test of labor, also called *trial of labor*. This is to see if you will go into labor and to see if the presenting part of the baby will descend into the pelvis.

This can be done by waiting for labor to begin on its own or with the help of medication that induces labor. If he chooses to induce labor, your doctor will administer medicine to stimulate uterine contractions when he believes your baby is mature enough to deliver and when he thinks your cervix indicates you are ready for labor. If you go into labor without being induced with medication, he will watch you carefully to see what progress you make.

The head is the largest part of the baby. If it descends into the pelvis and beyond the narrowest diameter of the pelvis, the baby will probably deliver, without difficulty, through the vagina.

TRANSFUSIONS

If a C-section is anticipated, your doctor may have a pint of your blood drawn a few weeks before your surgery. If transfusion becomes necessary, you receive your own blood, called *autotransfusion,* rather than blood from a donor. If the C-section is an emergency, blood from the laboratory is typed, crossmatched and held in readiness in case it's needed.

OTHER LABORATORY TESTS

Urinalysis and a complete blood-cell count are routine. Blood levels of certain electrolytes, such as potassium, are usually determined.

POST-OPERATIVE TESTS

In spite of estimated blood loss, it's always good to check hematocrit and hemoglobin or to take other tests as recommended by your doctor *after* your surgery. These tests will indicate if you need to take iron or any other medication.

WHERE IS SURGERY PERFORMED?

Some hospitals set up one or more delivery rooms with all the necessary equipment for C-sections and care of a newborn. Other hospitals perform C-sections in the major surgery suites on the surgical floor.

A Cesarean operation is considered major surgery and has not been relegated to the outpatient department. It is important for this major surgery to be performed where equipment and personnel are available for the safety of you and your baby. After adequate recovery time, you can be transferred to the obstetric floor.

HOSPITALIZATION AND DURATION

If you know you will have a C-section, you're admitted the day of surgery or the day before for lab tests, unless these are done before admission. This includes typing and crossmatching blood, complete blood count, urinalysis, complete history and physical exam.

In many instances, patients are admitted to the hospital on the morning of surgery. If special tests are required, or if there are other reasons, you may be admitted the day before surgery. In any event, take nothing by mouth after midnight the day before surgery.

You may be given an enema so your lower bowel is empty. This results in fewer gas pains because it may be a few days before you have a natural bowel movement.

You may be shaved in the pubic area because the incision will extend into this area or be completely confined to this area.

Your stay in the recovery room is important because you continue to waken from the anesthetic. Your blood pressure, pulse and breathing are carefully monitored. If you are disoriented, the recovery room attendant will help you by reassuring you surgery is complete.

You are checked carefully for bleeding, shock or other immediate complications. If you have an in-dwelling catheter in your bladder, it must be working. You are not released from the recovery room until you have responded from the anesthetic and can be safely cared for on the surgical or maternity floor.

With an epidural block, you can usually be sent from the recovery room to the obstetric floor as soon as you have been checked for bleeding and when your vital signs—blood pressure, pulse and respiration—are normal.

COMPLICATIONS

Perhaps the most common complication following a C-section is hemorrhage. This is often due to lack of complete contraction (atony) of the uterus. Normally the uterus clamps down on open blood vessels in the uterine wall. This bleeding can usually be controlled and stopped by massage of the uterus and with medication that causes it to remain in a state of contraction.

Fever, along with redness and tenderness in the incision, indicates infection. Slight elevation of temperature is common with a C-section. Temperature is checked every 4 hours, and your wound is inspected daily so any evidence of infection is noted early.

The amount and type of vaginal discharge is also charted regularly so any sign of hemorrhage or infection can be detected early.

It's best to get up as soon as you are permitted to do so. You'll be helped to your feet the morning after surgery. Soon after, you can get up to go to the bathroom by yourself.

Except for clear liquids by mouth, eating may be delayed until you have passed flatus (gas) by rectum, a sign your bowel has begun to function on its own. An enema may be given the third or fourth day if you have not had a bowel movement.

Following spinal or epidural anesthesia, you may be kept in bed for up to 24 hours after surgery. By the second post-operative day, most patients are walking.

The average stay in the hospital is about 3 to 7 days after surgery. Although shots for pain may be given the first 24 hours, they are often decreased by the second day and discontinued completely before the third post-operative day.

Women who have a C-section may nurse their babies if they wish and often start nursing, even in the recovery room after surgery. Milk flow is not impaired by the surgery, and nursing stimulates your uterus to contract, helping to decrease blood loss.

ANESTHESIA

Regional or general anesthesia may be used. The anesthesiologist will discuss this with you before surgery, unless your operation is an emergency. There may be reasons you *must* have a particular type of anesthesia, but your anesthesiologist and obstetrician will try to discuss it with you.

GENERAL ANESTHESIA

If general anesthesia is used, everything is ready for delivery of the baby before you are put to sleep. You are "prepped" and draped, a catheter is inserted and your obstetrician and assistants are scrubbed, gowned and gloved, so everyone is poised, ready to make the incision.

Then you are put to sleep. The reason for the delay in putting you to sleep is to avoid unnecessary drugging of the baby. The anesthesiologist usually gives you just enough barbiturate or other drug in your vein so you go to sleep quickly. After this, he puts a mask over your face for continuous anesthesia and oxygen. Within a few minutes, your doctor will have made his incision through your abdominal wall, through the wall of the uterus and the amniotic sac and will have extracted your baby from your uterus.

REGIONAL ANESTHESIA

Regional anesthesia may be epidural (anesthetic placed around the spinal canal) or spinal (anesthetic placed inside the spinal canal). Both are safe and produce numbing from the waist down. Each type allows you to be awake without discomfort and to observe the birth of your baby if you wish.

Spinal and epidural anesthesia each have special indications. Epidural is used for some normal vaginal deliveries, and a Cesarean section can be performed without the need for additional anesthesia, if complications arise that demand it. The use and availability of spinal or epidural anesthesia varies throughout the country and from one doctor to another.

In certain emergencies, the baby must be delivered rapidly by C-section, even before the anesthesiologist arrives. In such cases, your obstetrician may elect to inject xylocaine or other local anesthetic directly into the skin along the area to be cut so he can make his incision and proceed with the C-section without delay. This is called *local* anesthesia.

He could complete the surgery under local anesthesia if he had to but often waits only until the anesthesiologist arrives and can put you to sleep. Many babies have been saved by the immediate use of local anesthesia to deliver a baby in distress.

PROBABLE OUTCOME OF CESAREAN OPERATION

A Cesarean is regarded as a safe operation for the mother and baby. One must consider the number of babies that might survive vaginal delivery yet sustain injury because of a difficult forceps delivery. Lack of oxygen to the baby during a difficult vaginal delivery may also cause brain damage.

Physiologically, a C-section should not impair the ability of your uterus to implant and carry subsequent pregnancies to full term. Nor should a C-section interfere with the future normal menstrual function of your uterus. The outcome of a Cesarean section should be excellent.

POST-OPERATIVE CARE

HOSPITAL

Your doctor will order drugs to relieve pain and to cause your uterus to contract to prevent bleeding. The latter medicine may provoke cramps, but they are temporary until your uterus does its job to prevent hemorrhage. If you don't receive enough analgesic to relieve discomfort, tell the nurse. She can relay your needs to your doctor.

Food is usually withheld until your bowel is functioning, as indicated by the fact you pass gas. If you wait until that happens before you begin to eat, you'll probably have less discomfort from gas pains.

Drink all you can when you're allowed to start drinking. This helps your bladder begin to function. Some doctors insert a tiny drain into the bladder through the abdominal wall at the time of surgery to avoid the discomfort of an in-dwelling catheter in the urethra and to prevent bladder distention and infection. This drain is removed when you begin to pass urine on your own.

Exercise in bed. Move your arms and legs as much as you can. See HPBooks *Pregnant & Beautiful!* for post-partum exercises to do in your hospital bed. When you have permission to get up, walk around your room, to the bathroom and up and down the hall. Until you're steady on your feet, have someone help you so you won't fall.

Ask for an enema if you can't have a bowel movement on your own. Lots of fruit juice will help in this respect.

Holding or carrying your baby won't hurt you or tear open your incision. Bending won't hurt, either. Sufficient rest is important, but beware of those who want you to stay in bed while they do everything for you. Phlebitis (inflammation or clots in the veins of your legs) is a danger if you stay on your back too much.

If you bleed more than a normal menstrual period, notify the nurse or your doctor.

AT HOME

Exercise as much as you can without tiring. The more you exercise, the faster you'll recover your health, strength and endurance.

If you bleed more than an ordinary menstrual period, call your doctor. Your vaginal discharge is almost straight blood at first, but it gradually tapers off to a watery-white discharge. If the discharge becomes odorous or foul smelling, let your doctor know because it could mean infection.

A fever is not normal. Report a temperature to your doctor. Your wound should not be red, inflamed or sore. If in doubt, call your doctor.

Your breasts won't be different because you had a Cesarean operation. If they become sore, inflamed or red, check with your doctor.

You share the responsibility for your welfare with your doctor. He isn't a mind reader; he won't know there's something wrong unless you tell him. So be sure to call, day or night, if you have any problems.

DIET

You can eat the same foods you ate while you were carrying your baby. If you gained weight, you will normally lose some in the next few weeks.

If you're nursing, all it takes to make milk for your baby is plenty of liquid, mainly water. Rich, creamy foods are *not* necessary. Although there is less chance for conception while nursing, do *not* depend on it if you don't want to conceive. Ask your doctor about contraception.

MISCONCEPTIONS ABOUT CESAREAN OPERATION

A woman can have only a certain number of Cesareans.

There may not be a limit to the number of Cesarean operations you can have if they are performed properly, if the incision in your uterus has healed properly and if there are no other limitations, such as poor general health or post-operative infections that have weakened the incision site. The risks of further pregnancies can be evaluated with each C-section. There is more risk if a *classical* Cesarean operation has been performed.

Women should have a Cesarean to avoid pain.

It is unthinkable that any woman or physician would consider this as an alternative to vaginal delivery for such a reason. This is major surgery and more debilitating than a normal vaginal birth.

Having a Cesarean is "less womanly."

This is strictly in the mind. If C-sections are done only when *necessary,* there will be no such feelings. You have still conceived, carried and delivered your child.

ALTERNATIVES TO CESAREAN OPERATION

Vaginal delivery is the only alternative; the possibility of injury to, or even death of, the infant or mother must be considered.

Nearly 1 in 5 women are now delivered by C-section, and this increased rate is being reviewed to see if it can be reduced. While some Cesareans may not be necessary, we must study the final results to determine if more infants are being saved by jeopardizing the life of the mother with a major operation.

Results seem to justify an increase in the number of Cesareans. Whether we have gone overboard in performing as many C-sections as we do is a question that may require several more years for an unbiased answer.

CALL YOUR DOCTOR IF . . .

1. You feel uneasy about your condition. You can't put your finger on it, but you know something is wrong.
2. You have a fever. It is *not* normal to have a fever after surgery.
3. You have red, tender breasts, especially with fever.
4. Discharge becomes too heavy or too bloody. It could be the beginning of a hemorrhage. Don't wait to report it to your doctor. Measure your bleeding by the number of sanitary pads you use. Your doctor will want to know. Tell him how long it takes to soil one and how many you have already soaked.
5. Your vaginal discharge develops a foul odor. This is a sign the uterus may be infected, and it's important to treat an infection early.
6. Your incision becomes more tender instead of less tender, especially if it becomes red and swollen.
7. You have soreness in your legs, with or without swelling. It could be phlebitis.

QUESTIONS TO ASK YOUR DOCTOR

Tell me, in lay terms, why I had a Cesarean operation?
   You may live elsewhere the next time you are pregnant and will want to be able to report the reason for your Cesarean to your new doctor. You may also need a copy of the ultrasound test, X-rays, fetal monitoring record and a transcript of your records from your doctor's office and from the hospital.

Will I have to have a Cesarean operation next time?
   In some cases, "once a Cesarean, always a Cesarean." In others, this axiom is not necessarily true. Perhaps the baby was too large the first time, but the next baby may not be.

What kind of Cesarean did I have—a low-cervical or a classical type?
   It makes a difference. Low cervical allows the possibility to have babies vaginally the next time, if all goes well. Many doctors will give you a copy of the description of the operation as recorded in your hospital chart.

Did I have any complications I should know about?
   Fever, evidence of infection or other problems might demand a repeat Cesarean operation next time.

Are there any precautions to take because of my surgery? How much can I lift? What kind of tasks should I avoid?
   Your doctor will give you guidelines for your specific case.

How soon can I safely tolerate another pregnancy?
    If you are planning more children, ask your doctor this question. It will depend on your recovery after surgery and your general health. These are different for everyone.

Do I need to take iron, vitamins, calcium?
    You should know if you are anemic following your C-section.

Will my Cesarean prevent me from performing my job and for how long?
    This depends on the type of work you do. Check with your doctor first.

How soon may I resume intercourse?
    Most doctors prefer that you wait for 1 month.

How soon may I use internal tampons?
    As soon as vaginal discharge is light enough so a tampon will absorb it.

How soon may I resume exercises, such as jogging, golf, tennis, racquetball?
    At least 1 month, perhaps longer. See how you feel and how completely you've recovered by then.

D&C—
Dilatation and Curettage

DEFINITION OF DILATATION AND CURETTAGE (D&C)

Dilatation and curettage, or *D&C* as it is commonly called, means stretching (dilating) the opening of the neck of the uterus (cervix) and scraping (curettage) the inner lining of the uterus. Usually the cervical opening, also called the *cervical canal,* is only large enough to allow passage of menstrual flow. But this same opening stretches enough to permit passage of instruments used to remove tissue. See illustration on page 170. The process is called a *D&C.*

ABBREVIATIONS AND OTHER NAMES

The term "D&C" is the common term used for this female operation. Occasionally a woman says her uterus was "scraped" or "cleaned out" after a miscarriage. In a miscarriage, the fetus and some of the placental tissue have already been passed from the uterus; the cervix is open and the cervical canal does not have to be stretched or dilated, merely curetted or scraped.

When a diagnostic D&C is performed to determine the cause of uterine bleeding, it is almost the same as a biopsy to sample the tissue lining the uterus. Because it often cures the bleeding, it may be called *therapeutic.* In a diagnostic D&C, the canal of the cervix must be stretched.

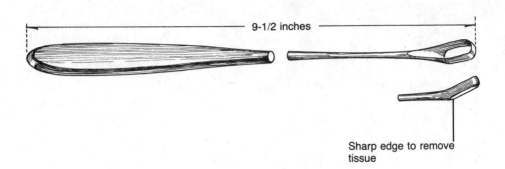

9-1/2 inches

Sharp edge to remove tissue

Sharp curette is instrument used to scrape the lining of the uterus in D&C.

PARTS OF BODY INVOLVED

The uterus and vagina are the only parts of the body involved in a D&C. The vagina is involved because we must approach the area to be scraped through the vagina.

If you are asleep for your D&C, your doctor will also examine you. This is called an *exam under anesthesia* or *EUA*. At this time, he can more easily feel your uterus, tubes and ovaries and possibly find other abnormalities, such as cysts on your ovaries.

COMMON REASONS FOR D&C

Since abortion became legal, over a million D&Cs have been performed every year for abortion alone. When combined with D&Cs done for incomplete miscarriages and those performed for diagnostic purposes, D&C is the second most common female operation performed in the United States each year.

In this section, we discuss only D&Cs performed for reasons *other* than abortion. Information on abortion is dealt with in a separate section, which begins on page 24.

"Miscarriage" is the lay term for an abortion that is a spontaneous, unanticipated loss of a pregnancy. This is in contrast to an induced abortion.

THREATENED MISCARRIAGE

In the first 20 weeks of pregnancy, if a pregnant woman begins to cramp and has less bleeding than a normal menstrual period, she is said to be "threatening to miscarry." The cervix hasn't begun to dilate nor has the woman passed any tissue. She could still carry the baby to term and is only threatening to miscarry. The woman is usually advised to take it easy, avoid intercourse and wait and see what happens.

Nature has a way of eliminating abnormal pregnancies, abnormally implanted pregnancies or those implanted in a uterus that is defective or one that has a defective cervix. For this reason, a couple who loses a pregnancy through miscarriage may take comfort in the fact that Nature may have been sorting out pregnancies that may have had or caused serious problems. The fact these women conceive once usually means they can conceive again.

INEVITABLE MISCARRIAGE

If the cervix has begun to dilate or if tissue has been passed, a miscarriage is inevitable. At this point, all attempts to save the pregnancy should cease. Usually the uterus quickly expels the fetus and placenta, and bleeding stops.

If bleeding persists or becomes heavier than a menstrual period, if membranes have broken or if the cervix has begun dilating, there is no reason to wait for the uterus to expel its contents. Waiting merely permits excessive, unnecessary loss of blood and a possible increase in the infection rate. It's better to perform a D&C and remove the products from the uterus. Then the uterus can begin contracting around the open blood vessels and stop the bleeding.

INCOMPLETE MISCARRIAGE

If the uterus has expelled part of the afterbirth and fetus, but continues to bleed, it is called an *incomplete miscarriage.* D&C is done promptly to avoid further loss of blood and to decrease the risk of infection. If all products of conception have been passed or removed, the uterus contracts and bleeding ceases. A medicine called *ergotrate* is often given to increase contraction of the uterus and decrease the blood loss.

COMPLETE MISCARRIAGE

When all products of conception have been expelled or removed by D&C, it is called a *complete miscarriage.* Some doctors feel no miscarriage is complete until a D&C has been performed, and they perform a D&C with *every* miscarriage. However, many miscarriages complete themselves spontaneously, bleeding ceases and no further treatment is necessary.

If bleeding continues after all tissue has passed, it may be due to failure of the uterus to contract. This is called an *atonic* uterus or one that has lost the tone in its muscular walls. Ergotrate usually helps the uterus contract and stop the bleeding.

MISSED MISCARRIAGE

Occasionally the fetus dies within the first 20 weeks of pregnancy, but for some reason the uterus doesn't expel it. If the products of conception are retained in the uterus, the condition is called a *missed abortion* or *missed miscarriage.*

A missed miscarriage may be a problem because the mother's body begins to lose its fibrinogen, and the blood does not clot. Intense bleeding can occur when the products of conception are finally delivered and the blood is unable to clot to prevent hemorrhage. Most doctors recommend a D&C to empty the uterus when this diagnosis is made.

HABITUAL MISCARRIAGE

For some couples, miscarriage happens many times. The term *habitual miscarriage* is used when three consecutive early pregnancies are lost. Additional medical testing is needed to determine the reason for the pregnancy losses. The woman has demonstrated she can conceive, and she should continue to do so in spite of the miscarriages. Many women eventually carry a normal pregnancy to successful full-term delivery in spite of frequent miscarriages.

SEPTIC MISCARRIAGE

With the legalization of abortion, the incidence of this problem has dropped dramatically. *Septic miscarriage* refers to a miscarriage complicated by overwhelming infection. Thanks to modern antibiotics, few women die of septic miscarriage, especially if they seek medical help early. A D&C is essential, along with antibiotics, and is the treatment of choice.

INCREASED AMOUNT OF FLOW

Most women experience a moderate variation from month to month in their menstrual flow. You may notice a heavier flow when fatigued or stressed, often with no obvious cause. If menstrual flow steadily increases in amount or if the amount is sufficient to deplete your blood, consult your doctor. Common causes of increased flow include endometrial hyperplasia, endometrial polyps, submucus fibroids, hormonal influence, cancer of the endometrium, endometriosis and other unknown causes. See illustrations on opposite page.

INTERMENSTRUAL BLEEDING

Bleeding between menstrual periods is not normal, although most women experience this type of bleeding at some time during their life. If it persists through more than one menstrual cycle, it should be investigated by a pelvic exam, a Pap smear and a D&C.

In younger women, the cause of spotting or bleeding between menstrual periods is less likely to be due to cancer, but it must never be ignored. Endometrial polyps, submucus fibroids, endometrial hyperplasia or cancer of the endometrium are the more common causes of bleeding between periods. All these can be diagnosed and many treated or cured by D&C. See illustrations on pages 174 and 175.

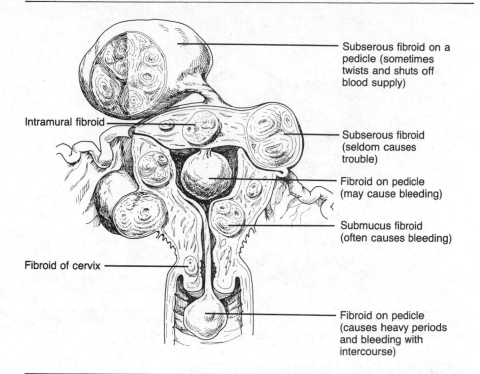

Subserous fibroid on a pedicle (sometimes twists and shuts off blood supply)

Intramural fibroid

Subserous fibroid (seldom causes trouble)

Fibroid on pedicle (may cause bleeding)

Submucus fibroid (often causes bleeding)

Fibroid of cervix

Fibroid on pedicle (causes heavy periods and bleeding with intercourse)

There are many locations for fibroid tumors of the uterus. Some cause bleeding, some cause pain and some cause pressure. Size and location often determine symptoms.

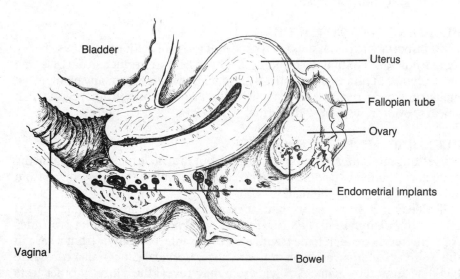

Bladder

Uterus

Fallopian tube

Ovary

Endometrial implants

Vagina

Bowel

Endometriosis is a condition in which pieces of endometrial tissue become implanted in other areas, such as on the ovary, behind the uterus, even in the bladder and bowel.

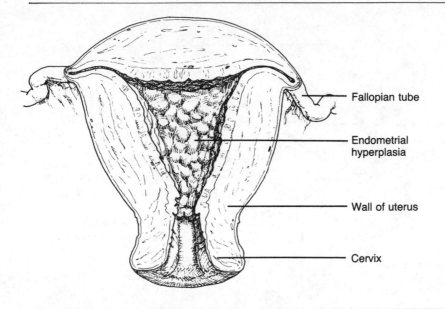

Fallopian tube

Endometrial hyperplasia

Wall of uterus

Cervix

Endometrial hyperplasia is an overgrowth of the lining of the uterus. Certain types of endometrial hyperplasia may become cancerous.

BLEEDING DUE TO EMOTIONAL STRESS

Emotional stress can cause heavier menstrual flow, an irregular menstrual period, menstrual bleeding between periods or total absence of flow. It's common to find some women miss a period because of death in the family or some other emotional crisis.

BLEEDING DUE TO CANCER

It's important to understand that cancer of internal genitals can cause heavy menstrual flow, continuous bleeding, slight or heavy intermenstrual bleeding or *no* change at all in the menstrual periods. For this reason, any change in a menstrual cycle *must* be investigated. It's also the reason for regular Pap smears, even in women with normal periods.

BLEEDING AFTER INTERCOURSE

Bleeding after intercourse is not normal, but the cause must be sought in the male *and* female. A specimen of semen can determine if the bleeding is from an internal source in the male.

If bleeding is from the woman, it could be due to cervicitis (also called *erosion* or *inflammation of the cervix),* a cervical polyp (growth that protrudes from the cervix enough to be traumatized with intercourse) or from a sore in the vagina. See illustration on opposite page. Cervical cancer also can cause bleeding from the vagina. A pelvic exam may reveal the cause. If other tests don't work, D&C should be done to help make the diagnosis.

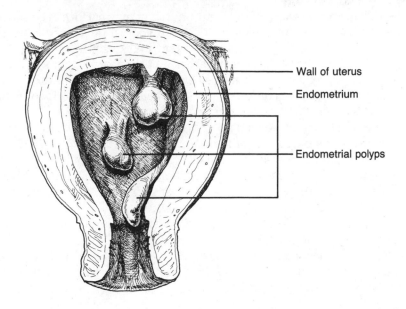

Wall of uterus

Endometrium

Endometrial polyps

Endometrial polyps can be single or multiple and are diagnosed by D&C. Some cause bleeding; others do not.

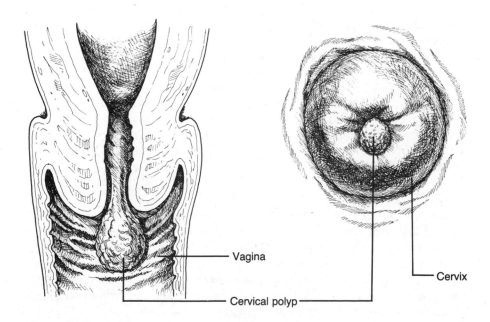

Vagina

Cervix

Cervical polyp

Cervical polyp hangs on a pedicle and protrudes from the cervix into the vagina. It often causes bleeding during intercourse.

SUSPICIOUS SMEARS

When a Pap smear is suspicious, your physician may perform a *colposcopy* in his office. A colposcopy allows the doctor to look at the cervix and vagina through a colposcope — a special instrument that magnifies the tissues. It also allows him to take biopsies of any areas that are abnormal or suspicious.

In some cases, removal of a cone of tissue from the mouth of the cervix is performed. This is called *conization*. A D&C may also be performed to make sure there is no problem with the lining of the uterus.

One question frequently asked is, *"When should a woman or her physician become suspicious enough of abnormal bleeding to consider a D&C?"* It's better to be overcautious than to overlook a condition that could be detrimental to your health. A Pap smear should be taken *before* any D&C is performed. A Pap smear may reveal early cancer of the cervix that would require a conization of the cervix, in addition to the D&C.

When there is a change in menstrual periods or if there is bleeding (even spotting) between menstrual periods, a D&C should be considered.

A woman past menopause should not have bleeding of any kind. A return of bleeding after several missed menstrual periods in a menopausal woman must be investigated by a Pap smear and D&C.

D&C FOR INFERTILITY

Microscopic examination of the lining of the uterus just before a menstrual period can reveal if you have ovulated; this is important in investigating infertility. This type of D&C may take the form of an endometrial biopsy.

An endometrial biopsy is a "partial" D&C in which a tiny metal or plastic tube is used. This tube can often be inserted into the uterine cavity in your doctor's office without stretching the cervix and without anesthesia.

Tissue is removed by gentle suction, combined with scraping, as the tube is pressed against the lining of the uterus during withdrawal. The procedure causes only a brief twinge of pain and is usually well-tolerated by the patient.

If tissue shows you are not ovulating, you can be given fertility medication (clomiphene, pergonal) that causes you to ovulate. Fertility drugs sometimes do their job so well that several eggs are released at ovulation, and a multiple pregnancy results. For this reason, these medications are used *only* under careful supervision.

EMBEDDED IUD

Occasionally an intrauterine device (IUD) becomes detached from the string that protrudes from the cervix. If it becomes embedded in the wall of your uterus, you may require a D&C to retrieve it. In other situations, an IUD may penetrate the wall of your uterus, causing problems such as inflammation, irritation, adhesions or even perforation of your bowel or bladder. In this case, you would require major surgery (laparotomy) to retrieve the IUD and repair the organ that has been damaged by it.

HOW COMMON IS D&C?

It is estimated about 1 in 5 women who have surgery undergo a D&C. This amounts to about 1 million D&Cs a year; in fact, D&C is the second most common of all surgeries performed in the United States. Often hysterectomies can be avoided by judicious use of a diagnostic or therapeutic D&C.

For example, you may find the gradual increase in your menstrual flow begins to deplete your hemoglobin and causes you to become anemic. Pelvic examination reveals an enlarged, irregularly contoured uterus that is typical of a fibroid tumor (usually benign).

Your doctor may be tempted to resort to a hysterectomy. However, D&C reveals endometrial hyperplasia, an endometrial polyp or some other benign cause of bleeding. If corrected by D&C, some of these problems may be solved without resorting to major surgery.

Many D&Cs show no abnormality, but this minor procedure avoids major operations in many instances.

FUNCTIONS INVOLVED IN D&C

Anatomy and physiology of the endometrium are discussed on pages 206 and 207. In general, only the lining of the uterus is involved when a D&C is performed, unless other parts of the uterus are encroaching on the lining.

A D&C should not scrape too deeply into the endometrium, or it can destroy the lining completely. A D&C is intended to remove the lining of the uterus down to the basal glands, without damaging them. If scraping is too vigorous, it may destroy some of these glands so they can't regenerate and prepare for the reception of a fertilized egg.

The time of the month when a D&C is performed is important. If investigating infertility, the doctor will want to perform the D&C just *before* the onset of menstruation to determine if you have ovulated and when you ovulated. If he is performing your D&C because of a bleeding problem, he prefers to do it immediately after your period to avoid interrupting an unsuspected early pregnancy.

HOW D&C IS PERFORMED

Most D&Cs are performed in the outpatient department of the hospital — you enter and leave the hospital on the same day of surgery. Occasionally, there is sufficient bleeding or some other reason to have you admitted to the hospital to stay overnight.

Some D&Cs, especially endometrial biopsies, can be performed without anesthesia. But the majority require a small amount of sodium pentothal or brevital.

If your D&C is planned, don't eat or drink after midnight because you may be given general anesthesia, especially if complications arise. An enema is not usually necessary prior to D&C.

Urinalysis and complete blood count are routine to rule out diabetes, anemia and infection. Your temperature, blood pressure and pulse are also recorded.

After the anesthesiologist puts you to sleep with an intravenous injection, you'll be placed on your back with legs spread apart in surgical stirrups. The skin and mucous membranes surrounding your vagina and the inside of your vagina are cleansed thoroughly with soap, water and an antiseptic.

The first thing your doctor does is re-examine you under anesthesia. Anesthesia produces relaxation of your abdominal muscles and permits a more thorough examination of your pelvic organs.

A weighted speculum opens your vagina and a hand-held speculum lifts the upper side of the vagina and exposes the cervix to view. Then a metal probe is carefully inserted through the cervical opening to determine the exact direction of your cervical canal and the depth and direction of the uterine cavity. This careful evaluation of the position of your uterus helps prevent perforation of the uterine wall during the operation.

Your doctor proceeds to dilate your cervical canal gradually, beginning with the smallest dilator. See illustration on opposite page. Your doctor uses larger dilators until the cervical opening is stretched enough to accommodate the necessary curette. After stretching the cervical canal, your doctor begins to curette the entire uterine cavity with long, gentle strokes, almost like raking a lawn. He carefully preserves the tissue he removes to send it to the laboratory.

Depending on the reason(s) for the D&C, your doctor may also use a "polyp" forceps to explore the cavity of your uterus. See illustration on opposite page. This is done to find and remove any polyps that may have escaped the curette.

Special precautions must be observed if the D&C is performed to remove retained tissue from a miscarriage. A pregnant uterus is softer than a nonpregnant uterus; its wall can be easily perforated by a uterine probe, a curette or polyp forceps.

VACUTAGE

Another method commonly used to remove tissue following miscarriage when a patient is still in her first trimester of pregnancy is called *vacutage.* Rather than a curette, a plastic suction tube, called a *suction curette,* is used, and the cavity of the uterus is vacuumed of its lining. See illustration on page 180.

There are several advantages to vacutage over the customary D&C with a "sharp" curette for early miscarriage. The cervix does not have to be stretched as much because the plastic suction tube has a smaller diameter than the curette. This is important because, in some cases, the cervix may be injured by stretching. The cervix may lose some of the tone necessary to keep it closed in subsequent pregnancies. This results in an *incompetent cervix* and could cause premature loss of pregnancies if the cervix is overstretched. Vacutage is usually the method of choice in performing early abortions. It is called a *menstrual extraction* or *menstrual regulation.*

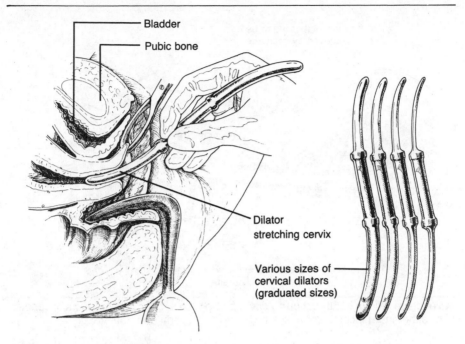

Bladder

Pubic bone

Dilator
stretching cervix

Various sizes of
cervical dilators
(graduated sizes)

Dilatation of the cervix. Before the uterine cavity can be scraped, the cervix must be dilated so instruments can enter.

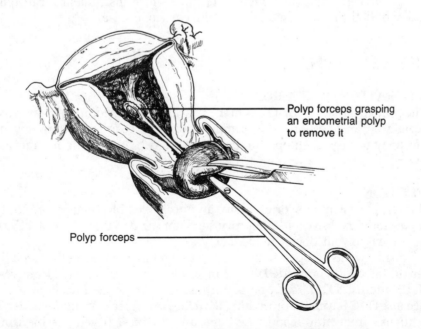

Polyp forceps grasping
an endometrial polyp
to remove it

Polyp forceps

Endometrial polyps are removed, when possible, by grasping them with an endometrial-polyp forcep.

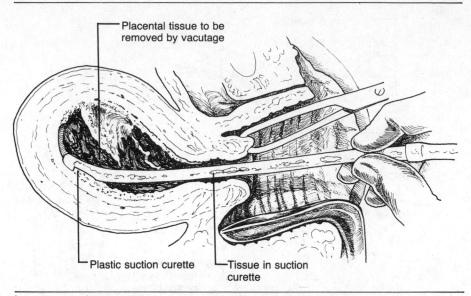

Placental tissue to be removed by vacutage

Plastic suction curette

Tissue in suction curette

In vacutage, doctor gently vacuums cavity of the uterus to remove products of conception, either in an incomplete miscarriage or for an early abortion.

But vacutage may not remove all the tissue. There may be a greater chance of continued bleeding due to retained placental tissue after a vacutage following a miscarriage. Your doctor will determine which instrument (or a combination of both) is more suitable in your particular case.

RISKS OF D&C

PERFORATION OF UTERUS
The principal risk of a D&C lies in the possibility of perforating the uterus, especially in an abortion. This complication may require laparoscopy or laparotomy to inspect the perforation to make certain there is no internal bleeding.

INFECTION
If fever, persistent pain or excessive and prolonged bleeding occur, notify your doctor. Excessive bleeding may also appear as large clots of blood. Report them to your doctor immediately!

No doctor wants to operate on a patient who has an infection, especially when the infection has invaded the organ on which he must operate. However, with the uterus, a D&C *must* be performed to clear up the infection.

Because D&C is a minor procedure, it can be performed even under adverse conditions. Frequently it must be done under stress. If you are bleeding heavily or if you are severely infected, D&C is an emergency and may be your only chance for survival.

AIR EMBOLUS

In the case of a D&C in which a pregnancy is involved, blood vessels are enlarged. There is always a chance for an air embolus, which is a bubble of air that enters an open blood vessel and is carried to another part of your body. This embolus could by transmitted to your brain or some other vital organ. This risk must be weighed against the urgency of stopping your bleeding.

INCOMPETENT CERVIX

Sometimes when the cervix must be stretched to accommodate the instruments used in D&C, tissues of the cervix don't return to normal size and tone. As a result, the cervix is rendered incapable of retaining a pregnancy.

A few months into a subsequent pregnancy, long before the pregnancy is mature enough to survive, the cervix begins to open. This may result in miscarriage or premature onset of labor with loss of the baby. This situation is called an *incompetent cervix.* It can be treated by an operation called a *cerclage,* in which a band of synthetic material is tied around the cervix like a purse string to keep it closed until full term. See illustration below.

The purse string can be cut when labor starts, or you can be delivered by Cesarean section. If the string is cut, you must undergo minor surgery to replace it for another pregnancy.

INJURED ENDOMETRIUM

Sometimes a too-vigorous D&C can result in damage to the inner lining of the uterine cavity. Usually only the superficial layers of the lining are removed

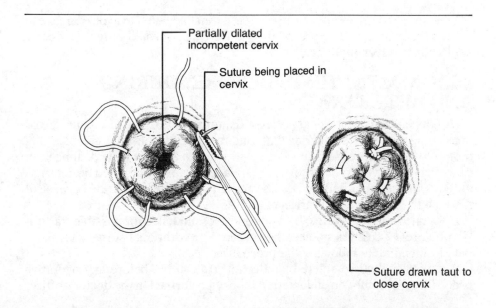

Partially dilated incompetent cervix

Suture being placed in cervix

Suture drawn taut to close cervix

Operation, called *cerclage,* is to correct incompetent cervix so a woman can carry a pregnancy to full term.

during D&C. This leaves the lower part of the glands to regenerate and function in subsequent cycles.

If a D&C removes too much of this glandular tissue, the lining is unable to regenerate itself. It can't thicken to produce a nutritious bed for a pregnancy to become implanted. It's possible some post-D&C patients have difficulty becoming pregnant or retaining a pregnancy for this reason.

ADVANTAGES OF D&C

A D&C may help avoid major surgery. It may help diagnose early cancer, stop hemorrhage, help cure infection, determine the cause of infertility, restore normal menstrual cycles and interrupt an unwanted pregnancy.

It is a minor surgical procedure, attended by minor risk, and is probably one of the most-valuable operative procedures we have. Some doctors believe it should be used more often prior to hysterectomy to improve diagnostic accuracy.

DISADVANTAGES OF D&C

It has few disadvantages, except for the rare occurrence of perforation of the uterus and occasional infection.

WHO OPERATES?

D&C is performed primarily by obstetricians and gynecologists. In some areas, family practitioners may perform this surgery if they have been trained to do so.

Even though D&C is minor surgery, care must be taken to avoid damage to the cervix or uterus. The procedure should be performed *only* by a doctor skilled in this technique.

DIAGNOSTIC TESTS BEFORE, DURING AND AFTER D&C

A Pap smear is performed before a diagnostic D&C because your doctor does not want to stretch a cervix that contains cancer. This might increase the possibility of its spread. Your doctor will want to know if he is dealing with cancer of the cervix. In the case of miscarriage, a Pap smear would be deferred until about a month after the D&C because it would be inaccurate because of the bleeding from the miscarriage.

It is unnecessary for you to be typed and crossmatched for possible transfusion before a D&C unless bleeding is severe or additional surgery is anticipated immediately following the procedure.

A urinalysis and complete blood count are routine before any operative procedure, except for an endometrial biopsy performed in the doctor's office.

WHERE IS SURGERY PERFORMED?

D&C is minor surgery, so it may be performed in a doctor's office if he has the equipment. Some emergency rooms are set up for D&Cs, while some hospitals refer D&Cs to their outpatient-surgery departments. If general anesthesia is used, the procedure will probably be done in the hospital or in an outpatient center.

If you're in critical condition, or if your D&C is preliminary to a major operation, such as a hysterectomy, the procedure is done on the operating table in a major-surgery suite.

HOSPITALIZATION AND DURATION

Unless the D&C is complicated by severe blood loss, severe infection, anesthesia complications or other problems, you can be released from your doctor's office, emergency room or outpatient department as soon as you awaken completely from the anesthetic.

When necessary, blood loss must be evaluated. If there is any infection, it must be cleared up before discharge from the hospital.

If perforation of your uterus occurs in the process of a D&C, laparoscopy is done to survey the damage and determine the need for abdominal exploration. Or you will be observed for a day or two for any evidence of complications due to the perforation.

ANESTHESIA

Anesthesia varies for D&C — from none at all for certain endometrial biopsies, mild sedation (such as valium) and intravenous sodium pentothal or brevital, to general anesthesia, depending on the severity and length of the procedure. Most D&Cs are done in a few minutes, so the anesthesiologist tries to administer as little anesthesia as possible. He may begin to wake you immediately after the D&C so you'll be able to go home quickly or be taken to your room in the hospital.

Spinal and epidural anesthesia are almost never used for D&Cs because sodium pentothal and brevital are simpler, shorter acting and easier to administer. There is risk of allergic response to the anesthetic, but a competent anesthesiologist knows how to deal with this complication.

PROBABLE OUTCOME OF D&C

The expected outcome of this surgical procedure is nearly always good. When skillfully performed, D&C is almost without risk, and the outcome is productive as a diagnosis or a therapeutic cure. Often, what was intended to be a diagnostic D&C, such as with an endometrial polyp or endometrial hyperplasia, becomes a bonus therapeutic D&C. The D&C makes the diagnosis and effects a cure by removing the problem.

POST-OPERATIVE CARE

No post-operative care is necessary in the average diagnostic D&C. A woman usually may resume all activities immediately or at least by the following day. But ask your doctor about specific activities, such as intercourse or use of tampons.

If your blood is depleted by hemorrhage, it might have to be replaced, and your convalescence could be delayed as you recover your strength. But the procedure of D&C itself doesn't impair your health or decrease your ability to function.

DIET

There is no special diet before or after D&C. When the D&C is scheduled ahead of time, you are asked to abstain from eating or drinking for 12 hours before surgery. This is routine when *any* anesthetic is administered. An empty stomach decreases the risk of aspiration of vomit into the lungs if vomiting occurs.

MISCONCEPTIONS ABOUT D&C

Early treatment won't necessarily help. I can really wait and see.

Some women put off investigation of symptoms until it is too late for early treatment that would give them a better chance for cure. Abnormal menstrual and non-menstrual bleeding should be studied early so your doctor can begin proper treatment. Often, treatment is minor and the cure almost certain. An avoidable tragedy is the situation in which bleeding is ignored until a cancer has spread when it could have been cured earlier with a D&C.

D&C is a major procedure.

D&C is a minor procedure, which is safe and painless, and it will not incapacitate you. It won't affect your menstrual periods, except in a positive way. It won't make you infertile or interfere with your response to sex.

ALTERNATIVES TO D&C

There are no alternatives to D&C when it is necessary. Watchful waiting is futile when there is abnormal bleeding. Delay can even be fatal, depending on your condition.

If your doctor suggests a D&C, and if he has good reasons for performing it, don't stand in his way.

CALL YOU DOCTOR IF . . .

1. You have chills or fever.
2. You have vaginal bleeding that is more than a normal menstrual flow.
3. You have pain — more than a few cramps.
4. You don't feel well and can't explain why.

QUESTIONS TO ASK YOUR DOCTOR

Explain why you think I should have a D&C.
You have a right to know what diagnosis your doctor suspects and what he hopes to accomplish by your D&C.

Will I be put to sleep during the D&C?
Most doctors use intravenous medication that has a very short action for a short, minor operation. Ask him about your anesthetic.

Will I have to stay overnight?
Most D&Cs are done on an outpatient basis. If you must stay overnight, it may be because of a special situation. Ask your doctor about it.

Will I have any pain afterward?
You should experience only mild discomfort following a D&C — probably only a few cramps.

Are there any restrictions on my activities after the D&C?
No intercourse, no douching and no tampons for at least 1 week. Most women return to work the next day unless there has been excessive blood loss.

Will this cure my problem, or do I need further treatment?
This varies according to your reasons for D&C. As mentioned earlier, a D&C is often diagnostic and therapeutic. It determines the cause of your bleeding and effects a cure at the same time.

Can I still get pregnant? (if near menopause or during menopause) Do I need to take precautions and for how long?
In general, if you have not had a menstrual period for over 1 year and you are 45 years or older, the chance is very low. But it is *not* impossible for you to become pregnant.

When can I resume tennis, golf, jogging?
As soon as you feel well enough. None of these sports should have any negative effect on you because you had a D&C.

How soon may I resume intercourse?
Some doctors have you wait for 1 month; others permit intercourse within a week. Ask your doctor about it.

How soon may I try to become pregnant?
Wait for at least one spontaneous menstrual cycle.

How soon may I return to work?
This varies with each patient. Some return to work the next day. Others require several days. If there has been severe blood loss, it may take longer to return to normal.

Ectopic Pregnancy

DEFINITION OF ECTOPIC PREGNANCY

Ectopic means you have a displaced pregnancy or a pregnancy that is located in an abnormal place. The pregnancy is implanted and growing *outside* the cavity of your uterus.

ABBREVIATIONS AND OTHER NAMES

When we speak about ectopic pregnancy, you may think of pregnancy in your Fallopian tube, but that condition is more accurately described as tubal pregnancy. A tubal pregnancy is the most common ectopic pregnancy and occurs more than 95% of the time. But pregnancy also occurs in other locations, and all these situations are referred to as *ectopic pregnancies.* See illustration on page 188. Ectopic pregnancy is also called extrauterine pregnancy.

Very rarely a pregnancy "aborts" out the end of the tube and becomes implanted in the abdominal cavity. In this case, it is called an abdominal pregnancy.

Pregnancy occurring in your ovary is called ovarian pregnancy, and one occurring in your cervix is called cervical pregnancy. Both conditions are extremely rare.

PARTS OF BODY INVOLVED

Ectopic pregnancy involves your Fallopian tube over 95% of the time, but if the pregnancy becomes implanted on your *omentum* (the apron of fatty tissue

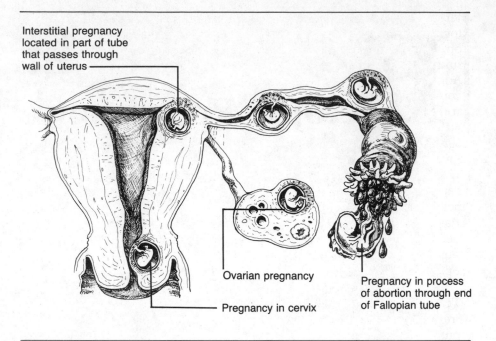

Interstitial pregnancy located in part of tube that passes through wall of uterus

Ovarian pregnancy

Pregnancy in cervix

Pregnancy in process of abortion through end of Fallopian tube

Various locations of ectopic pregnancies. Pregnancy in the cervix, ovary or abdomen are rare.

that hangs down over your bowel), it may involve your entire abdominal cavity and the organs in it.

The omentum is considered the "watchdog" of your abdomen because it polices your abdominal cavity. It is ready to wall off infection, the rupture of an organ or any other threat to the sterile environment. In ectopic pregnancy, your omentum attempts to wall off the pregnancy. In the process, it may provoke many adhesions, which are bands of scar tissue that form between raw or irritated surfaces. Only rarely are the ovary or cervix invaded by a pregnancy.

COMMON REASONS FOR ECTOPIC PREGNANCY

Anything that delays progress of the fertilized egg in its journey through your Fallopian tube to the uterine cavity may cause an ectopic pregnancy. This delay allows the fertilized egg to reach the stage in which it can erode its way into any organ and become implanted. If a fertilized egg, in this eroding stage, reaches other tissues, such as your Fallopian tube, ovary, cervix or abdominal cavity, implantation may occur at the site — the result is an ectopic pregnancy.

Specific causes of ectopic pregnancy are numerous. One cause is an extra-large embryo, due to rapid cell division. Extreme growth of the egg during external migration from an ovary to the opposite tube may also result in an ectopic pregnancy. Destruction of cilial cells lining the Fallopian tube, which propel the egg toward your uterine cavity, slows progress of the egg. As a result, the egg implants itself in your tube.

Adhesions in tubal folds form pockets into which the egg may drop and become trapped. These pockets and folds can be caused by endometriosis or scar tissue from gonorrhea or chlamydial infections in and around the tubes.

Stricture or narrowing of your Fallopian tube slows or prevents normal progress of the egg. It is believed some ectopic pregnancies are conceived in the week prior to menstruation.

The incidence of ectopic pregnancy increases almost 10 times if you have an intrauterine contraceptive device (IUD). This could be due to the fact pregnancies that would normally occur in the cavity of your uterus are prevented. But an IUD does *not* prevent an ectopic pregnancy.

Defective ovum or sperm, or a combination of the two, might result in ectopic pregnancy. This has been shown to be the case in over 50% of all ectopic pregnancies.

INTERSTITIAL PREGNANCY

Pregnancy can occur in the part of the tube lying inside the uterine wall. Rupture of a pregnancy in this area can cause massive, life-threatening hemorrhage. It may be so severe that an immediate hysterectomy may be necessary to control it.

OVARIAN PREGNANCY

A pregnancy attached to the ovary is extremely rare. Diagnosis may be confused with an ovarian cyst that twists on its pedicle (cord by which it hangs) or a cyst that ruptures and bleeds into the abdominal cavity. It is difficult to differentiate between an ovarian pregnancy and a tubal pregnancy until your abdominal cavity is opened or until it can actually be seen by laparoscopy. Only rarely does an ovarian pregnancy go beyond 2 months without diagnosis or rupture.

It's hard to understand how an ovarian pregnancy occurs. This situation almost always destroys the ovary, and removal of the entire ovary is necessary to control the hemorrhage. Ovarian pregnancy occurs in less than 1% of all ectopic pregnancies.

ABDOMINAL PREGNANCY

Abdominal pregnancy usually occurs when a living embryo aborts from its primary location in your Fallopian tube and becomes implanted somewhere in the peritoneal cavity. This occurs only once in about 3,500 pregnancies.

This is an impossible situation as far as delivery is concerned. The diagnosis may not be made until you reach full term and fetal movements produce nausea, abdominal pain and diarrhea.

X-ray and ultrasound in abdominal pregnancy reveal the fetus is lying crosswise in the abdominal cavity, with a small uterus lying in front of it. As soon as abdominal pregnancy is diagnosed, laparotomy is performed and your baby is removed. Because of the large blood vessels supplying your placenta, this organ is usually left in place to be absorbed slowly by your peritoneal cavity.

Fetal mortality ranges from 75 to 95%. Maternal mortality depends on the amount of hemorrhage or infection that goes along with separation of your placenta from your abdominal wall. In rare instances, mother and infant survive and do well.

CERVICAL PREGNANCY

A cervical pregnancy is very rare, and it is attended by the risk of severe hemorrhage. This type of pregnancy is implanted in the cervix. Usually a cervical pregnancy terminates before the fourth month and may require a hysterectomy to control hemorrhage.

HOW COMMON IS ECTOPIC PREGNANCY?

Ectopic pregnancy occurs about once in every 200 pregnancies. The rate of this type of pregnancy appears to be on the rise. From 1970 to 1978, the number of ectopic pregnancies more than doubled. Ectopic pregnancy is more common if you have a history of infertility, especially if you experience sterility after giving birth to one child.

Gonorrhea in the Fallopian tubes often causes complete sterility by blocking them. If it doesn't cause complete sterility, it may impair your tubes enough that when pregnancy does occur, the pregnancy is trapped by tubal adhesions, resulting in tubal pregnancy. Chlamydia infection is another major cause of tubal adhesions.

FUNCTIONS INVOLVED IN ECTOPIC PREGNANCY

Fertilization may occur normally — the sperm travel from your vagina through the uterine cavity, enter the tube and ascend against cilial cells lining the tube. After fertilization, your egg (now called an *embryo)* begins to grow by dividing. See illustration on opposite page.

If your growing fertilized egg is unable to navigate through a diseased, narrowed or adhesion-obstructed Fallopian tube, it may become trapped in the tube. In a short time, your embryo develops the ability to burrow into the wall of your tube and becomes an ectopic (abnormally placed) pregnancy.

Implantation of the fertilized egg in your Fallopian tube provokes the same response in the wall of the tube that it does in the lining of your uterus. The problem is the lining of your tube is unsuitable for development of a fertilized egg.

The tissue underlying the embryo, which normally develops into a placenta, is incapable of this type of development. Instead of burrowing into a nutritious bed of prepared tissue, the egg burrows into the ill-prepared wall of your Fallopian tube. It continues this erosive process until the tubal wall is perforated, with consequent hemorrhage.

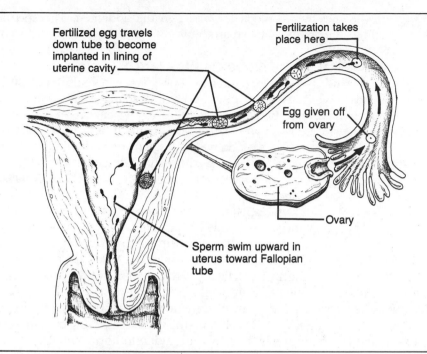

Fertilization takes place in the Fallopian tube, then the fertilized egg makes its way down the tube to become implanted in the lining of the uterus. If it becomes trapped on the way, a tubal pregnancy may occur.

After the embryo is implanted in the wall of your tube, the eroding process occasionally causes weakening of the tissue *over* it. The result is a rupture of the *inner* lining of the tube, which allows escape of the embryo into the cavity of the tube instead of directly into your peritoneal cavity. When the embryo is expelled from the tube, it is called *tubal abortion*.

When tubal abortion occurs, it may be accompanied by minimal hemorrhage that soon ceases, along with death and absorption of the tiny embryo by your peritoneal cavity. If associated with heavy hemorrhage (usually into the peritoneal cavity), the tubal abortion may produce shock from loss of blood. It could require surgery to stop the bleeding.

Let's define *shock*. The ordinary signs of shock are rapid, feeble pulse, falling blood pressure, cold sweat, pallid skin, shallow breathing, air hunger, restlessness and extreme anxiety, almost like a feeling of impending death. In this case, the signs and symptoms of shock are due to acute loss of blood. If you have any of these signs, call your doctor immediately!

HOW SURGERY FOR ECTOPIC PREGNANCY IS PERFORMED

Surgery for an ectopic pregnancy may be diagnostic *and* therapeutic. Diagnostic procedures may include D&C, laparoscopy, page 238, and culdocentesis. Culdocentesis is done with a long needle that is placed behind the cervix, into the abdomen, to look for blood in the abdomen. Therapeutic surgery includes laparoscopy or laparotomy.

D&C FOR NORMAL AND ECTOPIC PREGNANCY

A D&C may be used to look for evidence of pregnancy in your uterus, such as when a miscarriage is suspected, or to find typical changes that occur in the endometrium with ectopic pregnancy. If there is any chance of a normal pregnancy in your uterus and you want to be pregnant, a D&C will not be done. When you have a positive pregnancy test, lower abdominal pain or cramping with bleeding from your vagina, this may be due to a miscarriage or bleeding from your uterus due to ectopic pregnancy. Vaginal bleeding is common with ectopic pregnancy.

The lining of your uterus responds to hormones generated by any pregnancy, even if the pregnancy is not inside your uterine cavity. Bleeding may be the first sign of abnormality and is normally assumed to be due to miscarriage. But when a D&C is performed, the tissue doesn't reveal placenta or fetus but reveals the hormonal effect of pregnancy outside your uterus. Your doctor must then find the location of your pregnancy.

D&C may be used, along with laparotomy, for ectopic pregnancy if vaginal bleeding is extremely heavy. A D&C helps stop vaginal bleeding by removing the tissue that has built up inside your uterus due to hormonal effect.

LAPAROSCOPY AND LAPAROTOMY

Laparoscopy is frequently used in *diagnosing* an ectopic pregnancy. If ectopic pregnancy is suspected but unconfirmed, laparoscopy lets your doctor look inside your abdomen and actually see your uterus, tubes and ovaries. If an ectopic pregnancy is found, further surgery is usually required.

Rarely laparoscopy shows a tubal pregnancy that has aborted out the end of the tube; bleeding has stopped and no further treatment is needed. The aborted pregnancy is absorbed into the peritoneal cavity.

Assuming the diagnosis of ectopic pregnancy is established, then *laparotomy* is done immediately. You will be typed, crossmatched and a transfusion or blood-substitute I.V. started if blood loss has been severe or if you're in shock. If your condition is stable (no shock), an abdominal incision is made as soon as you can be prepped and anesthetized.

Internal bleeding is due to ruptured blood vessels in the wall of your Fallopian tube. Bleeding won't stop, and shock won't improve until bleeding vessels have been clamped.

It's futile to pour a lot of blood into you when you're in shock and expect your condition to improve while you're still bleeding from open blood vessels. Yet the moment bleeding vessels are clamped, shock begins to subside, blood pressure immediately begins to return to normal and your general condition improves. For this reason, life-saving surgery may have to be undertaken while you are still in shock. To combat shock while typing and crossmatching your blood, blood substitutes may have to be administered.

Surgery involves an incision through the abdominal wall from the navel to the pubic hairline for rapid access to the bleeding area or through a horizontal incision. A horizontal incision may be made within the pubic hairline. Women prefer a bikini incision that doesn't show when they wear a bathing suit, and surgeons prefer it for better post-operative support, with less chance of hernia. The type of incision used depends on individual preference and urgency of the situation or if you have a scar from previous surgery that can be used.

Fallopian tubes are inspected for rupture, and tiny instruments are used to clamp bleeding blood vessels. Tissue must be handled carefully to avoid unnecessary trauma to the tubes so their function is not impaired. If future pregnancies are anticipated, unnecessary injury to the tubes must be avoided.

In the past, the involved Fallopian tube would have been removed immediately if it had been ruptured by tubal pregnancy. Often the ovary was removed because the tube and ovary share the same blood supply. Today, attempts are made to preserve as much of your Fallopian tube and ovary as possible for future pregnancies.

If sufficient damage has been done to your tube by rupture of the tubal pregnancy, your surgeon may be forced to remove the injured tube to control bleeding, which can be life-threatening. If you desire future pregnancies, all attempts will be made to preserve as much of your tube as possible. This may require surgery at another time to repair the damaged tube.

In some cases, the opposite tube has been removed because of a previous tubal pregnancy or other disease, such as infection of the tube. In every case, the opposite tube and ovary should be examined and assessed at the time of surgery. If it is also impaired, every effort is made to preserve your tube after the bleeding is controlled.

If a large amount of blood is found in your abdominal cavity at surgery, it may be handled in one of three ways. It may be sucked out and discarded, which is the most common method. It may be sucked out, processed and reused by being transfused back into you. Or it may be allowed to remain in your abdominal cavity, where it is gradually absorbed, and its iron is utilized by your body to rebuild blood.

Depending on your age, condition and desire for future pregnancies, your involved tube may be surgically removed and your opposite tube tied off to prevent additional pregnancies. If your condition is stable, this surgery does not impose a risk.

If your pregnancy is located in the interstitial area (the part of the tube that lies within the uterine wall), damage to your uterus and the resulting hemorrhage may be so severe that hysterectomy is required. Each situation is different and calls for careful evaluation.

If your tubal pregnancy has not ruptured, a tiny longitudinal incision is made in your Fallopian tube. The embryo is carefully removed, and blood vessels are cauterized or tied with very fine sutures. The cut edges of the tube may be left open to heal by themselves or sewed back together.

After bleeding is under control, the emergency is over and careful inspection of your other pelvic organs is made. The appendix should be examined because it might be infected. Although your doctor would not subject you to unnecessary surgery at this time, it could be fatal to leave an infected appendix. Your surgeon may also inspect your gallbladder for stones, along with other abdominal organs, depending on your condition.

RISKS OF SURGERY
FOR ECTOPIC PREGNANCY

Ectopic pregnancy was identified over 1,000 years ago. It was first described by Albucasis, a famous Arabic writer on surgical topics. The case he described was not operated on; it became infected, abscessed and extruded through an opening in the abdominal wall when the abscess burst and drained.

A little over 100 years ago, a surgeon named Dr. Lawson Tait successfully operated on a patient in Birmingham, England, and removed her Fallopian tube and the pregnancy growing inside it. The patient survived. In 1894, Dr. Bussiere in France performed an autopsy on a female prisoner after she was executed and discovered an unruptured pregnancy in her Fallopian tube.

With the use of anesthesia, blood typing and crossmatching, antibiotic therapy and skillful surgery, the risk in ectopic pregnancy has gradually decreased over the years. In 1970, the maternal mortality rate due to ectopic pregnancy was reported at under 2% in the United States.

But the risk increases if your tube has ruptured, if hemorrhage is severe, shock is intense or there is a delay in diagnosis or facilities for emergency surgery are inadequate. If you're anemic, poorly nourished, have other illnesses compounding the problem or fail to report for medical help immediately, the outlook is less favorable.

The first sign of tubal pregnancy may be complete physical collapse. If this occurs, the outlook is less favorable. When the tube ruptures, the availability of paramedic help, emergency-room service, blood banks and physicians-on-call can help save lives in this life-threatening condition.

Everyone, including physicians, should be aware of the possibility of ectopic pregnancy in any woman who has sudden, severe, lower abdominal pain, followed by collapse, shock and failure to respond to simple stimuli.

Rupture of tubal pregnancy commonly occurs when you're straining to have a bowel movement. This is called the *bathroom sign*. The situation is urgent, so it's important to get to the hospital immediately! If no ambulance or paramedic facilities are available, get to the emergency room as quickly as possible. To save your life, time is of the essence in a ruptured tubal pregnancy.

The incidence of ectopic pregnancy has more than doubled in recent years and has become a more common cause of maternal death. It now accounts for about 12% of maternal deaths, up from 6% in 1975.

Tubal pregnancy is more common in women who have had difficulty getting pregnant. This may be because the Fallopian tube is diseased or damaged. The most common condition found in women is *salpingitis* (infected tubes), either acute or chronic, with or without adhesions.

Tubal pregnancy is increasing because of the greater incidence of multiple sexual partners, with its greater incidence of infection in the Fallopian tubes, earlier sexual experience (for the same reason) and greater frequency of gonorrhea and chlamydial infections that attack the Fallopian tubes. One-third to one-half of all ectopic pregnancies reveal residue of pelvic inflammatory disease.

According to research reported in the May 1983 *Current Problems in Obstetrics & Gynecology,* gonorrhea is one of the principal agents involved in most primary tubal infections. The risk of transmission from an infected male may be as high as 90%. Chlamydia is also one of the most common causes.

One of the most distressing things about a gonorrheal infection is only 10 to 20% of all infected women have the typical signs and symptoms that accompany infection of the uterus, tubes or peritoneal cavity. For this reason, insist on a culture for gonorrhea if you are at all sexually active and have unusual symptoms, such as painful urination, excessive vaginal discharge or abdominal pain.

If you've had several sexual partners and have any of the above symptoms, ask for a culture for gonorrhea when you go in for your annual Pap smear. It could be important for future pregnancies and to prevent damage that could prevent pregnancy or cause a tubal pregnancy.

What about chlamydial infection? In the September 1984 issue of the *The Female Patient,* Dr. Hugh Barber states that sexually transmitted chlamydial infection is more common than gonorrhea and may be causing problems in the Fallopian tubes.

Although a chlamydial infection in your pelvic organs causes less-acute symptoms, the symptoms last longer. This infection may produce more scarring in your tubes than a gonorrheal infection. If you have an infection in your vagina, consider the possibility that it involves your internal organs, including scarring of Fallopian tubes.

Be aware of the possibility of tubal pregnancy. Any woman of childbearing age with lower abdominal pain might be suspected of having a tubal pregnancy until proved otherwise. As many as 85% of all ectopic pregnancies are diagnosed *after* the tube has ruptured. Some of these might be diagnosed *before* rupture if the patient and doctor were more aware of the possibility of tubal pregnancy.

The outcome is more serious if the Fallopian tube has already ruptured. It's important to make the diagnosis *before* rupture when possible.

BEFORE RUPTURE

Before rupture, there is a vague, difficult-to-describe discomfort, perhaps only a soreness, similar to cramps. There may be no pain at all. There is no fever, no elevation of your white blood-cell count and no signs of severe pain when your abdomen is pressed by the doctor's hand. It doesn't hurt because there has been *no* bleeding in the peritoneal cavity at this point. There may or may not be a mass alongside the uterus for your doctor to feel, but it is small. It takes an alert, perceptive doctor to diagnose a tubal pregnancy before it ruptures.

DURING RUPTURE

The period during rupture of a tubal pregnancy is critical because things happen quickly. It is essential that diagnosis be made and treatment instituted as rapidly as possible.

An episode of acute pain is often followed by temporary relief when tension on your Fallopian tube is relieved by the rupture. Examination of the pelvis reveals a sensitive, painful cervix that hurts when it is touched or moved because the tube is also moved and stretched at the same time.

Vaginal bleeding may become constant, which can be confused with a miscarriage. Tenderness is marked, demonstrating there is free blood in the peritoneal cavity. On pelvic examination, there is a tense, tender mass felt next to the uterus.

AFTER RUPTURE

Diagnosis of tubal pregnancy is easier after rupture because the pain is agonizing. It is localized on one side, with signs of internal hemorrhage (positive culdocentesis and rigid, tender abdomen) followed by increasing shock. Your condition may deteriorate rapidly if transfusions and surgery do not begin soon.

Culdocentesis consists of inserting a needle into the lowest part of the peritoneal cavity, called the *cul-de-sac,* to check for the presence of blood. See illustration on opposite page. In this case, blood would be due to a ruptured ectopic pregnancy. See page 198 for more information on culdocentesis.

About half of all tubal pregnancies become subacute (less severe symptoms), chronic (longer-lasting, with mild pain) or atypical (unusual, not typical of usual tubal pregnancy). With or without the signs and symptoms, bleeding may stop. Blood present in the peritoneal cavity may become walled off, causing decreasing, persistent discomfort. The situation often becomes a diagnostic dilemma that can't be solved until laparoscopy is undertaken, often only after some other tentative diagnosis has been made.

If tubal pregnancy develops into a chronic situation, the risk becomes less, but you continue to have pain and wonder what is wrong with you. Months sometimes pass before the situation is understood and the problem is resolved by surgical exploration.

INTRAUTERINE DEVICE (IUD)

Having an intrauterine device (IUD) is a situation that is common to tubal pregnancy. An IUD effectively prevents pregnancy in the uterine cavity, but it does *not* prevent a pregnancy in your tube. There is still some question as to whether the IUD increases inflammation and infection in the Fallopian tubes, which may cause the tubal pregnancy.

It's difficult to prove an IUD actually causes tubal pregnancy, but the incidence of tubal pregnancy is 10 times greater when an IUD is present. It is

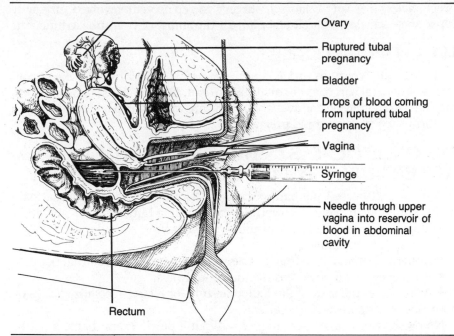

Ovary

Ruptured tubal pregnancy

Bladder

Drops of blood coming from ruptured tubal pregnancy

Vagina

Syringe

Needle through upper vagina into reservoir of blood in abdominal cavity

Rectum

Culdocentesis in a ruptured tubal pregnancy in which blood accumulates in the lowest part of the periotoneal cavity. A valuable test to prove bleeding is to withdraw some of this blood through a needle placed through the vagina.

possible normal intrauterine pregnancies are usually prevented by the IUD, so we are more aware only of tubal pregnancies. While this debate goes on, understand that tubal pregnancy occurs more often if you wear an IUD. If you suspect tubal pregnancy, perhaps the diagnosis can be made early and emergency treatment begun. If you have an IUD and develop abdominal pain, have a pregnancy test. If the test is positive, ectopic pregnancy must be ruled out.

ADVANTAGES OF SURGERY FOR ECTOPIC PREGNANCY

The only treatment for tubal pregnancy is immediate surgery. There is no alternative treatment once the diagnosis has been made. Early suspicion, early diagnosis and early surgery produce less risk, lower mortality and possibly less unfavorable impact on future fertility.

DISADVANTAGES OF SURGERY FOR ECTOPIC PREGNANCY

There is *no* alternative to surgery. We might say there are no disadvantages, but there are some. The Fallopian tube is already impaired, so it might have to be removed, which further decreases your chance for additional pregnancies. If it isn't removed, surgery to repair your involved tube may cause some adhesions and further impair the ability of your tube to function.

WHO OPERATES?

It is usually your obstetrician-gynecologist who performs this operation, but most general surgeons are qualified to do it. In some areas, family doctors may be the only physicians available; many are well-trained and competent to perform surgery for ectopic pregnancy.

DIAGNOSTIC TESTS BEFORE, DURING AND AFTER SURGERY FOR ECTOPIC PREGNANCY

We have discussed the bathroom sign — sudden lower abdominal pain while straining to have a bowel movement. In addition, there are other symptoms that raise suspicion of tubal pregnancy:
- Any lower abdominal pain.
- Abnormal vaginal bleeding (not necessarily a missed menstrual period).
- Pregnancy test may be positive but not always.
- A "mass" in the area of the Fallopian tube or ovary, recognized only by your doctor by *pelvic examination.*

No doctor would consider surgery without a pelvic exam, but it must be done gently to avoid increased hemorrhage.

In only half of reported cases are all three signs or symptoms present. But if you are a sexually active woman of childbearing age with any of these signs, your physician should evaluate you to rule out tubal pregnancy. Any woman in shock — low blood pressure, unsteady pulse with cold perspiration and pallor — should be suspected of ruptured tubal pregnancy.

CULDOCENTESIS

In the presence of any of the above symptoms, a valuable test can be performed in your doctor's office or in the emergency room. It is called *culdocentesis.* A needle is inserted through the top of the vagina, just behind the cervix, up into the cul-de-sac of the peritoneum to test for the presence of blood in the abdominal cavity.

Nearly 85% of all ruptured tubal pregnancies and some unruptured tubal pregnancies cause enough hemorrhage into the peritoneal cavity to show up in this test. A ruptured, bleeding corpus luteum cyst, occasionally caused when an egg is extruded from your ovary at the time of ovulation, can also cause lower abdominal pain and bleeding into the peritoneal cavity. However, this imitator of ruptured tubal pregnancy is less common. Occasionally it demands surgery, but usually the bleeding is minimal and stops by itself.

Your doctor will keep in mind that tubal pregnancy may also be present even when no blood is found on culdocentesis. This procedure may cause you some discomfort, but it is not severe. Culdocentesis is a useful diagnostic test and is worth the time and discomfort because it increases the accuracy of diagnosis. If positive, it rapidly diagnoses your internal hemorrhage and hastens your treatment.

HUMAN CHORIONIC GONADOTROPIN TEST

Another test for tubal pregnancy is the amount of human chorionic gonadotropin (HCG) present in your blood or urine. This is the same hormone that gives a positive pregnancy test with urine or blood. Ectopic pregnancies usually have a detectable level of HCG — they will give you a positive pregnancy test. If the test is positive, the diagnosis of tubal pregnancy can be questioned.

In a normal pregnancy, the level of HCG doubles every 2-1/3 days. If it is not an emergency situation, you can be observed for a week or so. If the level of HCG does *not* increase, tubal pregnancy or miscarriage must be considered.

To differentiate between miscarriages and tubal pregnancy, ultrasound exam is valuable and may show an intrauterine pregnancy sac as early as 5 to 6 weeks after your last menstrual period. If ultrasound shows an empty uterus when the pregnancy test is positive at 5 to 6 weeks of pregnancy, ectopic pregnancy must be considered. Ultrasound also shows fluid in your abdomen (probably blood), which indicates a possible ruptured ectopic pregnancy.

LAPAROSCOPY

If you're not in serious condition, laparoscopy may be performed to confirm the diagnosis of ectopic pregnancy. In this procedure, two 1/4-inch incisions are made in your lower abdomen. A laparoscope and a probe can be inserted through the incisions. With these instruments, the surgeon examines your tubes and ovaries and confirms or rules out tubal pregnancy.

In many instances, this minor procedure can save you major surgery by *ruling out* the possibility of tubal pregnancy.

In addition to the possibility of miscarriage, your doctor must also differentiate a tubal pregnancy from appendicitis, bladder infection, salpingitis, a bleeding ovarian cyst, a cyst that is twisted on its pedicle, a tumor of the muscle wall of the uterus that could be twisted on its pedicle, a threatened or inevitable miscarriage and other conditions.

Several laboratory tests, including complete blood count and urinalysis (to eliminate urinary infection), help rule out some of these conditions. When your doctor orders all these tests, be thankful he's thorough.

WHERE IS SURGERY PERFORMED?

Diagnostic tests can be performed in your doctor's office or in the emergency room. But the actual surgery for tubal pregnancy is done in an operating room, where blood is available, with adequate anesthesia and skilled personnel present.

HOSPITALIZATION AND DURATION

Outside of diagnostic tests, surgery for ectopic pregnancy requires about 1 to 1-1/2 hours, depending on how much reconstructive work must be done. We have already discussed the need for care in repairing a ruptured Fallopian tube so future pregnancies may occur. In many cases, this requires microsurgery and time-consuming, painstaking care. If bleeding is excessive, microsurgical repair will be delayed until another time.

You remain in the recovery room until your condition is stable. Hospital stay is about 5 days, unless your convalescence is complicated by anemia, fever, infection or other conditions. Ruptured ectopic pregnancy is an emergency, so transfusion must come from a donor. If abdominal bleeding is severe, some of your own blood may be processed and retransfused to you. Usually, blood from a blood bank is required immediately to stabilize your condition and to combat shock.

The possibility of transfusion reaction is real if massive amounts of blood are necessary. The most common complication of ectopic pregnancy is infection. Because of the amount of blood left in your abdominal cavity and risk of infection, antibiotics given at the time of your surgery may be advisable.

ANESTHESIA

A general anesthetic is usually administered because of the urgency of the situation. Before the arrival of an anesthesiologist, your surgeon may begin surgery by injecting a local anesthetic along the line of incision. In dire emergencies, the entire operation may be carried out under local anesthesia by injecting deeper tissues with the local anesthetic as the doctor approaches them. But today, adequate anesthesia, including skilled personnel, is readily available in most areas.

Only in rare situations are spinal or epidural anesthesia used for tubal pregnancy surgery. If you or your doctor prefer regional anesthesia, if you are allergic to gas anesthesia or if you have lung disease, your doctor will use spinal or epidural anesthesia.

PROBABLE OUTCOME OF SURGERY FOR ECTOPIC PREGNANCY

Ruptured tubal pregnancy is a serious emergency condition that carries a risk of 1 to 2% mortality. The greatest danger lies in the fact that it may not be recognized and treated early enough.

When diagnosed early and treated adequately, the operation is safe and the outcome uncomplicated. Ectopic pregnancy recurs in the opposite tube in about 8% of all patients, usually because the disease that produced the ectopic pregnancy probably involved both Fallopian tubes.

In the past, about 1/3 of all women who had a tubal pregnancy could expect to be infertile, 1/3 would have a subsequent normal intrauterine pregnancy and 1/3 would have a miscarriage or another ectopic pregnancy. Recent reports of improved microsurgical techniques indicate rates of successful subsequent pregnancy at 50 to 85%.

Two factors influence the likelihood of future normal pregnancy — the health of the other tube and whether diagnosis was made *before* or *after* rupture of the involved tube.

POST-OPERATIVE CARE

Post-operative care is about the same after surgery for ectopic pregnancy as it is following an appendectomy or other uncomplicated abdominal surgery. You'll be encouraged to get out of bed the day after surgery. You'll be helped to the bathroom and can usually pass urine on your own.

You receive only clear liquids by mouth until your bowel resumes activity, as shown by active bowel sounds (heard by stethoscope) or until you pass gas by rectum. When you can drink adequately, you'll no longer need intravenous fluids.

Your blood count shows whether you need further transfusions. It is better to allow you to manufacture your own blood if possible, rather than take the risk of transfusion. You may need iron tablets to help rebuild your blood.

DIET

There is no special diet necessary after surgery for an ectopic pregnancy because the bowel was not involved, unless bowel adhesions were present or if extensive bowel manipulation was necessary because of adhesions. Ordinarily, you may quickly resume a normal diet following surgery.

MISCONCEPTIONS ABOUT ECTOPIC PREGNANCY

If I have an ectopic pregnancy, I won't be able to conceive again.
With modern microsurgical techniques, an ectopic pregnancy does not always mean you'll lose the involved Fallopian tube or that you can't conceive again, even if your involved tube required microsurgery.

Doctors don't know what causes ectopic pregnancy.
The most common cause of ectopic pregnancy is infection of the Fallopian tubes, most often by gonorrhea and chlamydial disease. Consider asking for a culture of the cervical and vaginal discharge, in addition to a Pap smear, when you visit your doctor.

It's dangerous to have an ectopic pregnancy, and surgery can be hazardous.
Although surgery for ectopic pregnancy is serious and urgent, it is fairly safe. Few complications arise if you and your physician are aware of its possibility and act promptly!

ALTERNATIVES TO SURGERY FOR ECTOPIC PREGNANCY

If a diagnosis of ectopic pregnancy is made, there are *no* alternatives to surgery. Keep in mind these signs and symptoms:
- abnormal menstrual period
- lower abdominal pain

- tender cervix
- possible mass alongside the uterus

There are diagnostic tests available — culdocentesis, HCG (pregnancy test), ultrasound, laparoscopy and D&C. Seek help early!

CALL YOUR DOCTOR IF . . .

BEFORE SURGERY

1. You have sharp lower abdominal pain, especially with a missed or abnormal menstrual period.
2. You have the bathroom sign, and there is the possibility you are pregnant.
3. If you are unsure about your condition, but you have lower abdominal pain, feel faint and may or may not have missed a menstrual period.
4. If you have had an ectopic pregnancy before and have similar symptoms.

AFTER SURGERY

1. You have chills or fever.
2. You have redness or tenderness in your wound.
3. You have a bloody or foul-smelling discharge from your wound.
4. Your wound separates.

QUESTIONS TO ASK YOUR DOCTOR

BEFORE SURGERY

How certain are you that I have a tubal pregnancy?
Although the pregnancy test is not always positive, culdocentesis should be positive, or ultrasound should show no pregnancy in the uterus. Consultation may be necessary to confirm suspicious laparoscopy.

Do you know that I have (or have not) had my appendix removed?
It is often difficult to differentiate between appendicitis and tubal pregnancy. Both are surgical emergencies, but laparoscopy may help with the diagnosis.

Is it necessary to perform culdocentesis?
If other signs and symptoms are positive, perhaps not. Some doctors prefer laparoscopy, but culdocentesis is a simple, quick office test to see if there is internal bleeding.

Will you have to remove my Fallopian tube? Could it be saved by microsurgery?
With modern microsurgical techniques, most tubes can be saved. Ask if your doctor is familiar with microsurgical techniques. The best time for microsurgical repair may be at a later time. Surgery done at the time of the ectopic pregnancy may be life-saving; it may attempt to save as much tube as possible for future microsurgical repair.

Are you going to remove my ovary?
Unless the blood supply of the ovary has been damaged by the ruptured tubal pregnancy, all normal ovaries are saved.

Will you check my appendix, gallbladder and other organs while you are at it?
These organs can be checked by feeling them with a gloved hand. It does not increase your risk, yet it gives your doctor valuable information about the condition of your other organs.

AFTER SURGERY

Please review exactly what you found and what you did at surgery.
You have the right to know all about your surgery and what was done.

Will I still be able to conceive and carry a pregnancy?
Your doctor can tell you about the condition of your female organs. He can only guess as to your chances for future pregnancies.

What are my chances of the same thing happening again?
Tubal pregnancy recurs in the opposite tube in 8% of all women. The incidence after microsurgical repair following a tubal pregnancy depends on the damage to the tube and the technique used in its repair.

How was my tube on the opposite side? Normal?
You want to know if your other tube appears to be normal in case you desire future pregnancies.

Did my ovaries appear normal?
Ask about cysts, endometrial implants, evidence of chronic infection and any other problems.

Did my appendix appear normal?
Your doctor can inspect your appendix while your abdomen is open.

Did my gallbladder appear normal?
Ask if it contains stones. They would not be removed at this time, but in case you have symptoms of gallbladder pain, it would be beneficial to know.

Were there any other abnormalities you found at surgery? Any adhesions?
Your doctor should tell you of any abnormalities he finds.

Are there any special precautions to take following this surgery?
In general, there are no special precautions, but be aware that you have an 8% chance of ectopic pregnancy in the opposite tube. Give yourself time to heal, perhaps a month, before you return to normal activities, lifting, sports and anything else that is strenuous.

How soon may I begin to think of pregnancy again?
Your doctor may have special reasons, but wait until you regain your strength. Most doctors suggest waiting for 3 months.

How soon may I resume sexual intercourse?
Wait until after you have had your checkup a month after surgery.

Will I have any bowel or bladder problems?
As soon as you are eating normally, your bladder and bowel functions should return to normal.

Will I need to take iron or other medication after I get home?
Your doctor will check your blood and give you iron if you need it.

How soon can I douche?
There is no danger in douching at any time after surgery for ectopic pregnancy, unless a D&C has been done as part of your surgery. Ask your doctor about douching.

Is it all right to take an enema if I can't have a bowel movement? Laxatives?
Take an enema if you feel you need one. If you drink sufficient amounts of water and fruit juices, you shouldn't need an enema or laxatives.

When should I return to have my stitches removed?
Stitches are often removed in 5 days, before you leave the hospital. Otherwise, your doctor will tell you when to return.

Do I have Rh-negative blood? If so, do I need RhoGam?
Whether it is a tubal pregnancy, a miscarriage or a normal pregnancy with an Rh-positive baby, you probably will need RhoGam if your blood is Rh-negative. Ask your doctor.

Surgery for Endometriosis

DEFINITION OF ENDOMETRIOSIS

The tissue lining the uterine cavity is called *endometrium;* when this tissue is found in a place other than the lining of the uterus, the condition is called *endometriosis.* Endometrium is the tissue that, through hormonal stimulation, prepares each month to receive and nourish a fertilized egg. When fertilization does not take place, superficial layers are sloughed away (plus some blood) as your menstrual flow.

In some cases, endometrium can become misplaced, which we cover in this section. Misplaced endometrium continues to function as endometrium regardless of where it is located because it continues to respond to hormones as though it were inside the uterus. It may cause symptoms severe enough to require surgery to remove it, or it may cause infertility. Although benign, endometrium spreads locally and distantly, infiltrating and even crowding out normal tissue.

The phrase "endometriosis" was first coined by Dr. John Sampson in 1922, but the disease has been around for a long time.

ABBREVIATIONS AND OTHER NAMES

Endometrioma, chocolate cyst, tar cyst, mulberry spots, even "powder-burn lesion" are terms for endometriosis. *Internal endometriosis* (now called *adenomyosis)* is limited to infiltration of your uterine wall. *External endometriosis* encompasses all other locations of the tissue and is called *endometriosis.*

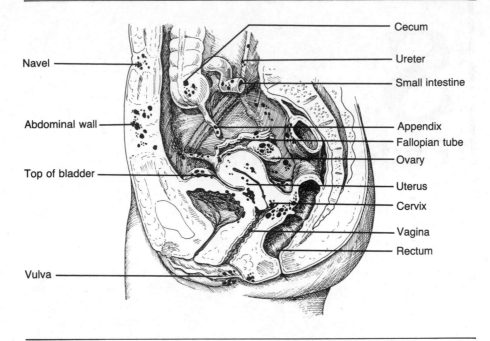

Navel

Abdominal wall

Top of bladder

Vulva

Cecum

Ureter

Small intestine

Appendix

Fallopian tube

Ovary

Uterus

Cervix

Vagina

Rectum

Sites of implantation of endometrium in endometriosis. Implants can occur almost anywhere.

PARTS OF BODY INVOLVED

Endometriosis most often spreads to the ovary, uterus, peritoneum and Fallopian tubes. Occasionally it spreads as far as the lungs, arms or legs. See illustration above.

OVARY

The most common site of endometriosis is the ovaries, and it usually involves both of them. You may have only tiny powder-burn lesions (named because they look like brown spots), or the misplaced endometrium may gradually form cysts called *endometriomas* or *chocolate cysts* of the ovaries. These cysts are full of old blood that has a chocolate appearance. One of the first signs of endometriosis may be an endometrial cyst in the ovary that is discovered during a routine pelvic examination.

UTERUS

The next most common site for endometrial implants is the back surface of the uterus, adjacent to the rectum, that extends along the utero-sacral ligaments (supporting ligaments behind the uterus). These implants often form small nodules that your doctor can feel during a pelvic exam and are very tender. It is not uncommon to have pain in this area with a bowel movement or with intercourse. Pain with intercourse is called *dyspareunia.*

PERITONEUM

The shiny membrane that lines the entire abdominal cavity and the outside of most abdominal and pelvic organs is called *peritoneum*. In the pelvic area, this membrane is frequently dotted with endometrial implants that cause pain and may cause adhesions.

FALLOPIAN TUBES

Whether the implants are large or small, they can cause distortion and impaired function in the Fallopian tubes. This can result in infertility or, if pregnancy occurs, a tubal pregnancy. Whether located in the tube or any other organ, pain seems to be characteristic of endometriosis.

OTHER LESS COMMON AREAS FOR ENDOMETRIAL IMPLANTS

Bowel (appendix, small and large intestine), bladder, ureter, cervix, vagina, navel, old scars, lungs, diaphragm and even arms and legs, although rare, have been recorded as sites for endometriosis.

CAUSES OF ENDOMETRIOSIS

There are many theories about what causes endometriosis, but we don't really know its cause. Dr. Sampson, who named the condition, thought the menstrual flow regurgitated backward through the Fallopian tubes and spilled into the peritoneal cavity. There, some endometrial tissue became implanted on the ovaries, the back of the uterus or some other surface. No one has ever observed the actual implantation to be sure of its origin.

COMMON REASONS FOR SURGERY FOR ENDOMETRIOSIS

The only way to diagnose endometriosis is to "see" it and biopsy it. However, there are typical symptoms that make your doctor *suspect* you have it.

PELVIC PAIN

This is the most common symptom and is found in 60 to 80% of all patients. This is the symptom that causes you to see your doctor and insist on relief. Characteristically, the amount of pain has little to do with the extent of the endometriosis. Tiny implants can cause severe pain, yet extensive endometriosis, including endometrial cysts (endometriomas), may cause no symptoms.

Usually, the pain becomes more severe with the onset of menstruation and disappears as the menstrual period ends. Pain may begin as a slightly more painful menstrual period, gradually increasing until your pain is constant and severe the entire month.

PAINFUL INTERCOURSE

Pain during intercourse may be the first sign that something is wrong. This symptom is also progressive and reaches the point that either you or your partner insists on medical examination and relief.

Dyspareunia (pain with intercourse) may be more severe just before the onset of your period and is likely to be more severe if the implants are on your ovaries or the back of your uterus. They are disturbed by the thrusting of your partner's penis during lovemaking.

If your primary problem is painful intercourse, your doctor may search for tiny nodules that he can feel behind your uterus. These nodules are suspicious of endometriosis.

PAINFUL BOWEL MOVEMENT

When endometriosis is located close to the rectum, you may have pain when passing a bowel movement. Physical findings are much the same as with dyspareunia. Small nodules of endometrial implants are located behind the uterus and can be felt by your doctor on rectovaginal examination.

We don't know why endometriosis causes so much pain, but many believe there may be an increased amount of the hormone prostaglandin, which is known to cause menstrual pain. Endometriosis may be relieved in many instances by an anti-prostaglandin that blocks the action of the prostaglandin.

HEAVY UTERINE BLEEDING

There is at least 30% chance of heavy bleeding if you have endometriosis. It may be heavy bleeding with your period or between periods. Or you may have irregular bleeding. Endometriosis may cause bleeding because it often affects the ovaries. It may interfere with your ovarian function, or it could interfere with your ovary's relationship with your pituitary gland.

A normal menstrual period results from a delicate balance between your pituitary gland, ovary and uterine lining. Any upset in these organs, such as endometriosis, can cause a change in menstrual flow. In this case, it causes heavier flow.

INABILITY TO BECOME PREGNANT

Infertility is one of the more distressing symptoms of endometriosis. This condition is more common in women who delay or defer pregnancy, so it is often difficult to know whether it causes infertility or infertility causes it. Some medical experts estimate that at least 30% of all women with endometriosis are infertile. It appears that if you defer pregnancy until your 30s, you are more likely to develop endometriosis.

Just how endometriosis causes infertility is unknown. You may have only a bit of endometriosis but be infertile. Extensive endometriosis may cause distortion of your tubes and destruction of large segments of your ovaries, yet have no negative effect on your ability to conceive. Endometriosis will not harm a pregnancy, unless tubes are blocked and an ectopic pregnancy occurs.

UNUSUAL SYMPTOMS

Painful blue areas in scars after abdominal surgery appear rarely and may be due to endometrial implants within the scars. Rarely, the symptom of coughing up blood accompanies your menstrual cycle. This may occur if you have endometriosis in your lungs.

HOW COMMON IS SURGERY FOR ENDOMETRIOSIS?

Endometriosis is not a new disease. In 1600 B.C., Egyptian records describe a condition typical of endometriosis. Modern medical history has recognized this disease for over 100 years.

Although it is found routinely in 30% of all women who have major surgery, the incidence of endometriosis might be higher because it could be microscopic in size and easily be missed unless your doctor and the pathologist are looking for it. Endometriosis is more common in women 25 to 40 years of age, but because symptoms are not always related to the extent of the disease, it is difficult to definitely diagnose.

Endometriosis has been called the "career woman's curse" because it occurs more often in women who defer their childbearing until later in life. It is rarely found in women under 20 years old. Endometriosis does not occur before periods start, but it has been found in teenagers. Although it is commonly associated with infertility, it is found in fertile and infertile women.

Pregnancy seems to suppress endometriosis and temporarily halt its progression, yet endometriosis can keep you from becoming pregnant. It is believed years of menstruation without pregnancy encourage the development and progression of endometriosis.

FUNCTIONS INVOLVED IN SURGERY FOR ENDOMETRIOSIS

The endometrium is a dynamic, constantly changing tissue that becomes the final target of the entire menstrual cycle. The many changes in the endometrium begin in the brain, with hormones from the pituitary gland stimulating the ovary, which stimulates the development and preparation of the endometrium. These hormonal changes have the ultimate goal of preparing your endometrium for pregnancy.

Any interruption in this process interferes with conception and your ability to conceive. It is not known how, but endometriosis upsets the cycle enough to cause infertility in many instances. The exact reason for infertility isn't known, but there are many theories, and it may be a combination of many factors.

Endometrial tissue is benign, and its menstruallike change each month provokes many symptoms of endometriosis. Part of the endometrial tissue, along with some blood, forms a menstruum (the menstrual flow). It can't escape as it does when it lines the uterine cavity, so the menstruum accumulates, forms cysts and causes irritation, adhesions and pain.

HOW SURGERY FOR ENDOMETRIOSIS IS PERFORMED

Endometriosis is not life-threatening. Because symptoms vary from none at all to those that are almost disabling, each situation must be evaluated individually. If the diagnosis of endometriosis is made, discuss the condition with your doctor. Keep in mind endometriosis is not malignant and doesn't have to be treated just because it exists.

If it causes sufficient pain, heavy bleeding or keeps you from becoming pregnant, it might have to be treated. If you're young, it is important to preserve your childbearing ability. But frequently anything short of a complete hysterectomy and removal of your uterus, tubes and ovaries will not cure the condition. It will merely relieve the symptoms temporarily, perhaps long enough for you to have a family.

If you're fortunate enough to conceive, in spite of endometriosis, you'll find pregnancy suppresses the disease, and you'll have fewer symptoms after each pregnancy. If you're close to menopause, you may want to defer any treatment. Menopause usually puts an end to endometriosis and its symptoms.

There are many methods of treatment for endometriosis. Every attempt is made to relieve symptoms with pain relievers, assurance and pregnancy, if this is your goal.

Hormonal therapy for the condition is *very* expensive and costs about $150 each month! Danazol is the treatment of choice in most cases, however less-expensive therapies include the use of birth-control pills or progesterone.

LAPAROSCOPY

Laparoscopy is very useful in diagnosing and treating endometriosis. Endometriosis is not life-threatening, so you may be observed for a while. But if pain is severe or infertility is a problem, the cause should be determined by laparoscopy and biopsy. The treatment chosen depends on your desire for pregnancy and the extent of your disease. For more information on laparoscopy, see information beginning on page 237. In addition to diagnosis, laparoscopy may be the method of treatment and evaluation after treatment.

With increased use of laparoscopy, more extensive procedures are being used to cauterize, cut and evaluate the endometrial implants and adhesions.

CONSERVATIVE SURGERY (LAPAROTOMY)

Conservative surgery means removing endometrial implants when possible without removing pelvic organs. With this method, your doctor tries to preserve your female organs and your childbearing ability.

The incision for conservative surgery is a 3- to 4-inch hairline (bikini) incision. The doctor inspects your pelvic organs to determine the extent of endometriosis and looks for adhesions or any other abnormalities of your pelvis.

Adhesions may have to be cut to inspect your pelvic organs. Next, the sites of endometriosis are destroyed by cutting with a knife, cautery or laser beam.

If you have chocolate cysts on your ovaries, the cysts will be removed. Every effort is made to preserve the function of your ovaries. The same care is exerted to preserve your Fallopian tubes so they will function as normally as possible.

If adhesions bind your uterus backward into the pelvis, your uterus may have to be suspended in the forward (normal) position to prevent formation of more adhesions that pull it backward. In the process of removing a chocolate cyst, if your ovary is found to be too badly involved, it may have to be removed.

In general, even conservative surgery is reserved until medical treatment of endometriosis has failed. If you can't tolerate medication to relieve symptoms of endometriosis, conservative surgery will be tried.

RADICAL SURGERY

If your pelvic organs are too involved with endometriosis to save them — especially if symptoms of pain and bleeding have been severe — your doctor may believe all your pelvic organs must be removed to give you relief. Discuss this possibility together before surgery! It would be foolish to leave diseased organs in your pelvis, especially if they cause you serious problems.

If your ovaries are removed at surgery, you probably will have no more pain. Removal of your uterus or both ovaries also takes care of bleeding problems.

You may wonder why one ovary could not be left so you would still have a chance to conceive and not go through a surgical menopause when both ovaries are removed. As long as there is hormonal stimulation from one ovary, endometrial implants, even though microscopic, can cause pain.

LASER

One of the newest methods of treating endometriosis is by laser. Laser is an acronym for "light amplification by stimulated emission of radiation," and it is being used in almost every branch of medicine. Although medical use of lasers is being practiced in many parts of the country, there are still many areas in which it is not available. Doctors must be specially trained to used it.

Laser has many advantages, especially in the treatment of endometriosis. The laser beam is a high-energy light that can be directed and controlled with pinpoint accuracy of location and depth. The energy of the beam is absorbed by water in the cells, which causes them to vaporize. See illustration on page 212.

Endometriosis is usually located on the surface of the organs it affects. It can be destroyed easily, accurately and safely with a laser. Only the endometrial implant is destroyed, leaving normal tissue almost untouched.

Healing after laser surgery is rapid. Laser surgery has been adapted for use with laparoscopy or laparotomy, and its use may replace cautery (burning tissue by passage of an electrical current through tissue between two electrodes). We are still learning about the laser and its applications in various fields of medicine.

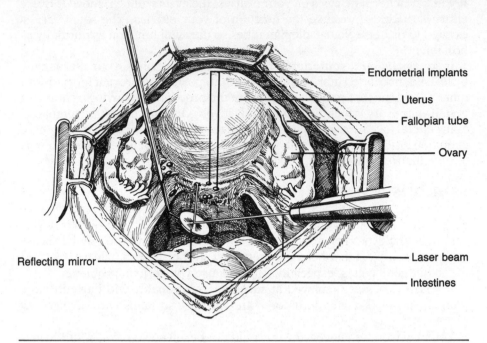

Endometrial implants

Uterus

Fallopian tube

Ovary

Reflecting mirror

Laser beam

Intestines

Vaporization of endometrial implants with laser beam, which can be focused accurately to destroy endometriosis.

SURGERY AND HORMONE TREATMENT

Occasionally a combination of conservative therapy (preservation of organs) and hormone therapy relieves symptoms enough to allow you to become pregnant. Pregnancy often relieves the symptoms of endometriosis, although relief is usually temporary.

Surgery removes most of the implants, then birth-control pills or danazol cause them to shrink further. If you desire a pregnancy, try immediately after completing the treatment because your fertility is increased for a short time afterward. Pregnancy is most likely to occur within 12 months of treatment.

RISKS OF SURGERY FOR ENDOMETRIOSIS

Risks of surgery depend on the extent of the endometriosis, the number of adhesions and their thickness, and whether other organs besides pelvic organs are involved. In addition to the usual risks of general anesthesia, the chance of bowel obstruction following surgery for extensive endometriosis can be significant. The risk of damage to ureters is also greater with endometriosis surgery.

Even laparoscopy carries some risk because of the presence of adhesions. Adhesions prevent proper inspection of the organs; there is more danger of perforation of other organs while attempting laparoscopy in the presence of adhesions.

When an adhesion is separated at surgery, you're left with two raw areas instead of the adhesion. This provides twice as much chance to form additional adhesions. Part of the surgery is to cover these raw areas to prevent adhesion formation. Medications, such as antibiotics, also are used to prevent formation of adhesions.

There is a small risk of burn injury to your bowel, bladder or other organs when implants are cauterized, but careful use of cautery usually avoids this complication. Risk also depends on your general health, state of nutrition, your ability to heal, your weight and your alcohol, tobacco and drug consumption.

ADVANTAGES OF SURGERY FOR ENDOMETRIOSIS

Surgery can remove most of the endometriosis, so it may relieve your pain and bleeding and may restore your fertility. If the medication does not relieve pain, bleeding or infertility, you may find surgery gives you the relief you desire. Bowel obstruction from adhesions is also a threat if endometriosis is severe and *not* operated on.

DISADVANTAGES OF SURGERY FOR ENDOMETRIOSIS

Besides the risks of major surgery, there are other disadvantages to surgery for endometriosis. You may develop more adhesions and experience more pain after surgery than you had before, but this is unlikely.

Surgery may restore fertility, but it can also increase infertility because it tends to form adhesions after surgery. Even conservative surgery may decrease your fertility, depending on the way you heal inside.

Removal of all pelvic organs may relieve distressing, disabling symptoms of endometriosis, but it can also cause depression and a sense of loss of femininity. This is something you must consider. All these disabling symptoms must be weighed carefully against your pain, bleeding, dyspareunia and infertility. Discuss it thoroughly with your doctor before surgery.

WHO OPERATES?

Endometriosis may be extensive, even with minor symptoms, and it may affect your ability to conceive. You may want to consult a specialist about your problem. Even laparoscopy should be performed only by someone skilled in this procedure because of the possibility and increased risk of adhesions.

If laser treatment is available in your community, ask your doctor about this treatment.

DIAGNOSTIC TESTS BEFORE, DURING AND AFTER SURGERY FOR ENDOMETRIOSIS

If you're considering surgery for endometriosis, the most important test may be a biopsy of the lesions performed by laparoscopy. This is the only way you can be sure you have endometriosis. It would cause needless pain and suffering to subject yourself to major surgery without a definite diagnosis if the disease can be confirmed easily by laparoscopy. Sometimes malignancy, adhesions or no abnormalities are found. You can avoid unnecessary surgery or the wrong type of treatment by having laparoscopy first.

Routine tests, such as urinalysis, complete blood count and any other tests your doctor orders, should be performed *before* surgery.

Ultrasound is being used as techniques improve. It sometimes shows chocolate cysts of the ovaries, and it can also monitor shrinkage of certain implants of endometriosis due to hormone treatment.

Following surgery, your blood will be checked to see if it is normal or if you need iron. Your doctor will also want to know how much relief you obtain from symptoms following surgery.

WHERE IS SURGERY PERFORMED?

LAPAROSCOPY

This is an outpatient procedure and does not require admission to the hospital. You go to the outpatient department early in the morning after fasting since midnight, spend 30 to 90 minutes in surgery, then remain in recovery for another 40 to 60 minutes or until you are awake.

You are carefully checked until you can walk around and you feel reasonably well. When your vital signs (blood pressure, temperature and respiration) are normal, you'll be released to go home. It's usually unnecessary to take any pain medicine after laparoscopy.

LAPAROTOMY

Laparotomy requires admission to the hospital the night before or the morning of surgery. Uncomplicated surgery requires about 1-1/2 hours. Adhesions on Fallopian tubes or ovaries can prolong surgery time by many hours.

An hour or so in recovery allows stabilization of your blood pressure and pulse so you can be returned to your room. The average hospital stay is 4 to 7 days.

HOSPITALIZATION AND DURATION

Hospitalization will vary depending on the extent of your surgery. Laparoscopy is an outpatient procedure. You will be operated on in the outpatient surgery department, recover and go home the same day.

Laparotomy is major surgery and requires more time to recover. You will be in the hospital 4 to 7 days. Recovery at home can take 4 to 6 weeks.

ANESTHESIA

Laparoscopy is usually performed under general anesthesia, although under some circumstances, physicians may choose to use local anesthesia for this procedure. Spinal and epidural anesthesia are seldom used and only in special circumstances.

Laparotomy requires general, spinal or epidural anesthesia. See pages 18 to 21 for more information on these types of anesthesia.

PROBABLE OUTCOME OF SURGERY FOR ENDOMETRIOSIS

Endometriosis can be a difficult problem to resolve, even for the most skilled surgeon. Extensive adhesions may have impaired function of any or all pelvic organs and your bowel or bladder. If you are young and anxious to overcome infertility, the challenge for your doctor is even greater.

But if you have suffered a long time from pain, bleeding or dyspareunia, with or without infertility, you may welcome *any* relief. In general, relief is prompt, and the outcome of your surgery should be good.

POST-OPERATIVE CARE

LAPAROSCOPY

No special post-operative care is necessary after laparoscopy. You should be able to return to work or your regular activities the day after surgery. If you have laparoscopy performed in the outpatient department, have someone drive you home.

You'll probably rest for the remainder of the day after your surgery, but you should require only over-the-counter remedies for pain relief. Resume exercising gradually. Although you have only a small incision, check it daily for discharge, redness or tenderness. Return to your doctor to have stitches removed on the designated day.

LAPAROTOMY

After laparotomy, you'll be in the hospital 4 to 7 days, and your doctor will write orders regarding your diet, activity and medications. You will be up to go to the bathroom the day after surgery, walking up and down the hall by the second day and be home within a week.

Average recovery time is about 6 weeks, including return to work, resumption of intercourse and full exercising.

DIET

Before any surgery, you are asked to refrain from food and drink after midnight. This is suggested even for laparoscopy because there is always the possibility of complications and the possibility of general anesthesia.

Following major surgery, you'll receive intravenous fluids until you're able to sip enough water. Liquids are steadily increased until you can pass gas by yourself, which is evidence your bowel is beginning to function. Solid foods are added gradually until you are eating a full diet.

MISCONCEPTIONS ABOUT SURGERY FOR ENDOMETRIOSIS

Endometriosis is contagious or cancerous.
This is untrue. Endometriosis is not contagious or cancerous. It cannot be diagnosed by D&C. You can have severe endometriosis without symptoms, or a tiny amount can cause intense pain, dyspareunia, heavy uterine bleeding and infertility. The cause of endometriosis is unknown, but it could come from implantation of bits of cast-off endometrium in menstrual fluid that flows in the opposite direction. These bits find their way out the ends of the Fallopian tubes and into the pelvic part of your abdominal cavity.

Endometriosis surgery requires a hysterectomy.
This is incorrect. Technology is helping conservative surgery (trying to preserve fertility and pelvic organs) so abnormal tissue is removed or destroyed while your uterus is retained.

ALTERNATIVES TO SURGERY FOR ENDOMETRIOSIS

The first alternative is to wait, watch, observe and evaluate your condition to see if anything must be done. If your symptoms persist and become severe, then the diagnosis must be established definitely by laparoscopy.

Most authorities believe that medical treatment should not begin without laparoscopic diagnosis. If treatment is begun before definite confirmation by laparoscopy, it should be limited to mild pain relievers or birth-control pills when symptoms are not severe and endometriosis is suspected. Danazol is effective to relieve endometriosis symptoms, but it is very expensive. It may cause your voice to deepen and cause hair to grow on your face. But danazol is of great value if you are young and anxious to have children.

Other than laparoscopy, surgical treatment of endometriosis is reserved for those cases in which symptoms are severe and unrelieved by medical means.

HORMONE TREATMENT
Diagnosis of endometriosis should be confirmed by laparoscopy. In general, there are two ways to treat endometriosis with hormones.
Birth-Control Pills—Birth-control pills suppress ovulation. Ordinarily if you don't ovulate, you don't have as severe menstrual pain or pain from endometriosis.

Unfortunately, birth-control pills don't always relieve the pain of endometriosis. You may want to conceive, and you can't conceive while taking birth-control pills. However, if you take birth-control pills for 6 months, you may suppress the endometriosis enough so pregnancy can occur. Your pregnancy may further suppress your endometriosis, giving you considerable relief, but this is usually only temporary.

Danazol — Danazol blocks the production of hormones by the pituitary gland, which in turn prevents the ovaries from being stimulated to produce hormones. These hormones from the ovary act on the endometrium. Danazol interrupts the cycle that produces the pain of endometriosis.

Danazol is especially indicated in younger women who require relief from symptoms and want their endometriosis suppressed to become pregnant. Unfortunately, danazol has some unpleasant side-effects.

One side-effect is masculinization. Although this is temporary, no woman wants a deeper voice or hair growth in unwanted areas. Never subject yourself to these effects unless the diagnosis of endometriosis had been definitely confirmed by laparoscopy.

Another drawback of danazol is that it is very expensive. It can cost as much as $150 or more a month.

CALL YOUR DOCTOR IF . . .

1. You have chills or fever.
2. Your incision becomes red, inflamed or it drains.
3. You have severe abdominal pain.
4. You have side effects from your medication.
5. You have any other symptoms or signs that seem abnormal to you.

QUESTIONS TO ASK YOUR DOCTOR

What did you find at surgery (laparoscopy or laparotomy)? What did you do at surgery? What did you remove?

Have your doctor use illustrations to show you where your endometriosis is and how much it has involved your pelvis and other organs.

Can I expect relief from pain, dyspareunia and heavy bleeding?

This depends on how extensive the involvement was and whether both ovaries were removed. If even a part of an ovary is left, it is possible you will still have discomfort with intercourse or any other symptoms you had because of the endometriosis.

What are my chances for pregnancy?

Most doctors allow their patients to conceive as soon as they feel well enough to have intercourse. Check with your doctor to see what his instructions are.

Will I need to take hormones?

If your ovaries are removed, you may expect to have hot flashes, some insomnia and maybe nervousness. When your ovaries are removed, hormone replacement (estrogen) can be used with only a small risk of growth of endometriosis again.

Hysterectomy

DEFINITION OF HYSTERECTOMY

Hysterectomy comes from two Greek words, *hystera,* meaning uterus or womb, and *ektome,* meaning to remove or cut out. *Hysterectomy* means to remove the uterus.

ABBREVIATIONS AND OTHER NAMES

Doctors often refer to the surgery as a "hyster," which is an abbreviation. Also TAH (total abdominal hysterectomy) or TVH (total vaginal hysterectomy) are common medical abbreviations for hysterectomy.

PARTS OF BODY INVOLVED

There are two parts of the uterus — a body (corpus) and a neck (cervix). The *cervix* is the part of the uterus that protrudes into the vagina and can be seen when your doctor looks into your vagina. It is from the opening of the cervix that your Pap smear is taken. The cervix stretches to permit your baby to pass from the uterus into the vagina in the process of birth.

The *body* of the uterus extends up into your abdominal cavity. In the lining of the cavity, tissue is prepared for implantation of a fertilized egg each month. When fertilization does not take place, the superficial layers of this lining are sloughed off and passed, along with some blood, as your menstrual period.

A fertilized egg implanted into this lining grows into a baby. The thick muscular wall of the uterus contracts during labor to produce an opening of the cervix so delivery of your baby can occur.

If only the body of the uterus is removed, it is called a *partial, subtotal* or *supra-cervical* hysterectomy. Usually the body and neck of the uterus are removed, and this is called a *total* hysterectomy. A total hysterectomy does not include removal of the ovaries. When the ovaries and Fallopian tubes are also removed, the procedure is called a *total hysterectomy with bilateral salpingo-oophorectomy.*

COMMON REASONS FOR HYSTERECTOMY

Although hysterectomy is a safe operation, deaths can occur — between 1 and 2 per 1,000 operations performed. Many deaths are due to anesthesia. It is estimated that over 900,000 hysterectomies were performed in 1985, with perhaps 1,800 deaths due to complications.

We suggest if you have any question about whether your surgery is necessary, insist on a second opinion. Many hospitals require this consultation before any major surgery can be performed.

Tissue or *chart-review* committees exist in most hospitals. Their responsibility is to make certain surgery is justified and the reasons for performing it are vindicated by the findings at surgery. These committees take their assignment seriously and conscientiously police their colleagues.

Some smaller hospitals are not so well-controlled, and unnecessary surgery may be performed. Statistics about unnecessary surgery can be misleading because, although the uterus is normal, it is removed along with diseased ovaries or Fallopian tubes, when a fallen bladder or rectum is repaired or when the uterus itself has fallen. If only the tissue removed at surgery was considered, rather than all the *reasons* for surgery, many hysterectomies would be wrongfully classified as unnecessary. Below are some common reasons for performing a hysterectomy.

FIBROID TUMORS

Fibroid tumors are not fibrous but originate in the muscle of the uterine wall. The correct term is *myoma* (short for leiomyoma) or *muscle tumor.* See illustration on page 220. Uterine myomas are the most frequent tumors found in the female pelvis. By the age of 50, nearly 40% of all women have a fibroid of some kind if they still have their uterus.

If you have myoma, it will probably become smaller after menopause. If you develop one fibroid, it's likely you'll develop others because these tumors are usually multiple.

A myoma is basically not cancerous; less than 1% become malignant. If they're benign, you may wonder why they figure so prominently as a cause for hysterectomy.

First, fibroids can be large or small, and they can be located anywhere in, or protruding from, the uterus. They may be large enough to exert pressure on your bladder or bowel. They may prevent the descent of your baby for delivery. Some may protrude into the cavity of your uterus and produce heavy menstrual bleeding, or they can hang by a cord and become twisted, cutting off their own blood supply and causing severe pain and possibly gangrene.

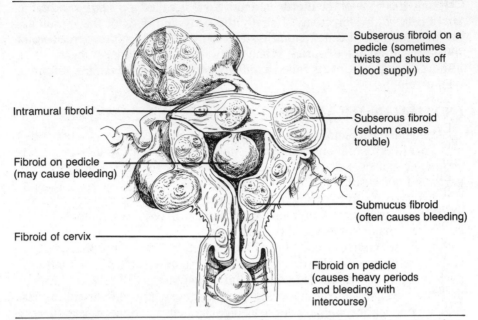

Subserous fibroid on a pedicle (sometimes twists and shuts off blood supply)

Intramural fibroid

Subserous fibroid (seldom causes trouble)

Fibroid on pedicle (may cause bleeding)

Submucus fibroid (often causes bleeding)

Fibroid of cervix

Fibroid on pedicle (causes heavy periods and bleeding with intercourse)

There are many locations for fibroid tumors of the uterus. Size and location often determine symptoms.

Fibroids in the uterus can cause increased bleeding, pain or pressure.

If a myoma on a stem or stalk lies inside the uterine cavity, it can cause bleeding between menstrual periods. This problem requires cancer be ruled out. If the tumor protrudes into the peritoneal cavity, it may become twisted because of intestinal motion. If twisting is severe enough, it shuts off the blood supply, causing gangrene or excruciating pain, correctable only by surgery.

Do all myomas require a hysterectomy? No. It is important not to operate on myoma unless necessary, especially in the childbearing age. If tumors are removed from the uterus, the incision into the uterine wall weakens it and makes it prone to rupture during labor. Cesarean delivery would probably be necessary. When symptoms demand surgery, only the fibroid is removed rather than the uterus, in case you desire more children. But the incision in the uterus for the myomectomy leaves your uterus more prone to rupture during labor.

Uterine myomas are not removed unless they cause such pain, pressure or bleeding that you demand something be done. Typically, fibroid tumors become larger during pregnancy (possibly due to hormonal influence) and decrease in size after pregnancy. Rapid increase in size, other than during pregnancy and after menopause, causes your doctor to suspect malignant degeneration of the fibroid, in which case immediate removal by hysterectomy is necessary to rule out cancer.

Some studies indicate that up to 30% of all hysterectomies may be due to fibroid tumors.

CHRONIC VAGINAL BLEEDING

Approximately 10% of all hysterectomies are performed for chronic vaginal bleeding that does not respond to medical treatment. One cause of bleeding is endometrial hyperplasia; see illustration below. Hysterectomy may be the final treatment when bleeding does not respond to hormone therapy or repeated D&Cs.

ENDOMETRIOSIS

Endometriosis is a condition in which endometrial tissue is located in areas where it should not be, such as the ovaries, Fallopian tubes, bladder, bowel or lining of the abdominal cavity. See illustration on page 222.

Endometrial tissue responds to ovarian hormones, regardless of where the endometriosis is located. It sheds blood and tissue each month, called *menstruum,* which produces irritation, inflammation, blood-filled cysts and adhesions. Endometriosis causes pain and often increased menstrual flow, and it may cause painful intercourse.

When any symptom, due to endometriosis, becomes severe enough that medicines (danazol, birth-control pills or analgesics) does not relieve it, hysterectomy may become necessary.

It's possible to operate and destroy endometrial implants by laser, cautery or surgical removal *without* hysterectomy. This treatment is often temporary and incomplete, and it is reserved for those women who desire additional pregnancies or those who have a record of infertility.

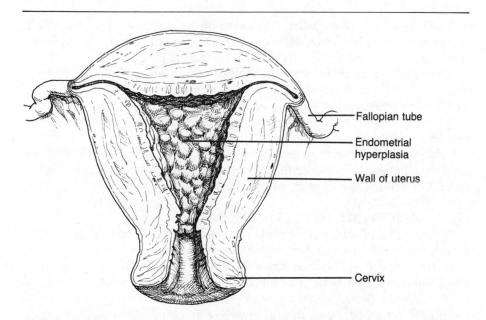

Fallopian tube

Endometrial hyperplasia

Wall of uterus

Cervix

Endometrial hyperplasia is an overgrowth of the lining of the uterus and may be corrected by hysterectomy.

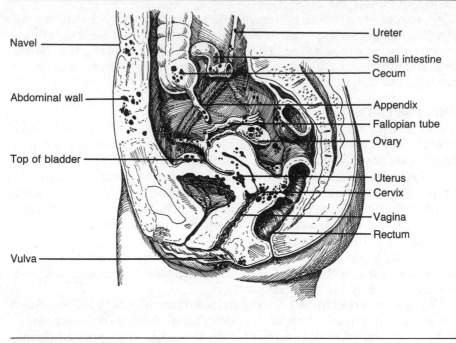

Navel

Abdominal wall

Top of bladder

Vulva

Ureter

Small intestine

Cecum

Appendix

Fallopian tube

Ovary

Uterus

Cervix

Vagina

Rectum

Sites of endometrial implants.

Endometriosis is often called "the curse of the career woman" because it occurs more often in women who defer pregnancy until later in life. Endometriosis may cause infertility but is lessened during pregnancy.

When endometriosis invades the wall of the uterus, it is called *internal endometriosis* or *adenomyosis*. Signs and symptoms are similar to endometriosis in other areas, except your uterus is often enlarged and tender. If danazol fails to relieve pain, hysterectomy may be indicated. The diagnosis of adenomyosis can only be confirmed by hysterectomy.

Because of adhesions from endometriosis, hysterectomy is usually through an abdominal incision, rather than a vaginal incision. For more information on endometriosis, see the section that begins on page 205.

LACK OF SUPPORT TO PELVIC ORGANS

Perhaps 25% of all hysterectomies are done because of loss of uterine, bladder or bowel support. Although a woman may inherit pelvic tissue with poor tone, the most common cause of loss of support in these organs is childbirth. Severity may be in direct proportion to the number of children you have delivered. See illustrations on opposite page.

Chronic coughing, often due to cigarette smoking, or sneezing, due to allergies, increase loss of support and increase symptoms. With a prolapsed uterus, you may have a feeling of "things falling out." If you have a *rectocele* (hernia or rupture of the rectum into the back wall of the vagina), you may

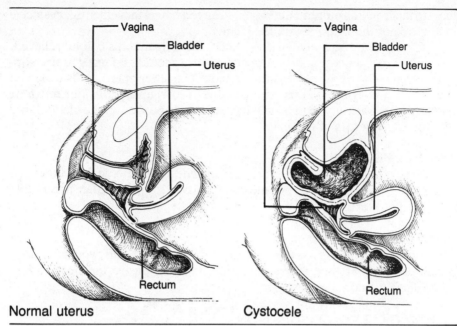

Normal uterus

Cystocele

Normal uterus, bladder and rectum with good support. Cystocele is hernia of bladder into vagina.

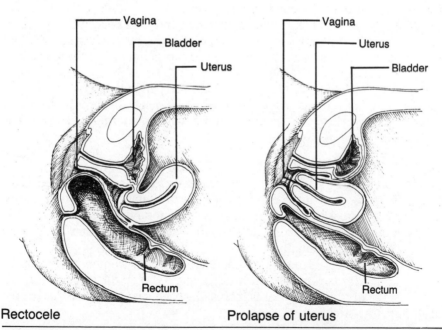

Rectocele

Prolapse of uterus

Rectocele is hernia of rectum into the vagina. Beginning prolapse of uterus. Uterus begins to descend into vagina. You may feel as though "things are falling out."

have to push on this bulge in the vagina to have a bowel movement. A *cystocele* is a hernia of the bladder into the vagina.

Unfortunately many women don't know these symptoms can be relieved. But failure to remove a poorly supported uterus could endanger future support of your bladder or rectum after repair. The latter operation is called an *A&P repair* (anterior and posterior colpoperineorrhaphy), *bladder repair* or *rectal repair*. With any kind of activity, the uterus pushes on the bladder and rectum, causing loss of urine.

PAINFUL PERIODS

Severe, intractable menstrual cramps, unrelieved by medical treatment (if you do not desire more pregnancies) may occasionally be an acceptable reason for hysterectomy.

STERILIZATION

About 9% of all hysterectomies are for sterilization. Usually you have other conditions present that, when combined with the desire for sterilization, probably justify the hysterectomy.

CHRONIC PELVIC CONGESTION

A condition that occasionally demands hysterectomy is chronic pelvic congestion. This condition is similar to varicose veins of your pelvis. Persistent aching in your pelvis, along with severe, nagging back pain and painful intercourse, are the most common symptoms.

This diagnosis has received much criticism and is not accepted by everyone. It has been refuted by some but supported by others. The diagnosis can be made only with surgery, laparoscopy or laparotomy, but there are still those who disclaim the diagnosis.

Only when you have extreme pain from chronic pelvic congestion, in spite of medication, is a hysterectomy considered. As a general rule, it's unwise to perform major surgery to relieve a symptom when no definite diagnosis has been made.

CANCER OF THE BODY OF THE UTERUS

Cancer of the body of the uterus is also called *endometrial cancer* because it almost always occurs in the endometrium of the cavity of your uterus. See illustration on opposite page. It is the most common type of cancer of female organs. It develops in about 28,000 women each year and claims the lives of about 4,000 women annually.

It's estimated that of the approximately 50 million women in the United States who are 35 years of age and older, about 700,000 will develop endometrial cancer. This type of cancer is increasing each year but when discovered early, it can be *cured!*

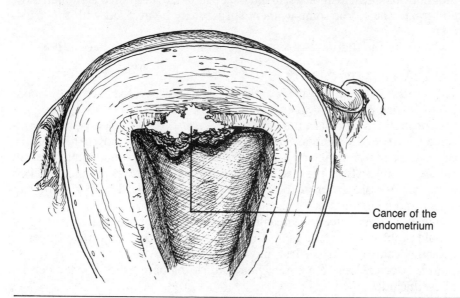

Cancer of the
endometrium

Cancer of the endometrium is cancer of the lining of the uterine cavity, commonly called *cancer of the uterus.*

Studies have shown the following groups are more likely to develop endometrial cancer:
- women with no children or few children.
- women who are obese, have diabetes or high blood pressure.
- women who experienced late onset of menstruation.
- women who have a history of skipping periods, irregular bleeding or polyps in the uterus.
- women who have a family history of cancer of the endometrium.
- women who have had a series of D&Cs for abnormal bleeding.
- women who have taken estrogens to relieve menopausal symptoms.

There are some things you can do to help detect cancer of the endometrium early and increase your chances for cure if you develop it. Report any *unusual* bleeding, excessive periods or spotting between periods to your doctor. Report any bleeding after menopause immediately!

Take female hormones *only* under the supervision of your doctor. See your doctor regularly — at least once a year — for a physical that includes a pelvic examination, breast exam and Pap smear.

There is a precancerous condition, called *adenomatous hyperplasia,* that often accompanies estrogen medication. It may or may not cause abnormal bleeding. Your doctor will follow this condition carefully; it may result in cancer. It is easily cured if detected early. The diagnosis of adenomatous hyperplasia is a red flag that sounds a timely, life-saving warning for you. Hysterectomy is not always necessary for this type of precancerous condition — a D&C frequently cures it. This also may be treated with hormones in a cyclical fashion for 10 days each month to help shed endometrial or abnormal tissue. For some women, surgery can be avoided with this treatment.

Cancer of the uterus is discussed in detail beginning on page 121.

CANCER OF THE CERVIX

About 20,000 cases of cancer of the cervix are discovered each year. About 7,500 women die each year of this disease.

Cancer of the cervix is a *preventable disease!* Since Dr. George N. Papanicolaou developed his famous Pap test, we have discovered most cancers of the cervix are slow-growing and can usually be detected early enough to prevent spread and death from the disease. In fact, over 40,000 cases of cancer limited to the surface of the cervix, before spread, are diagnosed each year by Pap smear and confirmed by biopsy.

Cancer of the cervix is decreasing in frequency, but it is still a prominent female problem. An annual Pap smear can greatly increase your chances of detecting cancer in its earliest, most curable stages.

Some women have a greater chance of developing cancer of the cervix. These include:

- women who begin sexual activity early in life.
- women who have multiple sexual encounters with many different male partners.
- women who have herpes infections or condyloma infections.
- women who have had several children.

There are no definite early symptoms that warn of cancer of the cervix, but any irregular or unusual spotting or bleeding after intercourse are suspect.

Cancer of the cervix is discussed in detail beginning on page 90.

Cancer-in-Situ — This cancer is limited to the superficial layer of your cervix. It has not spread or penetrated to the deeper layers of your cervix. The earliest type of cancer we can call cancer for certain, *cancer-in-situ,* is curable in nearly every instance.

Cancer-in-situ can be treated conservatively by local excision (called *conization),* by cryosurgery (freezing) or by laser if you are still in the childbearing age and desire more children. If you desire no more children, a hysterectomy will probably be performed.

Invasive Cancer of the Cervix — When cancer of your cervix begins to invade the tissue surrounding it, it demands *immediate* treatment. It is life-threatening, so you can't delay treatment even to wait for maturing of a pregnancy.

If invasion is confined to the cervix, treatment may consist of radiation therapy or surgery. If the cancer has progressed beyond your cervix, treatment is radiation only, and the outlook is less optimistic.

Any anticipated hysterectomy *must* be preceded by a Pap smear to rule out cancer of your cervix because a hysterectomy would remove the site where radium would be inserted to treat your cancer.

In certain cancers of the uterus, a radical hysterectomy is performed in which tissue adjacent to the cervix and body of your uterus, lymph nodes (to which the cancer spreads first) and the upper part of your vagina are removed in an effort to remove all the cancer.

CANCER OF THE OVARY

Cancer of the ovary has been called the *silent cancer* because it causes no bleeding and often gives no warning signs or symptoms until the disease has progressed. While it is true that ovaries produce vital female hormones that prevent menopausal symptoms, it is possible for you or your doctor to be overzealous about their preservation.

When hysterectomy is anticipated, you and your doctor must decide whether or not your ovaries will be removed. Weigh how many years your ovaries will serve you as a supplier of natural hormones versus the risk of cancer if ovaries are not removed.

If you are over 45, your doctor may recommend that your ovaries be removed. If you are under 40 and your ovaries are healthy, he will probably recommend they be left in place. If you're between 40 and 45, the decision is not so simple.

If hysterectomy is performed because of cancer of the body of the uterus or cancer of the cervix, ovaries may also be removed, but this varies and may not be necessary in younger women. If the procedure is done for a benign condition, such as endometriosis, your ovaries may also be removed because this may be the only way to guarantee relief of pain. If surgery is done because of lack of pelvic support or some other benign condition, your ovaries will probably be left in. Each case must be evaluated on its own merits. Your age and desire to retain your ovaries definitely influence this decision.

Unless the disease has progressed too far, treatment for cancer of the ovary is removal of tubes, ovaries (with as much tumor as possible) and uterus (complete hysterectomy), plus radiation and chemotherapy in most cases. Advanced cases may be treated only with chemotherapy or possibly chemotherapy and radiation therapy combined. Side effects with radiation have been found to be significant.

OTHER CANCERS OF FEMALE ORGANS
FOR WHICH HYSTERECTOMY IS PERFORMED

Cancer of the vagina and cancer of the Fallopian tubes are extremely rare but usually call for a hysterectomy as part of the treatment. Either condition may cause bleeding or a watery discharge from the vagina. Cancer of the Fallopian tubes, the rarest type of cancer of female organs, often causes abdominal pain.

HOW COMMON IS HYSTERECTOMY?

Over 900,000 hysterectomies are performed annually! As a female operation, it is surpassed in frequency only by biopsy, D&C and Cesarean operation.

FUNCTIONS INVOLVED IN HYSTERECTOMY

Hysterectomy removes the uterus, which houses a growing baby. It also means an end to menstrual periods and an end to your reproductive potential. For many women, this is a relief. Others feel they have been "desexed" and feel as if they have lost their femininity because they no longer can bear children. This feeling occurs even when they don't want any more children.

This vital function of childbearing is closely related to sexual feelings, so discuss your feelings frankly with your doctor *before any* surgery.

HOW HYSTERECTOMY IS PERFORMED

There are two principal methods to remove your uterus — through your abdomen and through your vagina.

ABDOMINAL HYSTERECTOMY

In an abdominal hysterectomy, the incision may be a vertical one, extending from your pubic bone to your navel, or a transverse one, which is confined within your pubic hairline. A *vertical incision* provides more room if your uterus is enlarged, if you have huge ovarian cysts or if you have had previous surgery (with possible adhesions) through a vertical incision.

A *transverse incision* provides better abdominal support with less chance of post-operative herniation of your wound. It is less obvious, and for this reason has been nicknamed a "bikini" incision.

If adhesions are anticipated (due to endometriosis, infection or previous surgery) or if your surgery is being done because of undiagnosed, but persistent, pelvic pain, an abdominal incision is preferred. It allows your doctor to explore your abdominal organs more easily and thoroughly.

Years ago, a vaginal hysterectomy was performed when urinary control had to be corrected. Modern surgical methods permit this condition to be corrected in many cases through an abdominal incision.

During surgery, pelvic and abdominal organs are carefully inspected. Blood vessels and ligaments that supply your ovaries and Fallopian tubes are identified, clamped, cut and securely tied with suture material. Meticulous dissection is continued on either side of your uterus, down to the blood vessels.

The bladder is dissected off the lower segment of uterus and upper vagina. Then an incision in your vagina is made. This amputates the uterus from your vagina but leaves the entire length of your vagina for future intercourse.

Behind the uterus are the uterosacral ligaments, which help support your uterus. They are sutured into the top of your vagina to give it additional support. The top of your vagina is closed, and the lining of the interior of the peritoneal cavity is used to cover the entire operative site. Closure of the abdominal wound in layers completes the operation.

Because of dissection close to your bladder, you may have difficulty passing urine for a few days. After filling your bladder with a saline solution to avoid discomfort, a tiny tube is inserted through your abdominal wall into the bladder to drain it as it fills. This tube drains your bladder until you are able to empty it by yourself through your urethra. The tube is then withdrawn, and the tiny hole heals by itself. If this method is not used, a tube (foley catheter) is placed through the urethra into the bladder for the same purpose.

VAGINAL HYSTERECTOMY

When hysterectomy includes repair of your bladder or rectum, the procedure is usually performed through your vagina. With the use of special instruments, your vagina can be stretched adequately to permit your doctor to remove your uterus, ovaries and Fallopian tubes and to perform needed surgery to repair your bladder and rectum.

Your uterus is removed by careful dissection, including clamping, cutting and tying blood vessels in the reverse order that is done in an abdominal hysterectomy. When removal of the uterus is complete, your bladder and rectum are repaired if necessary, and your vaginal hysterectomy is complete.

When a vaginal hysterectomy is planned, adhesions, large uterus, massive, undiagnosed ovarian tumors or other problems may require an abdominal approach to complete your surgery. The vaginal wound can be closed and an incision made in your abdominal wall to accomplish whatever needs to be done.

Your tubes and ovaries can also be removed through the vagina when necessary, but it may be more difficult. Some surgeons have been trained in vaginal surgery, while others prefer the abdominal route. There are advantages to both approaches. Ask your doctor to discuss these and give you his reasons for using the method he chooses for your case.

RISKS OF HYSTERECTOMY

The mortality rate in hysterectomy is about 2 in 1,000 operations. Surgery is performed in a hospital, where there are board-certified gynecologists, skilled anesthesiologists and blood banks. Some hysterectomies are emergencies and are performed where there is the greatest safety and supervision.

If your surgery is not an emergency, you may want to lose excessive weight, stop smoking, discontinue medication or build up your blood. Stressful situations may also need to be dealt with to improve the outlook for your postoperative recovery.

ADVANTAGES OF HYSTERECTOMY

One of the greatest advantages of hysterectomy is that it removes the site of some common cancers. If you have a hysterectomy, you shouldn't develop cancer of the cervix or cancer of the endometrium. These cancers carry considerable risk. If your ovaries are also removed, which is commonly done if you're over 45, the risk of ovarian cancer is also eliminated. A hysterectomy is not done only to remove the risk of cancer if there is none.

When your uterus is removed and ovaries are left intact, the only thing that changes in you is the lack of menstrual periods. If your uterus is removed but you still have your ovaries, you may continue to suffer from PMS (premenstrual syndrome).

You will eventually go through the change of life because you still have your ovaries. They continue to secrete their hormones, including estrogen. You may be 45 to 50 before you go through a normal menopause.

Another advantage to hysterectomy is that without your uterus, you may take estrogen without the risk of its causing cancer of the endometrium. There is no endometrium without a uterus.

DISADVANTAGES OF HYSTERECTOMY

Some women feel defeminized and castrated, even when their ovaries have not been removed. This feeling of "loss" can be very real and extremely distressing. Doctors should not ignore this possible aftereffect of hysterectomy. Some women feel so strongly about "keeping" their uterus that they are willing to put up with considerable discomfort.

A hysterectomy is a major operation and carries the same risk as any other major operation. There is the risk of anesthesia, infection, hemorrhage, shock, adhesions, bowel obstruction, separation of your incision, allergic responses to medication and the possibility you may have to take estrogen for a long time if your ovaries are removed.

WHO OPERATES?

This surgery is specialized and requires skill in surgery and gynecologic judgment. Hysterectomies should be performed by surgeons who have had special training and have a special interest in gynecologic problems.

DIAGNOSTIC TESTS BEFORE, DURING AND AFTER HYSTERECTOMY

A Pap smear is *always* done before surgery. It would be tragic to remove your uterus if there was an undiagnosed cancer of the cervix — cancer for which the best treatment is radiation therapy rather than surgery. The area in which the radium would have been placed — the uterus — is removed!

When hysterectomy is planned because of chronic vaginal bleeding, a D&C is done to rule out cancer and to see if the D&C might cure the chronic bleeding.

If the diagnosis is believed to be endometriosis, chronic infection with adhesions or ovarian cysts, laparoscopy can probably confirm the diagnosis *before* major surgery is undertaken.

The laboratory work that must be done includes complete blood count, a series of blood tests (performed on one specimen), a urinalysis to rule out bladder or kidney infection or other kidney disease, and type and crossmatch of your blood, in case transfusion is required. If your hysterectomy is not an emergency, a pint of blood may be drawn from you a couple of weeks before surgery and kept on hand in case it's needed. This avoids the risk of transfusion reaction, AIDS, hepatitis and other potential problems. Depending on your health, age and medical condition, additional tests, including chest X-ray, cardiogram or blood chemistry, may be required.

Assuming there are no complications, the only test that may be required after your surgery is a blood count to check for anemia.

WHERE IS SURGERY PERFORMED?

Hysterectomy is *not* an office or outpatient procedure. It is a major operation and requires hospitalization and skilled anesthesiologists. Adequate workup and preparation for your major operation are important.

HOSPITALIZATION AND DURATION

You may be admitted to the hospital the morning of surgery instead of the night before. If special preparations are necessary or there are medical problems, you may be admitted the day before surgery.

An average hysterectomy requires from 1 to 3 hours in the operating room, depending on whether adhesions, profuse bleeding, difficult dissection or other problems arise.

Recovery-room stay depends on the length of the procedure, the depth of anesthesia required and whether additional transfusions are necessary. If prolonged anesthesia is required to obtain adequate muscle relaxation, your recovery time may be longer.

If no complications arise, such as post-operative bleeding, your stay in the recovery room lasts from 1 to 1-1/2 hours.

Your average stay in the hospital ranges from 5 to 7 days. A vaginal hysterectomy incapacitates you less, permits you to be up sooner and recovery is generally faster.

You may have more difficulty passing urine after a vaginal hysterectomy because more surgery is performed around the urethra. A tiny tube, inserted into your bladder through the abdominal wall for bladder drainage, may be more comfortable than an in-dwelling urethral catheter. However, you may have fewer gas pains post-operatively following a vaginal hysterectomy because your bowel was less involved.

If bladder repair is required, the catheter remains in place for 3 to 4 days to allow healing and to regain bladder function. Occasionally, if there is difficulty in passing urine, your doctor may send you home with the catheter still in your bladder. You must return to the hospital or doctor's office to have it removed.

ANESTHESIA

LOCAL ANESTHESIA

This is rarely indicated or used in *any* type of hysterectomy. It might be employed in an emergency situation when the surgeon is awaiting the arrival of an anesthesiologist or in a patient who cannot tolerate general or spinal anesthesia.

SPINAL ANESTHESIA

Spinal anesthesia may be used in patients who cannot tolerate general anesthesia, such as those with lung, throat or mouth problems or allergy to gas anesthesia. The same general guidelines apply to epidural anesthesia as to spinal anesthesia.

GENERAL ANESTHESIA

General anesthesia is the anesthetic of choice for most hysterectomies. It permits adequate muscle relaxation and allows you to be asleep (preferred by most patients) during the surgery.

The anesthesiologist will visit you the night before or the morning of surgery and check for evidence of fever, infection, allergies, medicines you're taking, anemia, heart condition or other conditions. He also discusses the type of anesthesia he intends to use and answers any questions you may have.

Your anesthesiologist will administer intravenous (I.V.) premedication if you have not already had subcutaneous premedication in your room. He will make sure you are comfortably situated on the operating table.

After starting continuous I.V. solution in your vein, he will inject a drug into the I.V. tube to put you to sleep, usually sodium pentothal. Then he places the mask on your face for administration of the gas anesthetic. A tube is inserted into your trachea to ensure an airway after you are asleep, and it is removed before you are completely awake.

PROBABLE OUTCOME OF HYSTERECTOMY

The outcome is usually relief from pain, discomfort, bleeding or other symptoms you had before the operation. The outcome should be excellent. A hysterectomy is an excellent solution to certain problems; surgery shouldn't produce additional problems for you.

Be certain *before* surgery that you understand what organs your doctor is going to remove and what effect the surgery will have on you. Ask questions before surgery, and feel free to ask more questions after the operation.

POST-OPERATIVE CARE

Whether you have a vaginal or an abdominal hysterectomy, you will be up as soon as possible to avoid blood clots in your legs and other problems. Move about in bed. As soon as you are awake, move your fingers, toes, legs and arms. Begin regular exercises in bed.

Most doctors allow their patients to sit in a chair that night after surgery and be up and walking the first post-operative day with help. Your doctor will want you to walk (with help) to the bathroom. When you can, walk down the hall, but be sure you have someone steady you. Your rate of recovery may depend on your activity.

Doctors like to have their patients urinating and having a normal bowel movement before they send them home. You'll be surprised how quickly your appetite returns. Your doctor will probably withhold solid foods until your bowel recovers its function after the anesthesia.

Don't take more pain medication than you need because analgesia shots and pills may delay recovery of your bowel and bladder function. If you require a sleeping pill in the hospital, take one, but try to avoid taking sleeping pills home with you. They can be addictive and may develop into a habit that is difficult to break.

DIET

There is no special diet following hysterectomy. Eat whatever appeals to you until your appetite returns. Get back to three regular meals a day as soon as you can.

Some women believe they will gain weight after a hysterectomy. You may gain weight after *any* surgery because you have not eaten normally for a few days. When you are exposed to tempting food, with no physical activity, it's normal to regain your appetite and gain excessive weight if you aren't careful.

There is *no* physiological reason for you to gain weight after a hysterectomy. It has not upset your metabolism or anything else except your eating routine.

MISCONCEPTIONS ABOUT HYSTERECTOMY

Hysterectomy will make me masculine.
A hysterectomy won't make you grow more masculine.

Hysterectomy will make me fat.
You won't get fat if you don't eat too much.

Hysterectomy will make me nervous and upset.
There is nothing about a hysterectomy to change your emotions unless you expect it to. It may require a few weeks or months to regain your strength and stamina, but you should feel better after hysterectomy than you did before.

Hysterectomy will make me depressed and tired.
You should feel better and happier, but any surgery can cause you to become depressed. There is no reason why hysterectomy should cause this any more than any other surgery. If you understand about your hysterectomy and why you need one, you'll have fewer problems accepting the surgery and adjusting to it.

ALTERNATIVES TO HYSTERECTOMY

Alternatives depend on the reasons for doing the hysterectomy. For example, if a uterus has a fibroid tumor that is causing no symptoms, the tumor should be observed because fibroid tumors rarely become malignant (less than 1%).

If you lose your urine when straining, try Kegel exercises before you have surgery. Ask your doctor to describe them. These exercises strengthen the muscles that control urinary flow. If you're conscientious about doing the exercises, you may improve your urinary control enough to be able to avoid surgery on your bladder, with or without hysterectomy.

The drug danazol often controls the pain and increased flow that accompanies endometriosis, but it is extremely expensive and has side effects. Sometimes birth-control pills ease menstrual cramps and help diminish symptoms to the point hysterectomy is unnecessary.

CALL YOUR DOCTOR IF . . .

1. You have any bleeding from the vagina.
2. You have any foul odor or discharge from the vagina.
3. You have any redness, swelling, excessive drainage or separation of your abdominal wound.
4. You have chills or fever.
5. You don't feel well and know something is wrong.
6. You lose urine through your vagina.
7. You notice any fecal (bowel movement) odor or material passing from your vagina.
8. You notice any bulging from your vagina or through or around your abdominal incision.
9. Any swelling or redness appears in your legs or groin.

QUESTIONS TO ASK YOUR DOCTOR

Is there a medical, as opposed to surgical, way to treat my condition? Would you be willing to try it?

Is there minor surgery, such as D&C or laparoscopy, that could treat my condition so I don't need major surgery?

Because I'm 46 (or whatever age), do you think menopause could soon relieve me of my symptoms, without surgery?

After my hysterectomy, will I need to take estrogens?
This depends on several factors. If your ovaries aren't removed, you don't need estrogens. If you have had a cancer of the breast, *don't* take estrogens. Many advantages are being found from taking estrogens, such as avoidance of softening of the bones (osteoporosis) and a decreased risk of ischemic heart disease (heart attack). Each case is individual. If you're not at risk, your doctor will consider low-dose estrogens, even if there are no symptoms of menopause.

By biopsy, I know I have early cancer of the cervix. Tell me the advantages and disadvantages of hysterectomy versus radiation therapy.

- Cure rates are identical in the hands of a good surgeon or a good radiotherapist.
- Radiotherapy avoids the long convalescence of a radical hysterectomy.
- Surgery permits preservation of the ovaries if you're young. Radiation can destroy the ovaries.
- Surgery avoids the diarrhea, nausea, bladder inflammation or bowel obstruction that often accompany radiation.
- Radiation occasionally causes narrowing of your vagina to the point where it may cause painful intercourse.

What are my chances of cure if I develop cancer in my ovaries after hysterectomy?

This depends on several factors, but most cancers are treatable. Many can be cured. Here are some conditions that affect the cure rate:

- Type of cancer—whether fast or slow-growing.
- Extent of cancer.
- Delay between onset of cancer and beginning of treatment.
- Whether treatment was adequate.

How soon will I be able to return to work and regular activities?

Much depends on your condition before surgery, the reasons for surgery, whether you had complications and your general physical condition. Most women can return to work in 4 to 6 weeks, but individuals vary. It also depends on the type of work you do.

Why don't all doctors use the "bikini" incision? It seems better not to have an abdominal scar.

Some operations require a vertical abdominal incision, such as removal of a huge ovarian cyst or a large uterus or extensive adhesions. Occasionally adhesions are known (from previous laparoscopy, for example) to be severe. This type of hysterectomy might be easier and safer when performed with the wide exposure of a vertical incision. If cancer is suspected or known, a midline incision is used to better examine your abdomen and perform necessary surgery.

How soon may I resume sexual relations?

In general, 4 to 6 weeks after surgery. Ask your doctor for his guidelines. If you have any problems, discuss them with him.

What are the advantages and disadvantages of abdominal versus vaginal hysterectomy?

Advantages of Abdominal Hysterectomy
- Permits complete exploration of abdominal organs and removal of appendix.
- Permits easier, less time-consuming surgery in difficult cases in which there are adhesions, large tumors or other problems.
- Less risk of infection in post-operative period.

Disadvantages of Abdominal Hysterectomy
- Abdominal scar is visible and may be unsightly or painful.
- Longer recovery time, by as much as 2 to 4 weeks.
- Occasional hernia through incision.

Advantages of Vaginal Hysterectomy
- No visible scar and no hernia of incision.
- Shorter hospital stay and recovery time.
- Less operation time and shorter anesthesia time.
- Less chance of gas pains and bowel adhesions.
- Less post-operative pain and fewer analgesics needed.
- Better for high-risk patients.
- Enables surgeon to repair bladder, bowel and uterine prolapse.

Disadvantages of Vaginal Hysterectomy
- Cannot explore abdominal organs.
- Poor exposure for removal of large tumors.
- Cannot remove ovaries and tubes when bound by adhesions.
- May shorten vagina for intercourse.
- More post-operative infections.

Laparoscopy

DEFINITION OF LAPAROSCOPY

Laparoscopy is a minor operation in which your doctor inserts a slender, light-containing telescope into your abdomen to look at your pelvic organs and abdominal organs. It is used for diagnostic and therapeutic treatment. It is minor surgery, so it is usually performed on an outpatient basis.

ABBREVIATIONS AND OTHER NAMES

Laparoscopy, "scope the patient," diagnostic laparoscopy, therapeutic laparoscopy, "Band-aid surgery," celioscopy, peritoneoscopy and open laparoscopy are various terms used to describe this technique.

PARTS OF BODY INVOLVED

The parts of the body involved in laparoscopy vary according to what your doctor wants to see. Laparoscopy is performed through the abdominal wall. Through his laparoscope, your doctor can see your bowel, bladder, pelvic organs and other lower-abdominal organs. Using special instruments, he can look inside your abdomen and operate on your uterus, tubes and ovaries. Your vagina may also be involved — through the vagina a special instrument may be placed on the cervix to move your uterus into various positions to see into all areas of your abdominal cavity. This instrument may be used in diagnostic surgery, such as infertility laparoscopy, to inject fluids through the cervix, uterus and tubes to see if they are open or blocked.

Attempts may be made to see other organs of the body, such as the appendix, liver, spleen and gallbladder, depending on the particular purpose of the surgery.

COMMON REASONS FOR LAPAROSCOPY

The list of uses of laparoscopy continues to grow as improvements are made in equipment, technique and skill of surgeons. Laparoscopy gives your doctor a direct look at your internal organs and provides him with information that X-ray, ultrasound and other tests cannot give him. Uses for laparoscopy are both diagnostic and therapeutic (for treatment).

Laparoscopy is best used when your signs and symptoms indicate a serious enough problem that intra-abdominal organic disease must be ruled out, but your doctor doesn't believe your symptoms warrant major surgery.

INFERTILITY

Infertility may be one of the most common uses for laparoscopy (besides sterilization). It provides a direct look at your female organs. At the same time, your Fallopian tubes can be tested to see if they are open enough to allow travel of sperm toward the ovary and for a fertilized egg to pass in the opposite direction to the uterus. Your doctor injects a dye through your cervix, then watches through the laparoscope to see if the dye comes out through the ends of the Fallopian tubes.

Laparoscopy can detect endometriosis, adhesions and abnormalities, such as cysts and tumors of your ovaries. Many of these diseases can be *treated* by laparoscopy. Your ovaries can be biopsied, endometrial implants treated with laser or cautery and adhesions separated to enable you to become pregnant.

PRIMARY OR SECONDARY AMENORRHEA

This problem is a lack of menstrual periods and other hormonal problems besides infertility. A more common condition causing lack of periods and infertility is polycystic ovaries, also called *Stein-Leventhal Syndrome* or *SLS*. Polycystic ovaries involve ovaries that contain many small cysts and a thick outer shell. Polycystic ovaries can be diagnosed by laparoscopy.

ECTOPIC PREGNANCY

Ruptured and unruptured tubal pregnancies can be diagnosed by laparoscopy when other tests may have failed. A normal pregnancy, an ectopic pregnancy and early miscarriage may have similar symptoms, but the treatment of each is different. An undiagnosed ectopic pregnancy can be very serious, even life-threatening.

Through the wise and skillful use of laparoscopy in suspected ectopic pregnancies, diagnosis may be made *before* your tube ruptures, thereby allowing earlier treatment and possible preservation of your Fallopian tube. This treatment improves your chances for future pregnancies. For more information on ectopic pregnancy, see the section that begins on page 187.

UNDIAGNOSED PELVIC PAIN

Pelvic pain is another common reason for laparoscopy and is one in which laparoscopy finds its greatest value. Your diagnosis may be confirmed definitely by a direct "look" through a laparoscope. For chronic or acute pain, laparoscopy can often determine the need for further surgery, hospitalization or other treatment.

Pelvic inflammatory disease (PID) can cause acute or chronic pain. Many times patients are treated or even hospitalized with this diagnosis, yet it is never confirmed.

Experience has shown that for every 100 patients treated for PID *without* laparoscopic confirmation, 4 had an ectopic pregnancy and 3 had appendicitis. You wouldn't want to be treated for PID if you really needed an appendectomy. Furthermore, 20 of the 100 women with clinical diagnoses of PID were found to have no abnormality and should not have been treated for PID. This means you have a 25% chance of being treated for PID when you don't even have the disease. More liberal use of laparoscopy to aid in the diagnosis of these conditions could help avoid such mistakes.

PELVIC ADHESIONS

Adhesions are bands of scar tissue between organs — in this case your pelvic organs. They are a common cause of pelvic pain. They may be caused by previous surgery or pelvic inflammatory disease (PID), including previous infections such as gonorrhea or chlamydia that you were not even aware of. Pelvic adhesions can be diagnosed and treated by laparoscopy.

ENDOMETRIOSIS

In this condition, tissue that normally lines the cavity of your uterus is found outside the uterus, such as on ovaries, tubes or the surface of other pelvic organs. This tissue responds to ovarian-hormonal stimulation each month with swelling, bleeding and pain, just as though the tissue was in your uterus. Endometriosis may cause irregular or heavy periods and must be ruled out in cases of infertility and pelvic pain.

Endometriosis often causes painful menstrual periods, pain with intercourse and infertility. History and physical examination can only *suggest* a diagnosis, but laparoscopy can *confirm* the diagnosis of endometriosis.

D&C and ultrasound cannot make the diagnosis. It can be done *only* by biopsy or a direct look at the tissue. Laparoscopy affords your doctor the opportunity to look directly at your pelvic organs and to biopsy suspicious areas.

Some doctors make a tentative diagnosis, with laparoscopy, of endometriosis when they see the characteristic gross lesions on the ovaries or tubes. But it's always better if a biopsy is done to confirm the diagnosis. Treatment for endometriosis is expensive and time-consuming, so it's important for the diagnosis to be confirmed by biopsy.

Your endometriosis can often be *treated* effectively through the laparoscope. This will be discussed later.

TWISTING OF AN OVARY
Twisting of an ovary or tube is painful, and pain can imitate a ruptured appendix or an ectopic pregnancy. Because these organs are directly seen by laparoscopy, a definite diagnosis can be made *before* major surgery.

RUPTURED OVARIAN CYST
This type of problem can also imitate acute appendicitis or a ruptured ectopic pregnancy. After confirming the diagnosis, the necessary surgery to treat the condition may be carried out through the laparoscope, such as removal of fluid from a cyst or control of bleeding due to a rupture.

If bleeding is too severe or organs cannot be seen clearly enough by laparoscopy, then major surgery may be required.

UNDIAGNOSED MASSES
Undiagnosed masses in the tube, ovary or abdomen can be looked at, biopsied and often diagnosed or treated by laparoscopy. Your doctor can determine if your condition requires major surgery or other medical treatment. X-ray and ultrasound may be helpful, but there is nothing as certain as a direct look at the mass through the laparoscope.

UTERINE PERFORATION
Perforation of the uterus occurs most often when a D&C is done for abortion, but it can also occur when radium is inserted into the cervix in the treatment of cervical cancer or upon insertion of an IUD. When perforation occurs, your doctor may need to look at the perforation abdominally to assess the damage and see if major surgery is necessary or if you can be observed. Assessment is accomplished by laparoscopy.

INTERNAL HEMORRHAGE
Internal hemorrhage can be evaluated by laparoscopy to determine if emergency laparotomy (opening the abdominal cavity through a major incision) is necessary.

PERFORATION BY IUD
An IUD that has perforated the uterus can be located in the abdominal cavity by laparoscopy. Perforation may occur at the time the IUD is inserted or later on. If the IUD can be seen with the laparoscope, it can often be grasped with an instrument and removed, thereby avoiding major surgery.

USES IN CANCER
With cancer, there are two main uses for laparoscopy. One use is for aspiration of fluid from your abdominal cavity to examine it for cancer cells. The second is for biopsy of a suspicious area to examine it for cancer. It is also

used for "second-look" operations, in which the diagnosis is already known and has been treated. Evaluation of your progress is made by laparoscopy to determine if further radiation therapy, chemotherapy or surgery are necessary.

TUBAL STERILIZATION
This procedure is performed on more than half a million women each year. It has been nicknamed "Band-aid surgery" because incisions for laparoscopy are so small they usually require only a Band-aid to cover them.

There are several procedures that can be used for sterilization with a laparoscope. These are be discussed in detail in the section on sterilization, which begins on page 250.

ADHESIONS
Adhesions can be cut, cauterized or removed with a laparoscope. This is usually necessary because of pelvic pain or infertility. Adhesions result from previous surgery, endometriosis or pelvic infection due to gonorrhea or chlamydia. Biopsy of adhesions occasionally helps determine their cause.

Adhesions can be thin, filmy bands of white scar tissue that bend and distort the Fallopian tubes or bind your ovaries to the back of your uterus. In other cases, adhesions are so heavy and dense that pelvic organs can't be seen. In situations such as these, major surgery may be necessary to correct your particular problem.

Infertility may be due to blocking or distortion of Fallopian tubes by adhesions. When these bands are severed and the tubes released, the problem of infertility may be solved. Once the restrictive bands are broken, pain may also be relieved.

Adhesions can be an increased risk during laparoscopy because they may distort the normal anatomy of pelvic organs, including bowel and bladder.

LASER TREATMENT
Laser treatment of endometriosis by laparoscopy is new and not yet widely available. Tissue can be destroyed without damage to surrounding tissues as the laser beam heats the cell water to 212F (100C) and forms steam that expands and explodes the cell contents into vapor. There is no resulting debris, and bleeding is minimal. See illustration on page 242.

The technique of laser surgery is still being perfected and is not available at all hospitals, but it has already established its place in medicine. Only a tiny laser beam is required, and it can be effectively and accurately used through the laparoscope.

IN-VITRO FERTILIZATION
Retrieval of eggs from your ovaries or from your abdominal cavity for in-vitro fertilization (IVF) is a new and exciting application of laparoscopy. Success with IVF is improving, and it allows some couples who have previously been unable to conceive to begin and complete successful pregnancies.

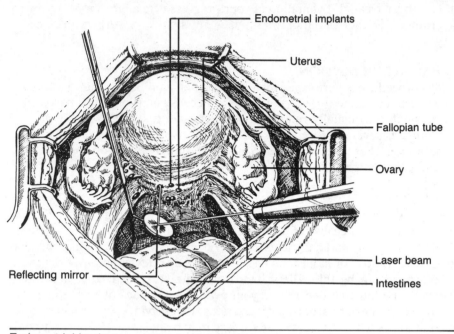

Endometrial implants vaporized with laser beam.

In IVF, ovaries are carefully monitored by ultrasound to watch for production of eggs. When the ovaries are thought to be ready, laparoscopy is performed, and eggs are removed and placed with sperm for fertilization. As IVF becomes more widely practiced, "harvesting" of eggs by laparoscopy will continue to be an important part of the treatment.

FLUID REMOVAL
Removal of fluid from the abdomen for diagnostic cancer tests or for relief of discomfort is occasionally performed with the aid of laparoscopy.

HOW COMMON IS LAPAROSCOPY?

Laparoscopy has been used for over 60 years. A surgical procedure, which was similar to laparoscopy, was used in 1805 in Germany. The procedure, called the *Lichtleiter,* was performed sporadically in Europe, where much of the equipment and techniques have been developed. Common use of laparoscopy in the United States began after 1950. Acceptance of this procedure has been slow because the medical profession has been waiting for more-effective equipment. The number of uses for the laparoscope continues to grow with improved equipment and skilled surgeons.

Over half a million sterilizations each year are performed by laparoscopy. If diagnostic and other laparoscopic procedures are included, it is one of the most common female surgical operations.

FUNCTIONS INVOLVED IN LAPAROSCOPY

No body functions are interfered with in laparoscopy. The procedure is usually minor and performed on an outpatient basis. It requires about an hour and does not require admission to the hospital.

HOW LAPAROSCOPY IS PERFORMED

The technique of laparoscopy varies from one surgeon to another and may depend on the equipment available. The three principal techniques are:
- one incision
- two incisions
- open laparoscopy

Whether you have one or two incisions depends on the reason for your laparoscopy and the equipment used. Some equipment permits a view of the organs and insertion of the operating instruments through the same incision.

If your doctor prefers the two-incision technique (because of his experience or the equipment available), he will use one incision for *looking* and the other for *operating* on or manipulating organs. The two-incision approach may be better suited for certain procedures, such as biopsy of your ovaries. Three mirrors might be used when a laser is used with a laparoscope.

Open laparoscopy requires special laparoscopic equipment and an operator who is experienced with this technique. The technique is believed to be safer when there are adhesions from previous surgery or when there is infection. A slightly larger incision is required (1/2 to 1 inch, as compared to 1/4 inch) as well as more time because the abdominal cavity is cut open before any scopes are put inside.

TECHNIQUE FOR ONE-INCISION METHOD

You are taken to an operating room and placed on an operating table. An intravenous needle (I.V.) is placed in a vein in your arm or hand. Through this you will be given fluid and medication as a part of your anesthesia. After you're asleep, you're placed in the same position as for a normal pelvic exam.

Your bladder is emptied with a catheter, and your abdomen and vagina are cleansed with antiseptic soap. Your doctor examines you under anesthesia to reaffirm his findings. An instrument is inserted through the vagina that grasps your cervix. It is used to manipulate your uterus, tubes and ovaries. Solution may be injected through the instrument to check for blockage of the Fallopian tubes.

Your head is lowered to permit your bowel to fall away from the pelvis. This aids your doctor as he examines your pelvic organs. A small 1/4- to 1/2-inch incision is made just inside your navel. A needle is inserted through this incision while you are in the head-down position. Carbon dioxide or nitrous-oxide gas are "pumped" into your abdomen to expand it like a balloon. This gives your doctor a better view of your pelvic organs. See illustration on page 244.

A larger needle, called a *trochar,* is inserted through the same incision after

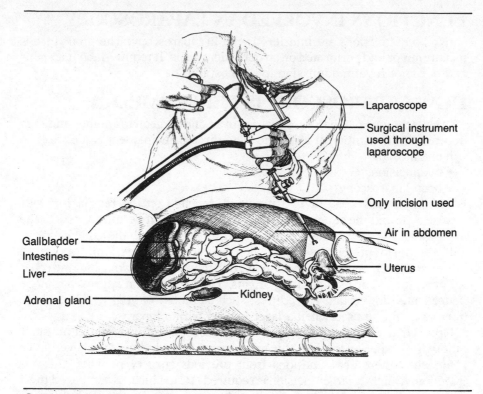

Laparoscope

Surgical instrument used through laparoscope

Only incision used

Air in abdomen

Gallbladder

Intestines

Liver

Adrenal gland

Kidney

Uterus

One-incision laparoscopy for exploration. Vision, light and instrument are all accommodated through the scope, so only one incision is necessary.

the needle is removed. It is through the trochar that an instrument containing a light is inserted. A general view of all your pelvic organs is now possible.

TECHNIQUE FOR TWO-INCISION METHOD

When using the two-incision technique, a second incision is made at the pubic hairline in the middle of your abdomen and a second trochar is inserted. See illustration on opposite page. Through this second trochar, laparoscopy instruments are inserted to biopsy, cauterize (for tubal ligation) or probe with a blunt instrument to obtain a better view of your pelvic organs. These same instruments, plus the laparoscope, can be inserted through the same incision in the one-incision technique.

The instruments described above, plus the clamp on the cervix through the vagina, enable your doctor to manipulate, inspect and perform laparoscopic surgery.

When your surgery is complete, the gas is allowed to escape through the trochar, and the instruments are removed from your abdomen and vagina. The tiny incisions are closed with sutures, and a small dressing or an adhesive bandage is placed on the incision(s).

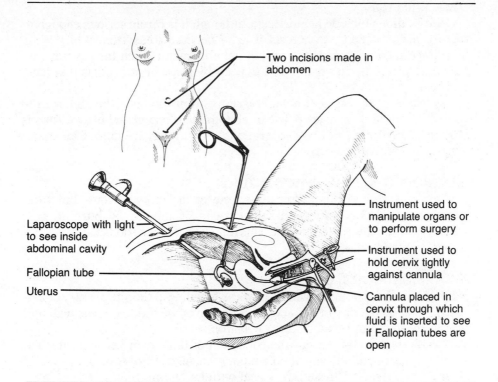

Labels on diagram:
- Two incisions made in abdomen
- Laparoscope with light to see inside abdominal cavity
- Fallopian tube
- Uterus
- Instrument used to manipulate organs or to perform surgery
- Instrument used to hold cervix tightly against cannula
- Cannula placed in cervix through which fluid is inserted to see if Fallopian tubes are open

Two-incision laparoscopy for tubal ligation. One incision is for laparoscope, which contains light, and the other incision is for the instrument used for surgery.

RISKS OF LAPAROSCOPY

The risks and complications with laparoscopy are extremely low. Most of the complications that occur are minor, such as infection of the incision. Complications rates are:

- Minor complications   1 to 6%
- Major complications   0.6% (6 in 1,000)

The risk in laparoscopy will probably be contraindicated in some conditions, such as severe heart or lung disease, intestinal obstruction, widespread cancer in your abdomen or severe infection in your abdomen with adhesions. Each situation is individual, and your specific risks will be considered.

Other conditions, though not serious enough to prevent laparoscopy, may make it more difficult or increase your risk of complications. These include gross obesity, large pelvic or abdominal mass or tumor, multiple previous surgeries with adhesion formation, previous anesthetic problems and shock or some other nervous condition.

HEMORRHAGE

Complications include hemorrhage, although it is rarely serious enough to require major surgery to control it. The general areas from which your bleeding can come include the wall of the abdomen (which the instruments may have pierced), an organ that has been biopsied or adhesions that have been cut.

In 7 out of 1,000 cases, it is necessary to surgically open the abdomen to control bleeding. If a major pelvic or abdominal blood vessel is torn (this is very rare; less than 1 in 10,000 operations), it may require immediate major surgery to control hemorrhage.

GASTROINTESTINAL-TRACT INJURY

Injury to the bowel and stomach is one of the more serious, but rare, complications. Your bowel and stomach can be injured by burning with cautery or when adhesions are cut. This injury becomes serious when it is not recognized immediately.

ABDOMINAL-WALL INJURY

Injury to your abdominal wall appears as bleeding at the site of entry or as a burn. Bleeding may be in the abdomen, or it may be hidden in the wall and form a collection of blood called a *hematoma*.

Blood loss is not great, but the collection of blood can become infected. Burns to the abdominal wall are often not recognized until several days after laparoscopy. Usually, these burns heal without any problems.

OTHER COMPLICATIONS

Pelvic infection occurs only 1 to 3 times in 1,000 laparoscopies and is easily treated with antibiotics. Infection of incisions is also rare and easily treated with antibiotics. Anesthetic complications are rare.

ADVANTAGES OF LAPAROSCOPY

It has taken several years for laparoscopy to gain wide acceptance in the United States and for equipment to reach the point where it now is one of the most common, safest and most valuable female surgical procedures. New advantages and new applications for laparoscopy continue to be found as more experience is gained.

The procedure is minor surgery and usually requires less than 1 hour to complete. Complication rate is low and recovery is quick — usually less than 1 to 2 days compared to several weeks for major surgery. In many instances, major surgery is avoided; treatment can be accomplished just as well by laparoscopy.

In nearly all instances, laparoscopy is an outpatient procedure and saves you the expense and emotional trauma of hospitalization.

Tubal sterilization has become much simpler and safer because of laparoscopy. Countless other uses make laparoscopy one of the most versatile minor surgical procedures of modern medicine.

DISADVANTAGES OF LAPAROSCOPY

There are few disadvantages of laparoscopy. The primary disadvantage comes when laparoscopy is used in place of more extensive major surgery. For example, extensive biopsies, exploration and treatment of cancer, widespread endometriosis and thick adhesions require a larger exposure than laparoscopy can provide.

WHO OPERATES?

Even though considered a minor procedure, this surgery requires training and experience. In most instances, this will be a doctor who specializes in obstetrics and gynecology.

DIAGNOSTIC TESTS BEFORE, DURING AND AFTER LAPAROSCOPY

Few laboratory tests are required prior to your laparoscopy. Routine tests for any general anesthesia include a complete blood count, urinalysis and some blood chemistries. You should have had a normal Pap smear within the last year.

If there are no complications, no tests are required after surgery.

WHERE IS SURGERY PERFORMED?

Most laparoscopies are performed in an operating room in a hospital, surgical center or outpatient surgical suite. Surgery in an outpatient facility or surgical center is used a great deal because it decreases costs.

HOSPITALIZATION AND DURATION

Laparoscopy is an outpatient operation, so only rarely is hospitalization required. Preparation, surgery and recovery take an average of 4 to 5 hours in an outpatient facility. If you have medical problems or complications, you may require admission to the hospital for additional care.

The average length of time for actual laparoscopy is 1 hour. Time spent in recovery is 30 to 45 minutes but will depend on your reaction to the surgery and anesthesia.

ANESTHESIA

Most laparoscopies are performed under general anesthesia, although surgery can be done under spinal or epidural anesthesia. Local anesthesia is being used more often for this surgery. You may want to discuss this with your doctor.

PROBABLE OUTCOME OF SURGERY

Laparoscopy may avoid a major surgical procedure for you. It may diagnose and even treat some problems, such as pelvic pain or infertility. This is done on an outpatient basis, at minimal cost.

POST-OPERATIVE CARE

Laparoscopy requires little post-operative care. It is best to have someone else drive you home after any anesthetic. You will have only a small dressing or adhesive bandage on your incision. Keep it dry for the first few days; it should be changed daily. You may require pain medication for minor pain for a few days. If an instrument is used to manipulate your cervix, you may have a little spotting that requires a sanitary napkin or internal tampon. You can go back to work or resume normal activities the following day. Don't rush it, but you should not require more than a day or two to recover.

Occasionally you may experience pain in your shoulders for a few hours. This indicates you have some air left in your abdomen, and it should go away in a few hours.

If you have been taking birth-control pills, complete your cycle. Make certain you are protected against pregnancy during the cycle when you have your surgery.

Generally there is no restriction of intercourse, although you might want to wait until bleeding has stopped.

DIET

There is no special diet before or after laparoscopy. Because of the anesthetic and the chance of complications, don't have anything to eat or drink after midnight the night before your surgery. After your surgery, gradually resume your normal diet.

MISCONCEPTIONS ABOUT LAPAROSCOPY

A hysterectomy, appendectomy or any other major surgery can be done by laparoscopy.

Untrue. These are major surgeries requiring a larger incision and extensive surgery.

If I have an ectopic pregnancy diagnosed by laparoscopy, I won't need further surgery.

No. Laparoscopy may only point out the need for further surgery if you are bleeding internally from an ectopic pregnancy. You will require more surgery.

ALTERNATIVES TO LAPAROSCOPY

Alternative approaches depend on your particular reason for surgery. If your surgery is "elective," you may want to wait and consider medical treatment, such as hormone therapy for endometriosis. Another alternative to laparoscopy is laparotomy (major surgery); your doctor will determine which is best for you.

CALL YOUR DOCTOR IF . . .

1. You have severe abdominal pain.
2. You have an unexplained fever.
3. You have swelling, redness, tenderness or drainage from your incision.
4. You have persistent vaginal bleeding.

QUESTIONS TO ASK YOUR DOCTOR

Why are you doing this laparoscopy? What do you hope to find?
    This is not an effrontery to your doctor's knowledge, skill or integrity. It is merely your desire and right to know all about your condition. This will give your doctor an opportunity to discuss with you, before surgery, his tentative diagnosis and to establish good communication.

Will I need further treatment? More surgery? Were you able to correct my problem?
    These are logical want to questions and your doctor will appreciate your interest and the fact you want to know about these conditions.

Sterilization

DEFINITION OF STERILIZATION

Sterilization has been used in one form or another for several thousand years. As early as 1200 B.C., a Chinese emperor had his servants and attendants castrated to make them sterile.

Babylonia, Syria and other cultures maintained control over their slaves by castrating them — they called the castrates *eunuchs*. They felt more comfortable when eunuchs looked after and protected their women. Other early civilizations mistakenly believed removing the ovaries of young girls would preserve their youth and attractiveness.

Early in this century, it was discovered that X-rays could sterilize men and women. But doctors soon learned of the harmful effects of radiation, so this method was abandoned.

Sterilization has been slow to gain popularity as a measure for birth control in the United States, although it has been used for many years in other countries. Even 20 years ago, it was a major undertaking to obtain permission from a hospital staff to sterilize a woman — the reason had to be critical to her health.

Today, over 1 million women a year select voluntary sterilization as their method of choice for limiting their family size. Tubal ligation in women is as popular as vasectomy in men in the United States. In Asia, by contrast, vasectomies have exceeded tubal ligations for many years. Over 6 million vasectomies were done between 1968 and 1972.

Sterilization in women usually refers to "tubal ligation." This means blocking or obstructing Fallopian tubes by one of several methods. We also discuss hysterectomy as a method of sterilization.

ABBREVIATIONS AND OTHER NAMES

Sterilization, bilateral tubal ligation, BTL, tubal occlusion, tubal resection and fimbriectomy (removal of the outermost end of the tubes) are all terms that mean sterilization.

PARTS OF BODY INVOLVED

Although sterilization usually involves blocking the Fallopian tubes, you will also be sterile if you have both tubes removed, both ovaries removed or if you have a hysterectomy. Anything that prevents the sperm from reaching the egg and fertilizing it or prevents your fertilized egg from becoming implanted in the wall of the uterus, prevents you from conceiving.

COMMON REASONS FOR STERILIZATION

Sterilization is an ideal, effective contraceptive, free of side effects. Men and women look toward sterilization as a permanent, non-reversible contraceptive method of birth control. You may consider this method because of health, age or economic situation or because you have as many children as you desire.

Until you want *permanent* sterilization, you may find contraception acceptable. When you definitely don't want any more pregnancies, sterilization may be the ideal choice for you. If you are over 40, many doctors suggest you not take birth-control pills. Even though they are convenient and have worked well for you for many years, you will have to select another form of birth control.

HOW COMMON IS STERILIZATION?

The table below gives you an idea of how sterilization has increased and certain contraceptive methods have decreased in the past 20 years.

METHOD	1965	1970	1975
Oral contraceptives	28.4%	35.4%	34.3%
Condom	22.0	14.8	10.9
IUD	1.2	7.5	8.7
Diaphragm	10.5	5.7	3.8
Foam	3.1	6.6	3.6
Rhythm	11.5	7.1	2.8
Withdrawal	4.0	2.3	2.0
Other	10.5	6.6	2.6
Wife Sterilized	4.7	6.8	16.3
Husband Sterilized	4.1	7.2	15.0

It is estimated that there are more than 1 million female sterilizations performed in the United States each year. This is an increase of almost 400% in the last 10 years. Vasectomy and tubal ligation are about equal in number in the United States at present. Sterilization seems to be more popular if you are over 30 or you have been married for more than 10 years.

FUNCTIONS INVOLVED IN STERILIZATION

If sterilization is performed by tubal ligation, there should be no interference with any bodily functions. Obstruction in the tube prevents the sperm from meeting the egg, leaving egg and sperm to be absorbed by the body. Unless the blood supply to your ovary is compromised by removing too large a section of the tube, you should continue to ovulate each month and produce hormones until menopause occurs. Your uterus is not affected in any way.

Menstrual periods should continue as usual, with regularity, duration and amount the same as before tubal ligation. The only difference you should notice is that you are unable to conceive.

If you have qualms about whether to be sterilized or not — wait. Don't have surgery unless, and until, you feel good about it. Regret, doubts and misgivings about femininity have no physiological basis, but they can be very real. For this reason, it's important to discuss with your doctor how you *feel* about sterilization. Take time to think it over and work it through. Be sure this is what you want and that you understand the operation will be permanent.

Your partner should also be considered. If your husband or partner cannot cope with sterilization — if he thinks it will change you or his feeling for you — you must take this into consideration.

HOW STERILIZATION IS PERFORMED

Although there are more than 100 variations in the technique of sterilization, there are five principal methods:
- laparoscopy
- minilaparotomy
- post-delivery tubal ligation
- vaginal tubal ligation
- hysterectomy

PROCEDURE FOR STERILIZATION

The same sterile precautions are taken, whether the incision is 1/4 inch or extends from your navel to your pubic bone. Your bladder is emptied by catheter, your abdomen is thoroughly scrubbed with soap, dried and painted with an antiseptic solution. It is then covered with sterile drapes.

LAPAROSCOPY

Laparoscopy is described in detail in the section beginning on page 237. Skill and safety in laparoscopy have reached the point where sterilization by this method is extremely simple. There are two principal methods of sterilization by laparoscopy — cautery and clips or rings.

In a laparoscopy, a tiny 1/4-inch incision is made through your skin, fatty tissue, fascia (heavy gristle layer covering muscles), through muscle and

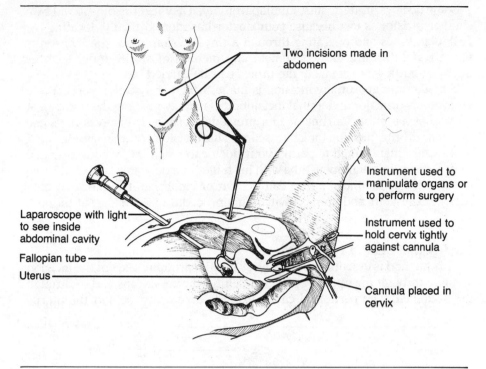

Two incisions made in abdomen

Instrument used to manipulate organs or to perform surgery

Instrument used to hold cervix tightly against cannula

Laparoscope with light to see inside abdominal cavity

Fallopian tube

Uterus

Cannula placed in cervix

Two-incision laparoscopy as a method of sterilization.

finally through the thin, shiny layer of peritoneum that lines your abdominal cavity. See illustration above.

Cautery — Cautery means *burning with electric current*. Sterilization by this method involves locating the Fallopian tube with the laparoscope, grasping it with the cautery instrument and turning the switch to apply heat.

Your doctor must be skilled at identifying your Fallopian tubes and making sure other organs are out of the way so only the tube is cauterized. After he burns a segment of the tube, he may cut through it to make absolutely sure no sperm can get through.

In skilled hands, cautery is a safe, sure method. But it is one of the most difficult to reverse if you change your mind.

Clips or Rings — Clips or rings block the tube mechanically by squeezing it together. A special applicator is necessary to place these devices accurately. Less tissue is damaged with clips and rings, so these operations can be reversed more easily and more successfully.

MINILAPAROTOMY

Minilaparotomy simply means a "small" incision into the abdomen. It is major surgery on the smallest scale. It was widely used before laparoscopy, and it is still used by some doctors, especially if they are not trained in laparoscopy.

Some doctors argue against minilaparotomy. They feel the time saved by a smaller incision is lost because your doctor has more difficulty locating the Fallopian tubes and operating through a tiny incision. Once the incision is made and tubes are located, almost any method of sterilization, such as burning, cutting or removing the tubes, can be carried out.

When a minilaparotomy incision is made, it is merely a miniversion of a laparotomy or major abdominal incision. It is usually made in the midline, at the top of the pubic hairline or in a previous incision. It involves the same layers as the tiny incision for laparoscopy. This incision varies in length from 1 to 2 inches, just enough to permit your doctor to reach into your abdominal cavity, grasp your Fallopian tube with his finger or a delicate clamp and bring it out through the incision. He can tie, cut or cauterize it to block it, then replace it in your abdominal cavity. This procedure is carried out on both sides.

VAGINAL TUBAL LIGATION

This method is essentially the same as minilaparotomy, except the incision is made through the upper vagina just behind the cervix, instead of through the abdomen. The peritoneal cavity extends downward behind the uterus

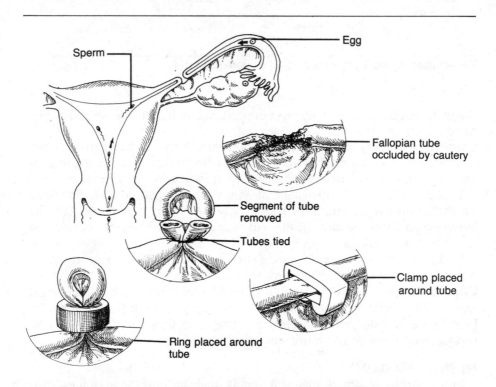

Some variations of sterilization by occluding (blocking) Fallopian tubes. Sterilization by tubal ligation makes it impossible for egg, coming from ovary, to reach sperm, coming from vagina.

where it ends in a blind pouch called the *posterior cul-de-sac*. With good exposure, this sac can be cut, giving immediate entrance to the peritoneal cavity and the Fallopian tubes. See illustration on opposite page

Some doctors are more familiar with vaginal surgery and prefer this method. But abdominal laparoscopy is rapidly becoming the method of choice for sterilization. This approach is easier if you have had several vaginal deliveries.

HYSTERECTOMY

There are many other simpler, safer methods—hysterectomy should not be performed only for sterilization. If there are other reasons for performing the hysterectomy, this procedure does prevent you from having more children.

If you have your bladder or a rectal hernia repaired, it's important not to have subsequent pregnancies. Delivery of a baby may cause ruptures to recur. This is one of the reasons your doctor performs a hysterectomy with the repair work on the bladder or rectum.

POST-PARTUM TUBAL LIGATION

Sterilization immediately after delivery of a baby has advantages and disadvantages. This is often called a *post-partum tubal ligation*. It is similar to a minilaparotomy tubal ligation.

Advantages of Sterilization After Delivery — You're already in the hospital, and you save the expense of another hospital admission. You also may avoid the extra risk and extra expense of another anesthetic if you have had a spinal, epidural or general anesthetic for delivery.

Your uterus is large, which means your tubes are more easily located and operated on. Your incision may be made a little higher in the abdomen than otherwise. If you've had a Cesarean operation, it requires only a few additional minutes to do a tubal ligation while your abdomen is open.

Disadvantages of Sterilization After Delivery — Assuming your condition is good, there is very little additional risk to do a tubal ligation but there is *some* risk.

The greatest argument against immediate sterilization is the fact that some problems in babies are not apparent at birth. It may take a day or two for them to develop. If the baby dies and you've already had a tubal ligation, you have no chance for another baby. This is the reason many doctors want you to wait for a least 48 hours to make certain your baby is all right and has a good chance of surviving before you are sterilized.

Be sure to discuss this matter of timing of sterilization with your doctor *before* your delivery if you are considering post-partum tubal ligation.

RISKS OF STERILIZATION

The risk to your life or health by sterilization is small. The risk of anesthesia is real and is discussed in the section that begins on page 18.

Minilaparotomy carries similar risks — infection, adhesions, hemorrhage, bowel obstruction — as any major surgery in which the abdominal cavity is opened, except on a lesser scale. Vaginal tubal ligation carries about the same risk.

Tubal ligation following Cesarean section does not seem to increase the risk enough to be significant. The risk of laparoscopy depends greatly on the skill of your doctor, but the risk is small.

Occasionally periods are heavier following sterilization. If you have been using birth-control pills and discontinue them after sterilization, you may notice heavier menstrual flow. This occurs because birth-control pills normally decrease your menstrual flow.

The risk of having depression following sterilization is not great but depends on your attitude toward tubal ligation and whether you sincerely wanted to end your fertility. If you've already worked through this, you won't feel guilty or have post-operative remorse. Sterilization won't affect your femininity or make you less of a woman. Sexually, you should feel the same or better because you don't have to worry about pregnancy.

Sterilization is permanent and cannot be reversed in most cases. Don't consider sterilization if you have any doubts about the procedure.

Another risk in sterilization is the risk of becoming pregnant. There *are* failures with any method. Failure rates (pregnancies) for various methods of sterilization are as shown below:

Cautery	2.3/1000
Band or rings	1 to 6/1000
Minilaparotomy	2/1000
Vaginal tubal ligation	3/1000

Skill of your doctor and the method he uses to sterilize you influence failure and success rates. Sterilization is an excellent method of preventing unwanted pregnancy when compared to failure rates of various methods of birth control. The chart below shows the theoretical use (if this method is used every day with no misses) and actual use (the way people actually use contraceptives, such as forgetting to use them or using them improperly.) Note the rates of pregnancy.

Type of Contraceptive	Theoretical Use	Actual Use
Oral Contraceptives	0.1%	2.0%
IUD	2.0%	5.0%
Condoms	3.0%	10.0%
Diaphragm	3.0%	13.0%
Foam/Cream/Jelly	10.0%	20.0%

ADVANTAGES OF STERILIZATION

If you have a life- or health-threatening condition, such as heart or kidney disease or systemic lupus, you can't rely on ordinary birth-control methods. You will require something that prevents pregnancy.

When you decide you have had enough children, you may wish to rid yourself of the threat of pregnancy and the inconvenience of birth control. Sterilization may be the answer to your problems.

For some other reasons, such as allergy to chemicals, side effects or other problems, if you can't use conventional birth-control methods, sterilization may solve your problem.

If you're over 40, especially if you smoke or have a history of phlebitis, you should not take birth-control pills. Unless you wish to use other birth-control measures, sterilization may be for you.

Peace of mind, one-time expense and the certainty of sterilization may be adequate reasons for you to consider this method.

DISADVANTAGES OF STERILIZATION

Sterilization is a permanent method of birth control. Although reversals can be done fairly successfully with newer microsurgical techniques, sterilization should never be done unless you are sure you do not want further pregnancies.

Sterilization is a safe, certain and relatively inexpensive minor procedure. By contrast, reversal of the procedure is major surgery, with greater risks, longer anesthesia and a relatively high chance of failure. Success of reversal depends on the method of sterilization and your doctor's skill at microsurgery.

If you are uncertain about sterilization — wait. Think it through, and discuss it with others. After you have worked through the various obstacles, including your own emotional response to infertility, you'll be better prepared for this safe, simple, sure method of controlling pregnancy.

Although sterilization is simple, safe and certain, it occasionally causes changes in menstrual flow — making periods heavier or lighter — and it may cause adhesions. If there is enough interference with blood supply to your ovaries (ovaries and Fallopian tubes share the same blood supply), the sterilization procedure can cause a premature menopause. While these complications are uncommon, they are a possibility.

WHO OPERATES?

In most instances, specialists in obstetrics or gynecology perform this surgery. But general surgeons and many family doctors in some areas have become skilled in this type of surgery. If your own doctor does not perform this surgery, he will refer you to a specialist who does. It's important to have a doctor who will discuss the problem with you, explain the various methods and help you decide if this is for you.

Many doctors are not familiar with laparoscopy, so you may have to settle for minilaparotomy. Minilaparotomy is a technique that is safe, sure and simple, and it may be best in your particular case.

DIAGNOSTIC TESTS BEFORE, DURING AND AFTER STERILIZATION

Before almost any surgery, you will have a urinalysis and complete blood count. Other blood chemistry tests may be required; your doctor will decide what tests you need.

It is wise to send any tissue removed to the laboratory for examination.

As more sterilizations are performed in outpatient departments and doctor's offices, this surgery becomes more routine. Post-operative infection and other complications are rare when precautions are taken.

WHERE IS SURGERY PERFORMED?

Most sterilizations, whether by laparoscopy, minilaparotomy or vaginal tubal ligation, can be performed in an outpatient setting. Outpatient departments have actually become minisurgical suites and are equipped with almost all the same facilities used in hospitals.

Some hospitals use their major operating rooms but admit patients for surgery and send them home the same day. Some patients with minilaparotomies and vaginal tubal ligations are kept overnight to relieve pain with medication and provide observation for 24 hours.

Hysterectomies and post-partum sterilizations are performed in the operating room. They require a post-operative hospital stay of 5 to 7 days.

HOSPITALIZATION AND DURATION

Laparoscopy is almost always an outpatient procedure. Surgery requires about an hour, plus an hour recovery before you are returned to the outpatient department. There you continue to recover, then go home.

Minilaparotomy and vaginal tubal ligation are more complicated than laparoscopy. They cause more discomfort, may require a little longer to perform and probably require that you remain in the hospital overnight.

Average stay for hysterectomy is about 5 days. Post-partum sterilization may add 2 days to your normal hospital stay after delivering a baby.

ANESTHESIA

Although most doctors still use general anesthesia for laparoscopy, local anesthesia is being used more often. Increased skill with laparoscopy produces less discomfort so your doctor can accomplish your sterilization under local anesthesia.

Spinal and epidural anesthesia are seldom used for sterilization procedures because most anesthesiologists prefer general anesthesia. They claim better control of your vital signs (pulse, blood pressure, temperature), better relaxation of muscles, fewer complications and better patient acceptance with intravenous general anesthesia.

PROBABLE OUTCOME OF SURGERY

Sterilization has an extremely low failure rate, and you can expect it to be successful in your situation. Your emotional outcome is less predictable but should be excellent if you have worked through it in your mind and asked your doctor all the questions that normally arise concerning this procedure.

POST-OPERATIVE CARE

LAPAROSCOPY

You can probably return to normal activities the day after your laparoscopic sterilization. You may want to schedule your operation before a weekend to give you a few additional days to get back to normal before returning to work.

A laparoscopy incision is small. It requires only that you watch for any undue redness or soreness.

MINILAPAROTOMY AND VAGINAL TUBAL LIGATION

Allow about a week to recover from minilaparotomy or vaginal tubal ligation. You won't have to stay in bed, but you'll want to rest when you're tired, and you'll probably want to stay near home.

An enema is not usually necessary prior to any of these surgeries because the procedures don't interfere with bowel function. You won't feel like straining so the chance of rupture of your incision is remote. Give yourself a chance to heal before lifting heavy objects.

If you have a minilaparotomy, you may want to cover your stitches with kitchen plastic wrap when you shower. Your pain may be greater than with other sterilization procedures, such as laparoscopy or vaginal tubal ligation, and you may require the strongest over-the-counter pain remedies or possibly mild prescription medications.

With a vaginal tubal ligation, you won't have stitches you can see. They are the absorbable type and don't have to be removed. You may have some bloody vaginal discharge for a few days. Intercourse should be deferred for 3 to 4 weeks, perhaps until you return to your doctor for your post-operative checkup.

DIET

No special diet or diet restrictions are necessary following laparoscopy. It might be a good idea to begin with fluids, then move to solids.

Minilaparotomy occasionally requires handling of the bowel to locate and operate on your Fallopian tubes. In this case, there is more chance of bowel upset, along with gas and nausea, following this operation. Begin eating chips of ice, then progress to sips of water, soups (bouillon) and finally semisolids. Your doctor will outline a diet for you, but you will also be able to tell what your stomach will tolerate.

Vaginal tubal ligation should not bother your intestines, and you should not have any changes in appetite. Anesthesia causes some nausea, but if you haven't eaten for 12 hours before surgery, you should have no problem.

MISCONCEPTIONS ABOUT STERILIZATION

Sterilization will make me masculine.
The operation will *not* make you masculine. And just because you can't conceive shouldn't make you feel as though you are less feminine.

Sterilization interferes with menstrual periods.
You should continue to have them with the same regularity, same duration and same amount of flow.

I won't have to go through menopause because of sterilization.
Menopause should come at the same time as it would otherwise.

If I'm sterilized, it can be reversed.
Sterilization cannot be reversed easily. Consider it a permanent procedure. It may be reversed, but this is an intricate, more complicated and expensive operation. It is not always successful.

My tubes will be tied with string.
Sterilization is spoken of as "tying tubes," but actually tubes are blocked by cautery, by tying with a suture or by putting a ring or clamp around them. Following this, a segment of the tube is often removed to be certain there is no way sperm can reach an egg given off at ovulation. In some methods, severed ends of the tube are buried in tissue to further assure that pregnancy does not occur.

ALTERNATIVES TO STERILIZATION

Birth-control methods, such as the pill, IUD, diaphragm, foams, jellies, creams, condoms or coitus interruptus can be used. Male sterilization (vasectomy) is also an alternative to your sterilization.

Silicone plugs in tubes are currently being used experimentally. They are placed in the Fallopian tubes, usually through the uterus, with the idea that they can be removed at a later date if you change your mind. This method requires more research to be sure it is effective and reversible.

Research has also been done with chemicals inserted through the uterus into the tubes to obstruct the tubes and prevent pregnancy. This method is also experimental.

There is a great deal of research going on to devise simpler methods of birth control. Some methods may eventually replace sterilization. In the meantime, for a simple, safe, sure, *permanent* method of birth control, you may find sterilization is the method you prefer.

CALL YOUR DOCTOR IF . . .

1. You have chills or fever.
2. Your incision becomes red, swollen or tender.
3. You have more abdominal pain than you think you should have.
4. You are unable to move your bowels or urinate.
5. You don't feel as well as you think you should.
6. You do not have a menstrual period within 6 weeks of sterilization.

QUESTIONS TO ASK YOUR DOCTOR

Do you feel sterilization is best for me? Why?

Hopefully you value your doctor's opinion. He may have special reasons he thinks a particular sterilization is best for you or not best for you. Ask him.

Which method of sterilization do you recommend? Why?

You will profit from his advice and reasons. For example, vaginal tubal ligation might be easier in an extremely obese patient because of her thick abdominal wall.

Is this method reversible?

Some procedures are more reversible than others. Clips and rings are easier to reverse. Cautery may be the most difficult to reverse.

How soon am I protected against pregnancy?

Immediately. Sterilization in a woman has no waiting period.

How soon may I resume intercourse?

As soon as you feel well enough. Most women feel free of discomfort within a few days. If you have a minilaparotomy, discomfort may last longer.

What kind of anesthesia is best for me?

Discuss this with your doctor and with the anesthesiologist to decide what is best for you.

Breast Augmentation and Reduction

DEFINITION OF SURGERY FOR AUGMENTATION AND REDUCTION MAMMAPLASTY

Mammaplasty means reshaping or recontouring of the breasts. There are two ways to reshape breasts according to what is desired:

- Enlarging is called *augmentation mammaplasty*. Information on this type of surgery begins below.
- Reducing is called *reduction mammaplasty*. Information on this type of surgery begins on page 270.

Our culture seems to pass through cycles in which breasts are emphasized or de-emphasized, displayed or covered by fashions. Look at some fashion magazines and catalogs from years ago to see how fashions have changed. Today, breasts are emphasized, and styles seem to be more breast-revealing. Although this trend could reverse itself at any time, styles have caused men and women to become breast conscious.

Because cosmetic breast surgery has become more skilled, safer and more available, some women now desire corrective surgery when they feel Nature has not endowed them with the particular breast shape or size they want. This type of surgery has become more common and less expensive.

SURGERY FOR ENLARGING THE BREAST

Augmentation mammaplasty means enlarging the breast by surgery. A few decades ago, it was common to pad brassieres to give women the size breast they desired. Possibly because of sexual attitudes, breast emphasis and improved surgery, women now want augmentation breast surgery. They want a better simulation of the real thing instead of the padded bra.

You may have inherited small breasts or you may have lost weight, and your breasts have gotten smaller. You may have noticed that your breasts have become smaller with each pregnancy. Whatever your reason, you now may enjoy the size breasts you desire through safe, simple, successful surgery, often performed in your doctor's surgical suite.

ABBREVIATIONS AND OTHER NAMES

Perhaps the most common term for augmentation mammaplasty is breast augmentation. Although it is now common to talk about breast surgery, you might be surprised to learn how many of your friends have had this type of surgery without anyone's knowledge.

PARTS OF BODY INVOLVED

There are two different areas in which artificial breasts (prostheses) can be placed. Surgery can involve only the breast, or it can involve the pectoralis muscles that lie immediately beneath your breast.

COMMON REASONS FOR AUGMENTATION MAMMAPLASTY

The most common reason for augmentation mammaplasty is to increase the size and contour of your breasts and improve your appearance. Occasionally a similar procedure is used to replace a breast that has been lost due to cancer or an accident.

Augmentation surgery improves your self-image and your sense of self-worth. You feel as good as you think you look. It's easy for someone who isn't bothered by tiny breasts to say, "Just be happy with what you have." But some women feel inferior and less feminine because they have small breasts. At least you should be offered the alternative of having augmentation mammaplasty if you want it.

HOW COMMON IS AUGMENTATION MAMMAPLASTY?

Some plastic surgeons claim this type of surgery represents most of their practice. Breast surgery is common and accepted as a logical alternative to undersized breasts. About 100,000 of these operations are performed annually in the United States.

FUNCTIONS INVOLVED IN AUGMENTATION MAMMAPLASTY

Breast function is usually not impaired or compromised by breast surgery. You can still nurse any babies you have after surgery. It is even claimed that examining breasts for lumps is easier than before because you can press your breast tissue against the smooth surface of the prosthesis rather than your uneven rib cage as you check for lumps, but there is debate about this.

HOW AUGMENTATION MAMMAPLASTY IS PERFORMED

Augmentation mammaplasty is performed by inserting an envelope filled with silicone gel, saltwater solution or a combination of the two into a "pocket" behind your breast. The device can be inserted through one of three common incisions, which are called *axillary, submammary* and *periareolar*. See illustrations below and on opposite page. There are also two places where your envelope can be inserted:

• Submammary placement. Insert the envelope directly under your breast tissue, between your breast and the pectoralis muscle.

• Subpectoral placement. Insert the envelope beneath the pectoral muscle that underlies your breast.

Some doctors prefer the submammary location because they claim it provides a softer, more breastlike feel. Others favor the subpectoral location because it is less likely to develop a hardened capsule around it — one of the frequent problems of this surgery.

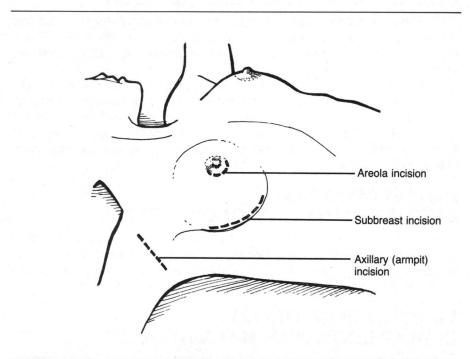

Areola incision

Subbreast incision

Axillary (armpit) incision

Three potential incision sites through which silicone-gel-filled envelopes can be inserted into breast.

Before surgery, you and your doctor will discuss the size and shape breasts you want. Within reasonable limits, you can actually choose the size and shape you want to have.

An incision is made in your skin and a "pocket" developed behind your breast or under your pectoral muscle. The silicone implant is inserted into this pocket. Implants come in various sizes and shapes.

After placement of the implant in the pocket, your doctor will close the incision and instruct you regarding post-operative care. Some doctors prefer to leave the dressing in place for 2 weeks, hoping for a reduced incidence of hardening around the implant. Others remove the dressing the next day, providing you with a good-fitting, well-supporting bra. After surgery, you'll be sent to recovery for about an hour, then you may go home.

There are several types of implants available. Your doctor may prefer one over the other, or he may recommend a certain type according to your specific needs. There are inflatable implants that contain saltwater. Others contain silicone gel, and still others are coated with polyurethane. Some can be inflated or deflated as desired. Some have double liners.

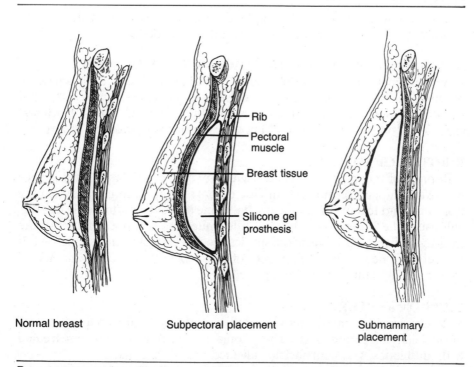

Normal breast   Subpectoral placement   Submammary placement

Breast augmentation with silicone-gel-filled envelope placed between breast and pectoral muscle or under pectoral muscle.

RISKS OF AUGMENTATION MAMMAPLASTY

INFECTION

Infection occurs in less than 1% of all cases and can usually be controlled by antibiotics. Only rarely will an abscess form and have to be drained.

HEMATOMA

A hematoma is an accumulation of blood that pools in one area after surgery. The condition occurs in about 1 to 2% of all women. Hematomas sometimes must be treated by draining. Sometimes they are allowed to be absorbed by the body.

HARDENED CAPSULE AROUND IMPLANT

Submammary implants are more likely to have a hardening around the implant. Reports vary widely about the number of women who develop this complication. Subpectoral implants seem to have a lower incidence of hardening — about 5 to 10%. This hardening can be troublesome. Attempted prevention is controversial at present, and each surgeon has his own preferences. If a capsule develops, your breast feels hard and can become deformed or painful. Surgery may be necessary if the hardness persists, but even then a completely soft breast can't always be achieved.

LOSS OF SENSATION

Loss of some sensation in the nipple may occur in up to 15% of all women. Usually this loss is temporary, but it can be permanent.

ABNORMAL APPEARANCE OR PLACEMENT OF IMPLANT

An abnormal appearance or placement of the implant is especially annoying because it makes your breast asymmetrical or lopsided. It requires additional surgery to correct it. This problem is usually associated with a hardened capsule and does not mean that the implant was placed improperly at surgery.

RUPTURE OF IMPLANT

Rupture of the implant can occur with any type of implant, but it is very rare. Most implant ruptures occur either from violent compression or simply from wear and tear over many years. If a saline implant ruptures or leaks, this will cause the breast to go flat. Gel-filled implants will not deflate but the long-term effects of free gel in the surgical pocket are not well-documented. If correction is necessary, replacement of the implant is the usual method of treatment. Implants cannot be repaired.

INCISION RUPTURE

Rarely your incision becomes infected or contains a hematoma that causes the incision to separate. If only a hematoma is present, you usually are treated with antibiotics, and your incision cleaned and sewed again.

UNSIGHTLY SCAR

For some unknown reason, certain people heal from any incision with a wide, thick, unsightly scar. Cortisone injections can help correct this, but occasionally the scar requires surgical revision to make it acceptable.

ADVANTAGES OF AUGMENTATION MAMMAPLASTY

Improved appearance is the objective, even when your breast is being replaced following amputation for breast cancer. Breast augmentation is safe and fairly simple.

DISADVANTAGES OF AUGMENTATION MAMMAPLASTY

The operation is expensive and will cause some temporary pain. More common, and even more distressing to you, is scarring around the implant. This scarring forms a fibrous shell that makes the breast hard to the touch. It may look all right on the outside, but it does not have the soft touch of a breast. There is no 100% successful way to prevent or treat this problem at the present time.

It is not uncommon to have to reoperate on your breast to try to obtain the proper feel and shape. Breaking the fibrous shell around the implant has been mentioned. Occasionally the implant is distorted by internal scarring, and your breast becomes lopsided. This deformity is usually corrected by additional surgery.

WHO OPERATES?

Usually a plastic surgeon performs augmentation mammaplasty, but general surgeons are beginning to perform more of them. Check your doctor's credentials by calling your local county medical society or ask the plastic surgeon about his training.

DIAGNOSTIC TESTS BEFORE, DURING AND AFTER AUGMENTATION MAMMAPLASTY

Other than urinalysis and complete blood count, it is important that you have no bleeding disorder that would increase the possibility of hemorrhage. Your doctor will order clotting time and any other tests he feels are necessary when indicated.

WHERE IS SURGERY PERFORMED?

To avoid hospital costs, many plastic surgeons now operate in their offices where they have elaborate, safe facilities or in outpatient surgical centers. Even if surgery is performed in a hospital, you should be in and out the same day.

HOSPITALIZATION AND DURATION

Only rarely is hospital admission necessary. Surgery requires 45 minutes to 3 hours, depending on your surgeon and whether complications arise. If surgery is performed under local anesthesia, recovery time is short, and you'll be sent home in a few hours.

ANESTHESIA

If performed in your doctor's office, anesthesia will probably be local, with additional sedation. In a hospital outpatient department, you may be given general anesthesia. If you have a preference, discuss it with your doctor before surgery. Your immediate recovery from surgery is shorter if you have local anesthetic.

PROBABLE OUTCOME
OF AUGMENTATION MAMMAPLASTY

Discuss the differences in surgical techniques with your surgeon, including placement of incision, type of implant, size and shape of implant, and type of anesthetic. If you are informed about all aspects of this surgery, your outcome should be good.

Complications do arise in augmentation mammaplasty, and you should realize that roughly 30 to 40% of all implants may become somewhat firm (develop a fibrous capsule around them). The result is a good outward appearance, but the consistency of your breast may not be as soft as you would want it to be. Rarely, you may have pain from constriction of the internal scar around your implant.

POST-OPERATIVE CARE

You may have binders or pressure dressings around your breasts, and you may have drains. If drains are used, they are usually removed after 2 or 3 days. Some doctors leave the binders in place up to 2 weeks. They hope to cut down on bleeding and scarring, and that in turn cuts down on constricting capsules around the implant.

Some doctors like the breasts to be massaged daily, sometimes beginning the day after surgery, to prevent capsule formation. This massage may be painful at first. Some doctors wait 5 to 7 days before beginning this massage.

Bathing and showering depend on whether dressings are removed early or late. Oral vitamin E may be used in the hope it might cut down on scarring.

Pain varies. Your pain may be minimal, but pain usually subsides after 3 to 4 days. It may persist for many weeks or months.

DIET

There is no special diet following breast surgery except possibly to use vitamin-E supplement.

MISCONCEPTIONS
ABOUT AUGMENTATION MAMMAPLASTY

There are no complications with augmentation mammaplasty.

Because this operation has become so common and because it may be performed in your doctor's office, you may be misled into thinking it has no complications. That is untrue. Augmentation mammaplasty occasionally fails, if you call formation of a hard capsule around the implant a "failure." The complication can sometimes be corrected, but it often involves more surgery and more discomfort. Other problems may arise, as we have discussed in the risks section.

The implants can feel colder than the rest of my breast.

Implants usually remain the same temperature as the body, but because they do not have circulation to warm them, some patients find their breasts get cold under certain conditions. For instance, if you go outside on a cold night in a low-cut dress, your breast implants may feel colder than the rest of your skin. But this is not harmful.

The implants may expand when I travel in an airplane.

Implants remain about the same size at all times. They are filled with material that does not expand significantly at low pressures, such as in an airplane, or compress significantly at high pressures, such as skin diving.

I won't be able to breast-feed after surgery.

Breast-feeding is still possible after augmentation because the breast ducts are not disturbed.

ALTERNATIVES
TO AUGMENTATION MAMMAPLASTY

The simplest alternative to this surgery is to be satisfied with what you already have. However, if Nature gave you small breasts, or if pregnancies or menopause have reduced your breasts to practically nothing, you have the alternative of augmentation mammaplasty.

The other alternative is to wear a padded bra. You can achieve the same effect without the pain.

CALL YOUR DOCTOR IF . . .

1. You have fever or chills.
2. You have hemorrhage or discharge from your incision.
3. You have redness around your incision.
4. You have sudden enlargement of your breasts. It could be hemorrhage in or under your incision.

5. You sustain any injury to either breast after surgery.
6. You notice increased firmness of either breast.
7. You notice any change in shape of either breast following surgery.

QUESTIONS TO ASK YOUR DOCTOR

What type of implant are you going to use?
There are several kinds your doctor can choose. You might want to ask why he is going to use the particular kind he selects for you. In view of the "hardening" that occurs around an implant, it will help you understand ahead of time why he is using the kind he does.

Which incision do you prefer? Why?
Many women prefer an incision in a specific part of their body.

Will you be implanting the prosthesis under my breast or under my pectoral muscle? Why?
There are advantages and disadvantages to both placement locations. Be aware of them so you can help make the decision.

What about massage of my breast after surgery? How painful will it be? How long will it be necessary?
You should understand what your doctor's post-operative program is. Have him detail *exactly* what he will be doing and what you should expect. You'll want to cooperate completely with him for best results.

What about future pregnancies?
If you aren't through having your family, discuss nursing with him.

Can implants cause cancer of the breast?
Implants do *not* cause cancer nor does any other surgery on your breast.

SURGERY FOR REDUCING THE BREAST

Reduction mammaplasty is any surgery to reduce the size of your breasts. If you have endured the discomfort of large, heavy breasts that cause your bra to dig into your shoulders and your back to ache, you can find relief! Typically you will ask, "Why didn't someone tell me about this operation sooner?"

If you have trouble buying clothes or playing sports because of your large breasts, you'll enjoy the freedom from discomfort. You'll be able to buy clothes, lie on your stomach and participate in athletics after you have this surgery.

ABBREVIATIONS AND OTHER NAMES

Reduction mammaplasty is not as common as breast augmentation. Breast reduction is the common term for this surgery.

PARTS OF BODY INVOLVED

Only the breast is involved in reduction mammaplasty, but relief is felt in many other parts of your body, such as aching shoulders and back. Other functions of your body may be improved by this surgery because you feel better about yourself. Occasionally it also reduces breast pain and skin irritation that occurs between the breast and underlying skin.

COMMON REASONS
FOR REDUCTION MAMMAPLASTY

Reduction mammaplasty is often performed to improve your appearance. But you may find relief from backache, shoulder pain and even what you may have believed was arthritis in shoulders and back.

Other factors also have their effect. You'll be able to select more styles of clothing. You'll be able to play sports without pain or ineptness. You will fit into styles without having to order special bras, special blouses and special dresses.

HOW COMMON
IS REDUCTION MAMMAPLASTY?

Reduction mammaplasty is becoming more common. It is unfortunate that more women don't consider it. We hope many of you will learn through this book that you no longer need to put up with the problem of oversized breasts.

It's impossible to estimate the number of women who have this type of surgery because many operations are performed in doctor's offices and do not show up on surgical records or surgical centers.

FUNCTIONS INVOLVED
IN REDUCTION MAMMAPLASTY

Except for the usual body functions affected by general anesthesia when it is used for this surgery, no other functions should be involved.

HOW REDUCTION
MAMMAPLASTY IS PERFORMED

Although reduction mammaplasty has been around for over 50 years, it is still not common. Many doctors are unaware of the benefits of this operation and do not suggest it to their patients who have oversized, uncomfortable breasts. See illustration on page 272. During the 50 years reduction mammaplasty has been around, many different techniques have been developed, and there are still many methods used to reduce the size of breasts. The method selected by your doctor depends on how large your breasts are, how much you want them reduced in size, how low your nipples hang, your age and probably your doctor's preference.

If your breasts are extremely large, your nipples may have to be cut off entirely, then moved up on your breast and grafted in place. If the distance is

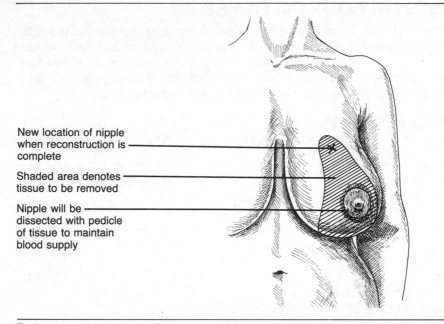

New location of nipple when reconstruction is complete

Shaded area denotes tissue to be removed

Nipple will be dissected with pedicle of tissue to maintain blood supply

Reduction mammaplasty. Breast is carefully measured by doctor, and new location for the nipple is determined. Shaded area shows amount of tissue to be removed.

not too great, your nipple can be left attached to a cord of tissue and moved up as part of the reconstruction of your breast. See illustration on opposite page.

An inverted-T incision is usually made in each breast, with the horizontal incision along the lower crease of your breast and the vertical part of the T extending up to your nipple.

Your nipple and its attached cord are cut free, and the nipple is pulled through a "keyhole" incision at a premarked place higher on your breast. There it is sewed in place. Excess breast tissue is removed, extra skin is trimmed away and the incision is closed with stitches. Drains may or may not be placed in the incision.

Supportive dressings are placed over your incision where they will compress the area that has been cut. This prevents any post-operative bleeding. Dressings must be tight enough for support, yet loose enough to allow adequate circulation to promote healing.

You may have to wear a specially fit brassiere to help shape your new contour and give correct support to your breasts and skin.

RISKS OF REDUCTION MAMMAPLASTY

The overall complication rate is about 25%. Some complications are serious; most are not. Some complications interfere with the final desired result, and others have no effect on the final outcome.

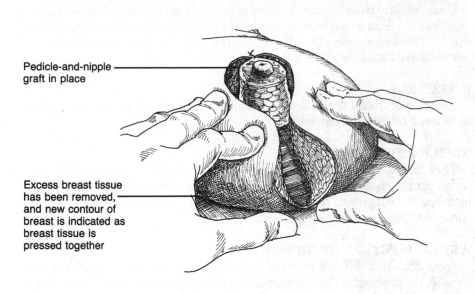

Pedicle-and-nipple graft in place

Excess breast tissue has been removed, and new contour of breast is indicated as breast tissue is pressed together

Wedge of breast tissue has been removed, cutting around pedicle graft of nipple. Nipple has been anchored in place at its new location.

HEMATOMA

A hematoma is an accumulation of blood trapped below the incision. It's the most common, most troublesome complication. If the hematoma is very large, it may require another operation to open the wound to remove blood and stop bleeding. If a hematoma is left untreated, it can enlarge enough to cause death of your nipple plus other skin areas because it interferes with their blood supply. It can also cause abnormal scarring.

NIPPLE LOSS

Although nipple slough occurs infrequently (less than 1% of all cases), it is a dreaded complication because the nipple may have to be rebuilt from other tissue (such as the labia) and grafted on your breast later.

SKIN SLOUGH

Usually any area of skin slough (death of tissue) is limited to 1 centimeter or less in size and occurs along the incision. These heal by themselves as your incision heals. If there is too much scarring, your incision can be redone at a later date, but the scars from breast reduction frequently cannot be made as fine as in other types of surgery.

DEATH OF FATTY TISSUE UNDER SKIN OF BREAST

Death of fatty tissue under the skin of your breast is usually due to dissection that can destroy too much of the blood supply to the fatty tissue. Usually this will drain for several weeks or months after the surgery. Sometimes a hard, scarred area may result.

INFECTION

Infection of breast tissue is uncommon, but it does occur. It usually heals with antibiotics and drainage.

NIPPLE RETRACTION

This means the nipple, in its new location, is pulled into the breast by scarring underneath it. If withdrawal is severe enough to deform the breast, it may require surgery to release it. As long as the blood supply is adequate, corrective surgery will be successful.

WRONG POSITION OF NIPPLE

Sometimes it is difficult to place your nipple in exactly the right position. Usually the problem is that the nipple looks too high on the breast. A common cause of this is the breast tends to slide down and out from under the nipple placement. Corrective surgery is difficult.

SCARS

You may heal by forming a keloid, which is a thick, unsightly, heavy scar. Cortisone cream or cortisone injections will usually improve its appearance, but it can also be surgically redone, if necessary, to try to improve its appearance.

CYSTS

Cysts sometimes occur in your breast due to blockage of the milk glands and ducts. These cysts usually resolve themselves spontaneously and disappear. Some may drain spontaneously.

SENSORY LOSS

You may lose sensation over areas of your breast after reduction mammaplasty, especially if breasts were large and required extensive dissection. Your nipples may lose their erectility and some of their sensitivity. In many cases, sensation returns, but in others the loss is permanent. Women with extremely large breasts often have lost much of the sensitivity even without surgery.

INABILITY TO NURSE

You may have a problem producing breast milk. In extensive breast reconstruction, many ducts are severed, and the milk system is disrupted. It is possible you will be unable to nurse a baby after this surgery.

ADVANTAGES
OF REDUCTION MAMMAPLASTY

You should find relief of discomfort due to heavy breasts, gouging breast straps, backache and pain in your shoulders and joints. You will have smaller breasts and a better appearance. You'll be able to wear normal clothing, and you will have an improved self-image.

DISADVANTAGES
OF REDUCTION MAMMAPLASTY

Scarring from the surgery may make it more difficult to examine your breasts for cancer. Scarring may also disrupt the pattern of your breasts, as shown on mammograms to detect cancer. Complications are not common but can be serious. They have been discussed in the risk section.

WHO OPERATES?

Usually plastic surgeons perform this type of surgery.

DIAGNOSTIC TESTS BEFORE, DURING
AND AFTER REDUCTION MAMMAPLASTY

A mammogram, complete blood count, urinalysis and a test for bleeding and clotting time may be performed before surgery. X-ray of back and neck also may be done, so if pain persists after surgery, you'll know if there may be some reason for the pain other than heavy breasts. Blood for autotransfusion is considered if dissection is going to be extensive or if a large loss of blood is anticipated.

WHERE IS SURGERY PERFORMED?

Breast reduction of large breasts is usually performed in the hospital operating room but can be done in a surgical center. General anesthesia is necessary, along with careful monitoring. This requires an anesthesiologist.

By contrast, breast reductions of smaller breasts can often be performed in an outpatient surgical suite or in a doctor's office.

HOSPITALIZATION AND DURATION

A normal breast reduction mammaplasty takes 2 to 6 hours. Nipple grafting usually takes less time than pedicle-type resection and transfer to a new nipple site.

Recovery room stay is 30 minutes to 1 hour, then you are returned to your hospital bed. Your recovery period is longer with a general anesthetic than with local anesthesia.

ANESTHESIA

Reduction mammaplasty involves more surgery and dissection than augmentation mammaplasty, so general anesthesia is almost standard. Some doctors perform surgery in their own surgical suite but only when they anticipate a smaller amount of dissection and only if they have well-equipped facilities with monitoring equipment.

General anesthesia may cause vomiting with the attendant threat of aspiration of vomit into your lungs. Drug sensitivity and shock are also unforeseen but occasionally occur with general anesthesia.

PROBABLE OUTCOME OF SURGERY

Relief from symptoms is remarkable, and nearly all patients are pleased to have lighter, more normal-sized breasts. As far as appearance is concerned, most patients are satisfied with the outcome. Occasionally patients will say they wished their doctor had removed more breast tissue.

Most dissatisfaction, if there is any, is due to the prolonged, persistent pain that lingers in some cases or to scars, which may widen and delay healing. You should be prepared for this possibility; discuss it with your doctor before surgery.

POST-OPERATIVE CARE

Your dressing must be supportive but not too tight. It is important to have post-operative contact with your doctor. It is not unusual to have the dressing adjusted and changed. If you have pain, you may appreciate being in the hospital where analgesics are readily available. However, your doctor will give you a prescription for pain relievers to take at home.

If drains are used, they are usually removed in 24 to 48 hours. Sutures around your nipples are removed in about 1 week, and all other stitches by 10 to 14 days. You will not want to exercise much before 4 to 6 weeks. After that time, you should be recovered enough to undertake almost any activity.

DIET

There are no special diets, but avoid excessive weight gain. The fat might be deposited in your breasts, creating the same problems you started with.

MISCONCEPTIONS ABOUT REDUCTION MAMMAPLASTY

Reduction mammaplasty will help me lose weight.
This is not a weight-loss method. If you have lost all the weight you can and your breasts are still extremely large, you might want to consider reduction mammaplasty.

Reduction mammaplasty is not complicated surgery.
This surgery involves a great deal of dissection and a lot of post-operative discomfort. It is accompanied by considerable scarring on your breasts. Complications can occur and must be dealt with.

Complications don't occur with plastic surgery.
Complications do occur. For a complete discussion of complications, see the information that begins on page 272.

Breast-feeding is still possible after I have reduction mammaplasty.
Breast-feeding is usually *not* possible after this surgery because of disruption of milk-producing ducts.

I won't have any scars after this surgery.
Scars are a result of incisions. They are permanent and may be quite apparent. Fortunately, the design of the operation usually places them in an inconspicuous position.

ALTERNATIVES TO REDUCTION MAMMAPLASTY

You can learn to live with your problems of extra large breasts. If you want relief, there is no substitute for surgery if you have reduced your weight to normal.

CALL YOUR DOCTOR IF . . .

1. You have fever or chills.
2. You have redness or swelling in your incisions.
3. You have bleeding or discharge from your incision.
4. You have blue discoloration around or under your nipples or in the skin along your incision.
5. You have any disruption of your incision (separation of the edges).
6. You have any injury to your breast, especially over the area of operation.

QUESTIONS TO ASK YOUR DOCTOR

How much can you reduce the size and weight of my breasts?
You need to have your doctor's opinion as to what he can do for you.

What do you think would be the best size for my breasts?
With his experience, he may be able to advise you as to what might look best for your build. Your desire of breast size is important, however, and you should make your wishes known to your surgeon.

How common are complications? How severe? Will they interfere with the end result?

You'll want to know about these things so there'll be no surprises and as few disappointments as possible. See the risk section, which begins on page 272.

How will you reposition the nipple? By grafting? By pedicle?

This is a common source of problems so you want to be informed about it. It usually depends on your breast size.

Tell me about costs, insurance, payment.

Reduction mammaplasty is occasionally necessary because of intolerable symptoms, such as backache, shoulder pain, fatigue, unsatisfactory appearance for work. Although you and your doctor may agree that surgery is medically indicated for these reasons, insurance companies often refuse to make this determination before the operation. They may refuse to pay benefits or may base their payment on the weight of tissue removed by the surgeon. Because of this, some surgeons ask to be paid in advance. To avoid unpleasant surprises, have a clear understanding *before* you have your operation.

One of my breasts is small and the other is quite a bit larger. Can anything be done for me?

Yes. This is called *breast equalization.* It is not uncommon for one breast to be larger than the other, but sometimes the difference can be extreme. Your breasts can be equalized by augmentation or reduction to make them more nearly the same size, even if they cannot be made to look *exactly* alike.

Face-Lift Surgery

DEFINITION OF FACE-LIFT SURGERY

Gravity may help you keep your feet on the ground, but it also exerts a constant pull on the rest of your body. Two of the obvious places in which gravity becomes your enemy are your face and neck. As you become older, gravity causes these tissues to sag.

Added to the sagging caused by gravity is the steady loss of fatty tissue in your skin. This is the reason you develop saggy wrinkles. You may also like to have that tanned, healthy look. Although tanning may make you *feel* more healthy, it actually ages your skin and promotes a leathery effect.

As if all of this were not enough, other things, such as smoking, also appear to age skin prematurely.

You can also inherit smooth, wrinkle-free skin or various degrees of wrinkling from your parents. There's nothing you can do to change heredity.

No one wants "old" skin, and no one wants wrinkles. With the stress placed on appearance today, it is only natural that women (and men) are turning more to face-lifting surgery. This type of surgery smooths the facial wrinkles and helps the face take on a younger, more youthful appearance.

ABBREVIATIONS AND OTHER NAMES

Face lift, rhytidectomy, removal of wrinkles, neck lift and facial cosmetic surgery all describe similar procedures designed to improve the appearance of your face.

PARTS OF BODY INVOLVED

Face-lift surgery involves only the head and neck. It is superficial, so it doesn't bother other organs.

Your age, state of mind, general health and inner reactions are reflected in your face. You are often judged by what people see, so you can understand why face-lift surgery is becoming more popular.

The most obvious areas of your face to show changes and aging are your neck, lips, eyes and forehead. A general fine wrinkling of your skin texture may also be in evidence. A classical face lift involves cheeks, neck, jowls and the part of your skin on the outer side of your eyelids—the part that reflects a smile, frown and other moods. See illustrations on opposite page.

In a way, wrinkles can be a barometer indicating the amount of fat or lack of it in your skin.

COMMON REASONS FOR FACE-LIFT SURGERY

Although plastic surgery may be necessary to correct scars from burns, accidents or war wounds, by contrast, face-lift surgery is designed to improve your natural appearance. It meets our needs and is intended to improve what Nature has taken away from us. A beneficial side effect is that face lift can help enhance self-image and self-esteem. People feel as young as they think they *look*.

Society is now demanding that we look younger. Many of us probably believe we'll act differently if we can stop time's telling on our faces.

HOW COMMON IS FACE-LIFT SURGERY?

In the past, face-lift surgery was often kept secret and not talked about. By contrast, today the media frequently reports when celebrities and politicians have face-lift surgery. Cosmetic surgery has become commonplace and is a familiar topic about which you're expected to be informed.

FUNCTIONS INVOLVED
IN FACE-LIFT SURGERY

No major body functions are involved in this surgery. But you should be ready to accept a change in facial appearance *before* surgery, or don't have the surgery. It's also important to discuss any questions and concerns with your family and your doctor *before* surgery.

HOW FACE-LIFT SURGERY IS PERFORMED

Face lifting is actually accomplished by making incisions in creases, and when possible, they can be hidden by hair. The skin in wrinkled, sagging areas is cut under, then stretched as tightly as is safe. Excess skin is trimmed away, and the incisions are closed with stitches. This sounds simple and

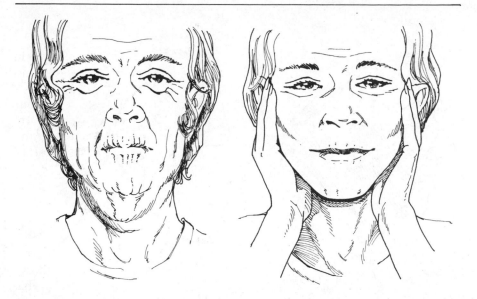

Patient's test for what face lift might accomplish. This test is partially accurate, but wrinkles around lips and nose will remain, to some degree. Jawline and neck will be improved the most.

uncomplicated, but it requires great skill and experience to know how to make it all turn out the way you want it. See illustration on page 282.

In addition to the classical face-lift procedure, which involves your cheeks, neck, jowls and skin near your eyes, there are procedures to correct other specific areas of your face. *Chemicals* peel the skin to minimize wrinkles on lips and acne scars on cheeks. *Dermabrasion* is a process in which wrinkles and acne scars are reduced by sanding, like sanding out the rough spots on a piece of wood.

One of the newer methods is the injection of collagen into the skin to smooth out wrinkles. In a sense, collagen replaces fatty tissue; the loss of the fatty tissue helped create wrinkles. In some patients, collagen seems to work well and last a long time; in others, it is less effective and seems to disappear in a few months.

Making special incisions in or behind the hairline to correct a wrinkled forehead is called a *browlift.* Another procedure corrects sagging, wrinkled eyelids and is called a *blepharoplasty.* Ears can be given a different contour or be drawn closer to your head. This procedure is called *otoplasty.*

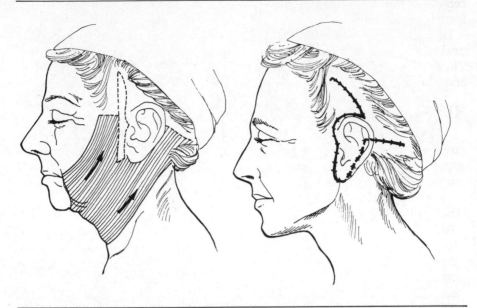

Shaded area shows skin that must be dissected free to pull skin tight to decrease wrinkles. Excess skin is removed in triangles above and on either side of ear.

PREPARING FOR SURGERY

Shaving some of the hair and preparing the skin may be done before you go into the operating room. You may have intravenous fluids and monitors, the same as with other surgeries. Local anesthesia, with sedation, or general anesthesia is used.

Incisions vary according to your needs and how extensive your face lift will be. Usually an incision is made in the crease of skin just in front of your ear, then the incision line is curved upward 1 or 2 inches into your hairline. One variation is to carry the incision just in front of your hairline to your ear.

The incision in front of your ear in the crease is carried down around your ear lobe and up behind your ear. This incision goes into your hair as far as necessary, usually about 1 to 2 inches. All the skin shown as shaded in the illustration above must be lifted off the underlying tissue so it can be stretched to remove wrinkles and sagging.

This is a long incision, but the only part that will show is in front of your ear. That incision will be disguised by the crease in your skin. Your doctor will determine how far your skin must be undercut, how tightly it safely can be stretched and how much skin should be trimmed away. Closure is then done as necessary to fix the skin.

When the operation is over, light-pressure dressings are applied to prevent bleeding and accumulation of excessive fluid under the flaps of skin that have been undercut. Your doctor will determine whether or not these areas will require drains in them to allow the fluid to escape, rather than accumulate and form a hematoma.

Be prepared to wear bulky head dressings for at least 1 day and nurse some bruised areas over your face for several days during the healing process. There are individual variations in technique, so don't be upset if your surgery and incisions differ from those described here.

RISKS OF FACE-LIFT SURGERY

Complications can and do occur in face-lift surgery. Although they are rarely life-threatening, they can be serious because they may affect your appearance. High blood pressure, smoking, heart disease, aspirin use and drug sensitivities add additional risks.

HEMORRHAGE

A great deal of skin must be undercut, so there is always the risk of bleeding under the skin. This is a troublesome complication that occurs in a small percentage of all cases. If bleeding is extensive, the incisions must be reopened to relieve the pressure. If extensive bleeding is left untreated, it can cause death of the overlying skin because skin is unable to establish blood supply and become reattached to the underlying tissues.

Bleeding may also lead to excess scarring, puckering and discoloration of your skin. Smaller collections of blood may go unnoticed until 5 to 7 days after surgery, when they feel like hard nodules beneath your skin. Another week allows them to liquefy automatically so they can be drained. When they are diagnosed, they must be treated so they will not cause the problems with your skin that are described above.

DISCOLORATION OF SKIN

Skin discoloration is called *hyperpigmentation* and is due to iron pigment (from blood) deposited in your skin after surgery. Although it is more common when there is excessive bleeding, it is also more prominent in brunettes.

HEMORRHAGE INTO SKIN

Occasionally the small blood vessels in your skin become enlarged and unsightly, almost like a birthmark. This could be due to the trauma of surgery. It is usually temporary. Most of the time it can be covered with cosmetics until it disappears.

SKIN SLOUGH

This is one of the most dreaded complications and may occur when your skin is stretched too tightly, when a large hematoma occurs or because of a lack of adequate blood supply to the skin. It is a rare complication, and when it does occur, it is usually located just behind, or in front, of your ears. If the resulting scar is unsightly, it usually can be improved by further cosmetic surgery after it heals.

INFECTION

Infection is rare, but it can occur. Because your facial skin has a rich blood supply, it usually heals well and fights off infection. If small areas of infection do occur along your incision, they can be drained without causing unsightly scars. Sometimes your doctor may give you antibiotics to prevent infection before it occurs.

LOSS OF HAIR

Loss of hair occasionally occurs when dissection of your skin is extensive. It is usually temporary and is more common if you have a tendency toward thin hair.

EXCESSIVE SCARRING

Some people have a tendency to form heavy scars (keloids), while other people heal with a hairline incision. It is true that certain techniques make for less scarring, but they may not be able to overcome your hereditary tendency toward keloid formation.

If scarring is severe, the scar usually can be redone surgically in such a way that it will be more acceptable. Cortisone cream and injections may also be used to reduce scarring.

NERVE INJURY

Nerve injury is frustrating, troublesome and sometimes serious. If a sensory nerve is damaged, the result is numbness. Numbness is most likely to occur over the skin in front of your ear and down your neck. Temporary numbness in these areas is normal following face-lift surgery.

If the nerve is a motor nerve, there will be loss of muscle function. The most common area of motor loss is over your facial muscles, especially your forehead and lower lip. Motor-nerve injuries are quite rare, and most will recover if left alone. But this may take several months.

DEFORMITIES

Sometimes unexpected irregularities in your face occur after face-lift surgery. Your face lift may look uneven or asymmetrical. Much of this could be due to swelling and may disappear in time. If the problem is severe and persists beyond 6 months, the area may have to be operated on again.

Even with the most skilled care, unexpected problems can occur. Your doctor will usually wait for at least 6 months for things to settle down before attempting to correct it with further surgery.

ADVANTAGES OF FACE-LIFT SURGERY

The advantages of face-lift surgery are most apparent in *before* and *after* photos. Self-esteem and confidence are some of the advantages of face-lift surgery. You'll feel better about your appearance and better about yourself.

DISADVANTAGES OF FACE-LIFT SURGERY

Although face-lift surgery may improve your appearance, it can't stop or reverse the process of aging. You may want similar surgery again in 5 to 10 years. Gravity and aging continue their pulling and tugging at your skin.

Complications have been listed, and you should consider these as you contemplate face-lift surgery. Weigh the cost, discomfort, risks, complications and lack of permanency. Discuss the surgery with your family and doctor. Only you can decide if the advantages outweigh the disadvantages.

WHO OPERATES?

This surgery is performed by a specialist — a plastic surgeon. Some plastic surgeons become more interested in face-lift surgery and become very skilled in this particular field.

DIAGNOSTIC TESTS BEFORE, DURING AND AFTER FACE-LIFT SURGERY

There are no special tests for patients undergoing face-lift surgery. Routine urinalysis, complete blood count and some tests for abnormal bleeding are routine. You may be asked to discontinue aspirin and other drugs because aspirin thins the blood and may cause excessive bleeding. You will also be asked about drug sensitivities and allergies.

WHERE IS SURGERY PERFORMED?

Face-lift surgery can be performed safely in a doctor's office if the office has a well-equipped operating room. If you have special problems, such as heart disease, high blood pressure, poor nutritional status or other chronic disease, your doctor may prefer to have you admitted to a hospital.

Today, face-lift surgery is often performed in an outpatient department, but you may prefer to have your surgery in the privacy of your doctor's office if it is properly equipped. You and your doctor can discuss this question when you talk of the safety features of each location and your particular needs.

HOSPITALIZATION AND DURATION

The average face lift requires 2 to 4 hours of surgery. If surgery is going to be prolonged, it may be safer for you to be admitted to the hospital, especially if you have other medical problems that might increase the risk.

ANESTHESIA

For minor face-lift changes, local anesthesia and sedatives are usually sufficient. If the surgery will be longer or more difficult, some surgeons prefer general anesthesia.

PROBABLE OUTCOME
OF FACE-LIFT SURGERY

A face lift must be done with skill and expertise from a medical-surgical point of view. But it must also be acceptable to you. Regardless of how perfect your surgery may be, if it doesn't please you, the outcome is questionable.

It's important for you to have before and after pictures to help you remember how you looked before surgery. In a way, face-lift surgery is similar to having new dentures in your mouth. It takes some time to get used to them, and you may forget how bad it was before you had the work done.

Your doctor is dealing with *appearance,* something that is very subjective. Think about it, talk it over and ask plenty of questions. Your doctor can promise to give you the best he can give, but he can't guarantee that you'll like the results or that it will be everything you expect.

POST-OPERATIVE CARE

Immediately following your surgery, bulky bandages are usually applied to the face and neck. These must provide enough pressure to help prevent bleeding under your skin, yet be loose enough to allow circulation of blood to the area. For about 48 hours after your surgery, limit your activity to prevent bleeding and development of a hematoma.

Tubes and drains, if they are necessary at all, are usually removed in 24 to 48 hours. After a few days, you won't have to wear any dressings. Your doctor will clean the incisions of all blood and ointments. It will feel good to be rid of the dressings.

Pain can usually be controlled by pain relievers, such as Tylenol with codeine. If you have more than moderate pain, call your doctor's attention to it. He'll want to check on you.

After 48 hours, you may gradually resume normal activity. Don't apply heat to your face. Numbness could cause you to burn the area. Ice and cold dressings are sometimes used to help control swelling.

Some sutures are removed beginning on the 5th day, and the last sutures may be removed as late as the 14th day after surgery. Sutures in your scalp are the last to be removed.

You'll want to shampoo your hair as soon as possible, but check with your doctor. Ordinarily you can on the 3rd day or up to the 5th day. Your doctor may give you permission to use ointments or creams on your face after about 2 weeks.

DIET

A non-chewable diet is preferable for at least 2 days after surgery. Gradually you can progress from a soft to a normal diet. Avoid moving your face and cheeks any more than necessary during the first few days after surgery.

MISCONCEPTIONS ABOUT FACE-LIFT SURGERY

Having a face lift is a problem solver.

Face-lift will not solve all your problems. Many people live well with what they have. Others can't cope with *any* problems, including their appearance. There are valid reasons why you may need face-lift surgery. If you have done your homework and given the procedure adequate thought, you know what to expect. Hopefully you know what face-lift surgery can and can't do, and you'll have a successful, satisfactory result.

Face-lift surgery needs to be done only once, and the correction of sagging and wrinkles will last a lifetime.

The aging process continues in spite of face-lift surgery. Although one face lift doesn't commit you to another one later, it is possible to repeat the operation at a later date if you wish.

There won't be any scars after surgery.

If you look for them, you'll see scars. But unless you point them out to others, they'll probably be unnoticeable.

There are no risks to face-lift surgery.

Complications aren't common, but they do occur. Unless you're willing to face this possibility, don't have face-lift surgery.

ALTERNATIVES TO FACE-LIFT SURGERY

One alternative is to have only the part of face-lift surgery done that is most necessary. Eyelids, eyebrows, noses, wrinkles and sags can be discussed with your doctor. Together decide how much surgery, if any, you should have done.

A chemical peel or collagen injections can help obliterate fine wrinkling. These procedures are less complicated and may be preferable to face-lift surgery. Talk to your doctor about these procedures.

CALL YOUR DOCTOR IF . . .

1. You have excessive pain.
2. You have excessive swelling.
3. You have bleeding from your incisions.
4. You have drainage from your wounds, unless you have drains.
5. You have chills or fever.
6. You are worried about your condition.

QUESTIONS TO ASK YOUR DOCTOR

Are you a specialist in plastic surgery?

It's best to have someone who has been trained in these techniques perform your surgery. There are few legal restraints on what a doctor may call himself, so someone who says he is a "plastic surgeon" or "cosmetic surgeon" may, in fact, have little or no training or experience with this kind of surgery. Although doctors in other specialties sometimes do cosmetic procedures, a reasonable guide to start with is certification by the American Board of Plastic Surgery or membership in the American Society of Plastic and Reconstructive Surgeons. Names of such surgeons in your community may be obtained from your local medical society office or by calling or writing the American Society of Plastic and Reconstructive Surgeons, Inc. The address and telephone number are:

233 N. Michigan Ave.
Suite 1900
Chicago, IL 60601
(312) 856-1834

How frequently do you perform face-lift surgery?

You may want to know if this is a regular practice of your plastic surgeon.

Do you feel that I need face-lift surgery?

Hopefully your plastic surgeon will be honest with you. He will tell you whether the surgery will help you.

Can you show me some before-and-after pictures of some of your patients who have had this operation?

It's always a good idea to see what kind of results other patients have had. It may help you realize what can and cannot be accomplished with this type of surgery.

What are the most common complications in this type of surgery? How common are they?

There is the possibility of complications with any surgery. For a complete discussion of complications, see the risk section, which begins on page 283.

How much improvement may I expect in wrinkle removal and correction of sagging?

Your doctor should be able to help you understand what results to expect.

Where will my scars be? Will they show?

Have your doctor answer this before your surgery. You should know where any scars will be, so you won't be surprised after the surgery.

Where will my surgery be performed?

Some doctors operate in their own surgical suites, and others use out-patient hospital facilities. Check this out with your doctor.

How long before the bruises will be gone?

This is different with every patient because of many personal variations. But your doctor should be able to give you some general answer to this question.

Are there other methods we should discuss besides face-lift surgery?

If there is any other method, in addition to surgery, discuss it with your doctor.

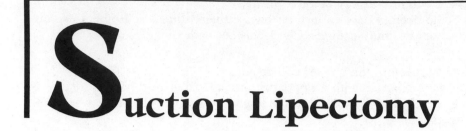Suction Lipectomy

DEFINITION OF SUCTION LIPECTOMY

Do you have an unwanted pad of fat you just can't seem to get rid of? Join about 100 million other Americans who have the same problem. Dieting and exercise haven't helped — lotions, potions and motions haven't helped either. Perhaps your fat has even become wavy, something faddists love to discuss as *cellulite.*

You may not really be fat — you aren't obese, except in one or two places, such as hips, arms, buttocks or a saggy, bulging stomach. There is a procedure that can "spot reduce" those areas; it's called *suction lipectomy.* Suction lipectomy means the removal of fat tissue from your body by means of a suction tube.

ABBREVIATIONS AND OTHER NAMES

Suction lipectomy is called fat suctioning, suction-assisted lipectomy, lipo-dissection and a few other medical terms. "Spot reducing" seems more appropriate, but the name smacks of quackery, which suction lipectomy is *not.* "Lipo" means fat, and "ectomy" means getting rid of it, whether by cutting, suctioning or other methods.

PARTS OF BODY INVOLVED

Although suction lipectomy can be done on men and women, the areas affected vary somewhat according to sex. As a woman, you probably have fat on your hips, especially on the outside of your thighs. You may be normal from

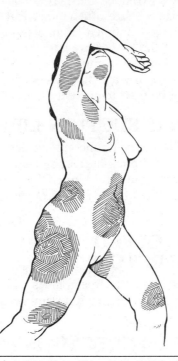

Shaded areas show places where fat will be removed during suction lipectomy. Hips and abdomen are most frequently involved in this surgery.

the waist up, but your hips are wide, far out of proportion to the rest of your body. This type of excess fat in one place is not often due to overeating. It occurs because that's the way Nature has chosen to distribute the fatty tissue on your body.

If you have this type of build and are unhappy with it, take heart! Suction lipectomy may be for you. The technique of fat-suctioning has become so skillful that almost any area of your body can be reduced in size. See illustration above.

COMMON REASONS
FOR SUCTION LIPECTOMY

It's important to know this technique is *not* for weight reduction and is *not* designed to replace dieting and exercise. Suction lipectomy finds its greatest use in removing fatty tissue from a *specific* area where it does not belong.

Like many women, you may have been successful in losing weight by dieting and exercise, but you have lost it from your breasts or face while your hips and tummy remain almost as before. Fat suctioning can help.

You may find one side of your body is larger than the other, or you may have fat that causes a bulge somewhere. Irregularities of contour, due to fatty tissue, can be corrected by this technique.

Fat suctioning is *not* used to reduce the size of breasts (except sometimes in males) or even to equalize the size of asymmetrical breasts. The standard methods of reduction or augmentation mammaplasty are preferred. For more information on equalizing the size of breasts, see the discussion on breast reduction and augmentation that begins on page 262.

If bone or muscle irregularities are the cause of your faulty body contour, suction lipectomy cannot be used to correct the defect.

HOW COMMON IS SUCTION LIPECTOMY?

This procedure is still relatively uncommon because it is new and few doctors are skilled in the technique. The technique was developed in Switzerland and France and was brought to the United States in 1983. Since that time, the technique has been refined further by surgeons in this country and in other countries.

FUNCTIONS INVOLVED IN SUCTION LIPECTOMY

The fat that is removed by suction lipectomy is relatively superficial on the body. There should be no interference with any body functions, especially vital functions.

HOW SUCTION LIPECTOMY IS PERFORMED

Until recently, the only method to remove fat surgically was to make wide incisions and remove moon-shaped sections of fat and skin, but this procedure left massive, unsightly scars. This also left occasional contour problems that were more unsightly than the original defect. See illustration on opposite page.

Now, through small, 1/4- to 1-inch incisions, the same amount of fat (or more) can be removed by the use of a wand or suction dissector attached by rigid tubing to a high-powered suction machine. See illustration on page 294.

Sterile technique is used, as with any other surgery. First the area is cleansed with a prepping and antiseptic solution. The definite areas from which you wish to have the fat removed are clearly marked. This may be done while you are still awake to make certain you and your doctor agree on these areas.

It is important for you and your doctor to communicate well for this procedure to be satisfactory to you. He must understand what you want, and you must understand what his limitations are. But you don't want him to remove the wrong amount of fat or take it from the wrong area.

Understand where the incisions will be, even though they will be small. You should know it is often impossible to obtain a "perfectly smooth" contour when fat is removed by suction lipectomy.

After making a tiny incision in your skin, the suction cannula is introduced into your fatty area. A series of long strokes are made almost parallel to each other, separated by strands of undisturbed tissue. The purpose of these strands of tissue connecting the skin with the underlying muscle is to preserve blood supply and tissue attachments, including skin nerves, which help your skin reattach itself to the underlying tissues and maintain sensation in these areas.

Your surgeon will try to taper the edges of the operative area so there won't be an unsightly rim. He prefers to err on the side of removing too little rather than too much fatty tissue. Any excess can be removed later, but a depression may be difficult to correct.

When he has removed sufficient fatty tissue, your doctor will close the small incisions in the skin. He may or may not place a drain in the area to remove excess blood and tissue fluids. Anticipate a tight compression-dressing — girdle, ace bandage, elastic adhesive tape — to enhance healing, prevent hemorrhage and keep swelling to a minimum.

RISKS OF SUCTION LIPECTOMY

Suction lipectomy has its share of risks; these become important because surgery is usually elective rather than necessary for your health. Suction lipectomy is cosmetic surgery. Much of its success depends on your youth and the texture and elasticity of your skin.

CONTOUR PROBLEMS

Unwanted dimples in strange places may appear post-operatively. Waviness of your skin sometimes occurs, but you must remember you may have had some of this *before* surgery. It is not uncommon to require some "touching up" at a later time to obtain a better final result.

SENSORY CHANGES

Sensory changes vary from itching to tingling to hypersensitivity. Occasionally numbness also occurs because some nerve endings have stopped working. Most of these symptoms usually disappear in 6 to 12 months.

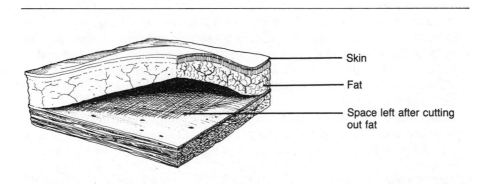

Skin

Fat

Space left after cutting out fat

Lipectomy with a knife leaves large area in which blood and tissue fluid can accumulate to form a hematoma or seroma.

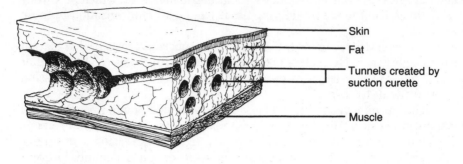

Skin

Fat

Tunnels created by
suction curette

Muscle

By tunneling with a suction curette, enough blood supply is left intact to ensure rapid
healing. Tunnels are less likely to permit hematomas.

SWELLING

You can count on *some* swelling, in spite of pressure dressings. This may be
proportionate to the amount of fat removed but not always. Swelling usually
significantly disappears within 2 to 3 months but may persist for more than 6
months.

BRUISING

It's normal to have some bruising because many tiny blood vessels have
been disrupted by the suctioning. Most of the bruises and the skin discoloration clear in 2 to 3 weeks. The change in skin color is due to the deposition of
iron in the tissues when bleeding occurs, so discoloration is rarely permanent.

HEMORRHAGE

There is always some blood loss; this is often proportional to the amount of
suctioning. Patients *do* vary in their ability to clot, the number of tiny blood
vessels in their skin and their ability to recover from blood loss.

If your doctor anticipates more-than-average blood loss, or if you have a
large area to be suctioned, he may have you donate your own blood 1 to 5
weeks prior to surgery. This will provide enough time for you to manufacture
a replacement in your body, then you can receive your own blood as transfusion at surgery, called *autotransfusion,* if necessary. Autotransfusion is an
excellent safeguard against hepatitis, AIDS and other diseases from transfused blood.

Compression dressings used post-operatively usually prevent undue
hemorrhage. Very rarely there is excessive bleeding during surgery, and
additional blood may be necessary.

HEMATOMA

A hematoma is an accumulation of blood that pools in one area after
surgery. A suctioned area may be difficult to compress all over, or it may be

impossible to maintain compression without strangulation of your tissue. A compression bandage, which is applied after surgery, shouldn't act like a tourniquet and shut off blood supply to that area of your body. But it does minimize the blood supply.

If hematoma occurs, the blood clot gradually liquefies and can be aspirated with a needle and syringe later.

SEROMA
Seroma is an accumulation of tissue fluids, other than blood. A seroma can be drained later in the same way as hematoma.

THROMBOSIS (PHLEBITIS)
This is a blood clot in the veins, often due to surgery or the anesthetic. It can occur with any surgery. It is infrequent in suction lipectomy. The danger lies in the fact that these clots can be dislodged and carried by your blood to the lungs.

FAT EMBOLI
Fat can get into the blood and cause injury to the lungs. The condition is rare in this type of surgery. It is more likely to occur in fractures of the long bones in the body.

SKIN SLOUGH
It is possible, but unlikely, that some of the skin overlying the area of fat suction might die due to lack of blood supply. Your doctor tries to keep suction deep enough so it won't interfere with the superficial blood vessels that lie beneath the surface of the skin.

DAMAGE FROM THE SUCTION CATHETER TO OTHER ORGANS
Normal precautions and skill should avoid damage to other organs from the suction catheter. Any vital organs can be injured if a suction apparatus is used in the abdominal cavity. Extreme care must be taken by the plastic surgeon to avoid this complication.

ADVANTAGES OF SUCTION LIPECTOMY
The principle advantage of fat suctioning is cosmetic relief for women who have conscientiously dieted and exercised, yet lost weight in the wrong places. Some even lose too much weight all over trying to correct a condition that *cannot* be corrected by dieting. When used skillfully to remove fat from certain areas only, suction lipectomy can bring happy relief to many women who have felt self-conscious because of body contour.

DISADVANTAGES OF SUCTION LIPECTOMY
Disadvantages include complications and the rare, sometimes prolonged, post-operative discomfort that accompanies this type of surgery. Although

skin incisions are small, the amount of dissection is great, possibly more than in most other types of surgery. It is impossible to estimate the amount of pain you will have. Sometimes pain is minor, but occasionally it is severe and persistent—even for months.

WHO OPERATES?

This type of surgery is reserved for plastic surgeons, and not all of them perform this specialized surgery. Techniques are improving, but experience is important. Choose a doctor who is interested in this subspecialty, has sufficient experience, performs the surgery frequently and will discuss your condition with you.

DIAGNOSTIC TESTS BEFORE, DURING AND AFTER SUCTION LIPECTOMY

The usual preoperative tests, such as urinalysis and complete blood count, are done first. You may be asked to donate your own blood for possible transfusion if the operation is to be extensive. Other tests are necessary if you have other medical problems.

WHERE IS SURGERY PERFORMED?

Unless the surgery is extensive, it can be performed in an outpatient surgical department or even in your doctor's office. If the suction area is large, you may want to be admitted to the hospital and remain overnight after surgery.

HOSPITALIZATION AND DURATION

Most suction lipectomies are outpatient procedures. It is unlikely you will be required to remain overnight in the hospital. You'll be asked to refrain from eating or drinking after midnight the night before surgery. This is to avoid aspirating food into your lungs if you vomit.

Depending on the amount of fat to be removed, surgery will take 1/2 hour to 2 hours. You'll stay in the recovery area until you are alert enough to leave for home. Recovery time varies according to the length of the procedure and duration of anesthesia. You won't be able to drive your car home, so make other arrangements.

It is unusual for you to have to remain in the hospital more than 24 hours.

ANESTHESIA

Unless the area is small, general or epidural anesthesia is used. If the area is small or if there is only a small amount to be redone from a previous suction lipectomy, local anesthesia is used.

Because you may have to be moved into various positions during surgery, spinal anesthesia is impractical.

Your doctor will mark the places on your skin from which he wants to remove fatty tissue before you are put to sleep. Then you can both agree as to the fatty areas that are to be operated on.

PROBABLE OUTCOME OF SUCTION LIPECTOMY

The outcome of your surgery should be excellent, but you must realize many variables enter the picture. Your general health, the particular way your tissues heal, your attitude and expectations — all combine with the skill of your surgeon to determine the outcome.

Discuss with your plastic surgeon what he intends to do. Be certain you understand his medical terms, and don't be afraid to ask questions before surgery.

Your self-esteem has much to do with the outcome. If you have a poor self-image to begin with, it's possible the outcome may not meet your expectations.

Don't allow yourself to be talked into this procedure if you don't want it. It is elective surgery designed to improve your appearance. You must be willing to accept its pain and inconvenience.

POST-OPERATIVE CARE

Perhaps most important fact in the post-operative care is your compression-bandage girdle. It is essential that the operated area have sufficient pressure to stop bleeding and reduce swelling without strangulating the tissue.

Blood vessels can't be tied off through such a tiny incision the way the doctor is able to do in open surgery. He must depend on pressure.

You may be asked to wear the compression garment for 2 or 3 weeks or longer. You may remove it for bathing, but must reapply it immediately after you finish.

You may be given antibiotics depending on the circumstances. You may need pain medicine, but your pain quickly lessens, and you may require only over-the-counter remedies. Avoid aspirin before and after surgery because it tends to cause bleeding.

Stitches are removed in 1 week, but you should contact your doctor before then, if necessary. Exercise is restricted for 3 to 6 weeks, after which you can begin massage and conditioning. You usually won't have to wear the compression garment after 3 to 4 weeks, unless there are special circumstances.

Most bruises disappear after 3 to 4 weeks. Most of the swelling is gone by 2 to 3 months but may take as long as 6 months.

Most plastic surgeons wait 4 to 6 months for complete recovery before performing "re-dos" or "touch-ups" on the operation to correct tucks, puckering, dimples, unevenness or ridges.

DIET

There is no special diet, except to caution you about gaining too much weight. Iron and vitamins may be prescribed only if you need them in addition to your normal diet.

MISCONCEPTIONS ABOUT SUCTION LIPECTOMY

This is a way to lose weight.
It is not. It's a method of removing fatty tissue from specific areas. Suction lipectomy is limited in what it can do; don't expect more. Discuss your case in detail with your doctor. He may be able to show you before-and-after pictures of other patients and their results to give a realistic expectation.

ALTERNATIVES TO SUCTION LIPECTOMY

You should not have suction lipectomy unless you have lost excess fat from the rest of your body by diet and exercise. Diet and exercise may not cure localized pockets of fat, and suction lipectomy won't cure obesity. This surgery is to improve contour, not to lose weight.

Some surgeons ask a patient to reduce down to her "ideal" weight before they perform this surgery so they see where fat deposits are. But this is not absolutely necessary.

CALL YOUR DOCTOR IF . . .

1. You feel faint or unusually weak. You could be bleeding into the wound and forming a hematoma.
2. You have any discharge from an incision.
3. You have chills or fever.
4. You have excessive swelling in any of the operative areas.
5. You lose sensation over any of the operative sites.
6. You have shortness of breath.
7. You notice any marked changed in your condition.

QUESTIONS TO ASK YOUR DOCTOR

Do you think I should have this operation?
In a way, this puts your doctor on the spot, but you certainly want to know if, in his judgment, this is the best treatment for you. If he's honest, he will tell you how he feels and why.

Can you show me some before-and-after pictures of other patients so I'll know what to expect?
These pictures give you an idea of the end result and may avoid your expecting too much.

Will you take pictures of me before and after, so I can compare the result of the surgery?
Your doctor may want to do this for his own protection.

What are the ordinary complications of this operation?
This gives you an opportunity to determine if you want to face these in this elective surgery. You may want to ask him how he handles these complications and how common they are in his practice.

Will this fat come back?
If you gain weight, it may return, so you also have a responsibility in the final result. Any weight gain may also cause fatty deposits in areas not previously affected.

How much pain may I expect and for how long?
Although it's difficult to estimate pain, it gives you an opportunity to face the problem and discuss it.

How long will my bruises last?
Bruising is inevitable, but you should be aware of them. It may take 6 to 8 weeks for some of the discoloration to disappear.

Tummy-Tuck Surgery

DEFINITION OF TUMMY-TUCK SURGERY

Deformities and unshapeliness of the abdomen are common but tend to be more common in women than men, perhaps due to pregnancy. Said one person, "The deformity is hereditary: women get it from their kids."

Saggy skin *is* inherited. Some women can have their tummy stretched by a dozen pregnancies and still have it return to normal after each one. Other women remain stretched and saggy after only one child.

A tummy tuck is a surgical method of correcting saggy abdominal skin and a bulging tummy. It is *not* a method of losing weight. If your skin has stretched enough so it hangs down over your pubic bone like an apron, the apron is called a *panniculus.* Whether you have sagging skin, distressing stretch marks or a pot belly, it probably can be corrected by a tummy tuck.

ABBREVIATIONS AND OTHER NAMES

Abdominoplasty, abdominal lipectomy, panniculectomy, repair of diastasis rectus muscle — all serve to tuck your tummy and get rid of the bulge. Tummy tuck is a name for abdominoplasty.

PARTS OF BODY INVOLVED

Although surgery is limited to your abdomen, it may involve only skin or it may extend to your entire abdominal wall. If you have a rupture (hernia) that extends through your abdominal muscles and fascia (tendonous attachment to muscles), the hernia must be repaired. Your navel may also be herniated

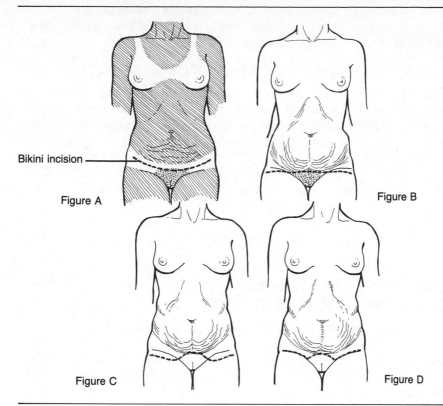

Bikini incision

Figure A

Figure B

Figure C

Figure D

Incisions used for tummy-tuck surgery. Figure A incision is a "bikini" type. Other incisions are variations, used according to distribution of fat and preference of surgeon.

and stretched and can be repaired at the same time as your tummy tuck is done.

The type of incision you have depends on your distribution of fat and the preference of your surgeon. See illustration above.

COMMON REASONS FOR TUMMY-TUCK SURGERY

Modern society is very conscious of appearance and critical of variations of the norm. For example, some Polynesian cultures prefer obese women — a large abdomen is a sign of good health. By contrast, in our culture women are expected to be thin, with flat tummies.

Fashions do not look good if you have a bulging stomach. Tight-fitting clothes look unsightly if your abdomen sticks out. Modern styles flatter you if you fit them, but they seldom allow for a sagging tummy.

It may be because of your attempt to fit yourself to these patterns that you consider a tummy tuck. You may have lost weight from everywhere else on your body, but your protruding stomach continues to protrude.

A tummy tuck may help backache, but it is presumptuous to blame your backache on an overly large stomach.

HOW COMMON IS TUMMY-TUCK SURGERY?

Tummy tuck is becoming more common, and this operation is frequently associated with other abdominal surgeries, such as tubal ligation or hysterectomy. You may be having major surgery anyway, so combining a tummy tuck with your tubal ligation or hysterectomy saves extra hospitalization, anesthesia and expense.

It is unwise to get pregnant after a tummy-tuck operation because it may stretch your abdomen again. It's wise to have a tummy tuck along with a procedure to prevent further pregnancies.

Tummy tuck is *not* a substitute for dieting, and it's not a method to lose weight. The procedure removes sagging and fat from an area that seems to be resistant to dieting.

FUNCTIONS INVOLVED IN TUMMY-TUCK SURGERY

No vital functions are involved. Except for the effects of general anesthesia on bowel and bladder functions, there should be no ill effects. If a large abdominal hernia is also repaired, you can expect the usual problem of gas pains and possible delayed bowel and bladder function that may accompany abdominal surgery.

HOW TUMMY-TUCK SURGERY IS PERFORMED

You are admitted to the hospital, usually on the same day you have your surgery. Your doctor may mark on your abdomen where and how extensively he intends to cut, showing how much tissue he will remove. He may do this while you're awake so you both agree as to what is to be done.

After sterile draping, you are put to sleep and your surgeon begins his dissection. If you have an abdominal hernia or a wide separation of your abdominal muscles called a *diastasis recti,* your doctor will repair this first. Your abdominal muscles and fascia (tendonous connections of your muscles) provide the support you need. Skin gives little support to your abdominal wall.

REPAIR OF LOWER-ABDOMINAL HERNIA

Instead of just saggy skin on your lower abdomen, if you have an actual bulge that is not due to obesity, you may have a lower-abdominal hernia or rupture. The most common cause of this rupture is a separation or weakness of your abdominal muscles, which extend from your ribs and breast bone to your pubic bone. These muscles provide most of your abdominal support. See illustrations on opposite page.

If you raise your head and look to see the baby immediately after delivery, a

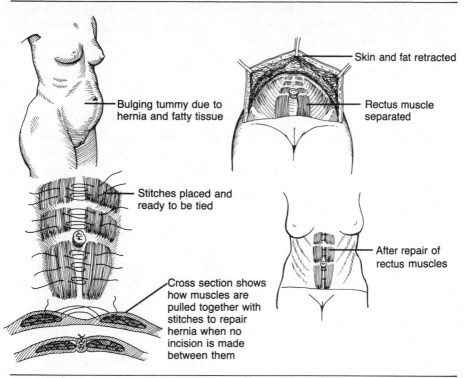

Repair of abdominal hernia (diastasis recti).

long 2- or 3-inch-wide bulge can develop between your navel and your pubic bone. This is a description of a midline weakness, which your doctor calls a diastasis recti.

This diastasis is repaired by sewing the rectus muscles together in the midline. When the extra skin is trimmed away, you have a new, improved contour to your previously poorly supported lower abdominal wall.

Excess skin and fat must be undercut before it can be trimmed away. As the excess skin and fat are trimmed from your abdominal wall, it's important to position your navel in the center where it belongs. Sometimes it must be transplanted, usually with a cord of tissue to maintain its blood supply.

Dissection during surgery is extensive, so some plastic surgeons place drains in the tissue to conduct excess fluid and blood to the outside of the incision where it is absorbed by bulky dressings or suction apparatus.

You may be fitted with a girdle or binder for support. You will be transferred to a bed that is bent in the middle to keep your wound from stretching. You will probably be left in this same bed in the recovery room, then transferred to your room.

RISKS OF TUMMY-TUCK SURGERY

BLEEDING

Bleeding may be the greatest risk in tummy tuck because of the large area that is dissected. If the blood pools in one place, it is called a *hematoma*. Most small hematomas can be drained by withdrawal of fluid with a syringe and needle in the post-operative period. Large hematomas require reoperation to stop the bleeding. If tissue fluid accumulates, the collection is called a *seroma* and is drained the same way as a hematoma.

INFECTION

Infection is always a possibility in any surgery; for this reason you may be given antibiotics to prevent infection before it starts. There is a greater risk of infection in tummy tuck because so much tissue must be cut. To prevent the accumulation of fluid that may increase the possibility of infection, your doctor may place drains in the area that has been dissected.

SEPARATION OF YOUR INCISION

Also called *dehiscence,* separation of your incision may occur if you strain or stretch excessively, such as with severe coughing episodes. Infection may also contribute to wound separation. Sometimes immediate repair can be performed, but at other times, a secondary closure may be necessary.

SKIN SLOUGH

Sloughing skin is uncommon but serious when it occurs. Loss of skin is usually due to a poor blood supply in your remaining skin or too much tension along the incision. Sloughing of abdominal skin can undo all that has been accomplished by surgery. Fortunately even this problem can be usually corrected by further surgery, which in some cases may include skin grafting.

NAVEL DISPLACEMENT

Displacement of your navel is a possibility but becomes a problem only if you intend to show off this part of your anatomy. In a bikini, it could be embarrassing if your navel is in the wrong place. When large sections of skin must be removed, especially when there is a sizable panniculus, your doctor could misjudge the final position of your navel.

NUMBNESS

Sometimes numbness results because nerve endings in your skin have been cut or stretched. This cannot always be avoided, but sensation usually returns in a few months. Some numbness may extend down on the thighs. You also may experience paresthesia (tingling sensation, pin and needles) in the dissected areas. These sensations are usually temporary.

EMBOLUS DUE TO PHLEBITIS

An embolus is a clot that is released from one area — usually a pelvic or leg vein — and carried by the bloodstream to another area of your body, often your lung. Symptoms vary with the size of the clot and the blood vessels that it occludes when it lodges. Fortunately emboli usually are uncommon, but they can be fatal.

DISSATISFACTION WITH SURGERY

This is a risk, but it can be avoided if there is good communication between you and your doctor before and after surgery. Pictures taken before and after surgery help you see what has been accomplished. Discuss with your doctor what results he hopes to obtain and what you may realistically expect from your tummy tuck.

ADVANTAGES OF TUMMY-TUCK SURGERY

The greatest advantage is probably cosmetic because it will give you a more desirable abdominal profile. You'll look better in pants, swimsuits and dresses. You won't have to compromise your appearance with loose-fitting, baggy clothing.

It'll feel good to feel supported in your abdominal area. You may lose some of your stretch marks, and you'll lose much, if not all, of your sagginess. As a bonus, you may have less backache, although this can't be guaranteed because there are many causes of backache.

A tummy tuck is often done with other abdominal surgery. This avoids separate hospitalization and anesthesia.

DISADVANTAGES OF TUMMY-TUCK SURGERY

This type of surgery is expensive, and the expense probably will not be covered by insurance. It is major surgery and carries the risks of major surgery and general anesthesia.

It is unwise to undertake pregnancy after tummy-tuck surgery because the resultant stretching may undo all that was accomplished by the tummy tuck. In fact, it is wise to be sterilized or use reliable birth control if you're going to have this surgery.

WHO OPERATES?

Plastic surgeons do most tummy-tuck surgery, although gynecologists and general surgeons may perform a tummy tuck with regular abdominal surgery if the patient desires it.

DIAGNOSTIC TESTS BEFORE, DURING AND AFTER TUMMY-TUCK SURGERY

Standard tests done before surgery include urinalysis, complete blood count, type and crossmatch of blood. A complete blood count is usually done to check you after surgery.

WHERE IS SURGERY PERFORMED?

Many tummy-tuck surgeries are performed at the same time as other abdominal surgery, so this becomes a hospital-based operation. If only a tummy tuck is to be performed, it sometimes can be done in the outpatient department. If you are sent home the same day as surgery, you may be accompanied by a nurse. The usual tummy-tuck patient remains in the hospital a few days because of the considerable dissection in this surgery.

HOSPITALIZATION AND DURATION

A tummy tuck and repair of an abdominal wall usually takes 2 to 5 hours, plus another hour in the recovery room. With this much surgery, it's unlikely you'll want to go home right after surgery. Plan on 1 to 4 days in the hospital, depending on the extent of your surgery.

If you have only a tummy tuck, your hospital stay depends on how much tissue must be removed and your general condition of health.

ANESTHESIA

Tummy-tuck surgery can be done under spinal or epidural anesthesia, but most patients and surgeons prefer a general anesthetic. Discuss the situation with your anesthesiologist and surgeon if you have a preference. He'll probably suggest a general anesthetic.

PROBABLE OUTCOME
OF TUMMY-TUCK SURGERY

This is planned surgery, so the outcome is usually very good. Abdominal contour will be improved, and you should be pleased. It's important to understand the limitations of surgery beforehand so you won't expect too much.

There are risks to any surgery, and unless you are prepared to face them, you should not have elective surgery, especially cosmetic surgery.

POST-OPERATIVE CARE

Following surgery, you'll be taken to the recovery room and will awaken there. Your vital signs will be carefully monitored; when your recovery condition is satisfactory, you'll be moved to your hospital room.

If you have any drains, they will be removed in 24 to 48 hours. Your most uncomfortable task will be to move around. It's important to get out of bed (with help) within 12 to 24 hours to avoid phlebitis in your legs.

You'll feel like staying doubled up because the tissues of your abdomen have been shortened. Your doctor may also leave orders to keep you from fully straightening up too soon — usually during the first week.

You'll be given pain relievers to take home with you. You will be encouraged to move around, but you'll be cautioned against excessively stretching. Resumption of full activity usually takes about 6 weeks.

DIET

When your abdominal cavity is opened, especially if intestines are involved, you may have some nausea or bloating after surgery. Your diet begins with liquids, then progresses to soft foods until your digestive tract returns to normal.

Be careful about gaining weight after surgery; you could quickly lose your new abdominal contour.

MISCONCEPTIONS ABOUT TUMMY-TUCK SURGERY

A tummy tuck will help me lose weight.

Tummy tuck is not a substitute for dieting and exercise. It is a way to lose the sagginess from your abdominal wall that does not disappear with dieting and exercise.

I don't have to worry about scars with a tummy tuck.

Scars — long ones — may be part of the procedure with a tummy tuck. There is no way to avoid them. You may even form a keloid, but this usually can be revised with minor surgery, or it can be treated with cortisone.

There aren't any complications with tummy tuck; it's like having minor surgery.

Tummy tuck *does* have complications because it involves a lot of tissue dissection. Most of these complications have little to do with the technique or skill of your doctor. Be prepared for possible complications.

I'll get rid of all my stretch marks with tummy-tuck surgery.

Surgery can remove some of your abdominal stretch marks but may not remove all of them.

ALTERNATIVES TO TUMMY-TUCK SURGERY

If you have already tried serious dieting and exercise with no improvement, the only alternative to tummy-tuck surgery is to do nothing. Lotions, ointments, exercisers, rollers, vibrators and massagers have no effect on a sagging tummy.

CALL YOUR DOCTOR IF . . .

1. You have questions that trouble you.
2. You have abnormal swelling in your incision. It could be blood tissue fluid or an abscess.
3. You have chills or fever.
4. You have excessive pain in your incisions.
5. You have redness around your incision.
6. You have excessive discharge from your incision.

QUESTIONS TO ASK YOUR DOCTOR

Do you think I should have a tummy-tuck operation?
If he is honest, he will tell you if he thinks you should *not* have this type of surgery.

Can you show me some pictures of other patients with before-and-after results?
This will help you to know what to expect.

Where will my scar be and how large will it be?
You should know how extensive your surgery will be. The incision for this surgery is not small.

Explain the various complications and risks. What has been your experience with these risks?
These are detailed in this section, but you need to understand them and be willing to face them because this is *elective* surgery.

Will my insurance cover these costs?
Tummy-tuck surgery is expensive and is usually *not* covered by insurance.

What about sterilization along with my tummy tuck operation?
A pregnancy may stretch your abdominal wall so discuss this with your doctor. You may want to make certain you won't get pregnant again.

Do I need to give blood ahead of time, in case I need a transfusion during surgery?
If you need a transfusion, it's better to receive your own blood, rather that take a chance on getting AIDS or hepatitis from a transfusion from someone else.

Will this bulge recur?
If you watch your weight and exercise abdominal muscles, the loss of support should not recur. Aging does cause skin to sag and muscles to lose their tone, but exercise helps prevent this.

Glossary

Abdominal hysterectomy—Hysterectomy performed through the abdominal wall.

Abortion—Electively terminating a pregnancy.

Adenomyosis—Internal endometriosis.

Adenosis—Benign cellular change of the cervix. It is extremely common in DES offspring.

Adhesions—Bands of scar tissue that form between any raw or irritated surfaces.

Afterbirth—Source of nourishment for fetus during growth in the uterus. Also called *placenta.*

Atelectasis—Condition in which baby's lungs fail to expand or inflate with air at birth.

Atonic uterus—Uterus that has lost tone in its muscular walls.

Atypical pain—Pain different from usual acute signs.

Augmentation mammaplasty—Surgically enlarging breasts with an implant.

Autotransfusion—Donation of own blood weeks *before* surgery; if blood is needed during surgery, patient will be given her own.

"Bathroom sign"—Rupture of tubal pregnancy with sudden lower abdominal pain while straining to have a bowel movement.

Band-Aid surgery—Common term used for laparoscopy.

Benign—Non-cancerous.

Bikini incision—Incision made just inside the pubic hairline in a slightly elliptical fashion. Also called *pubic hairline incision* or *pfannenstiel incision.*

Blepharoplasty—Plastic-surgery procedure that corrects sagging, wrinkled eyelids.

Breech presentation—When baby comes feet or buttocks first during delivery.

Browlift—Special incisions in or behind the hairline used to correct a wrinkled forehead.

C-section—Cesarean operation.

Cancer cells—Nuclei of cells become larger, darker in color and irregular in shape. Material inside the nucleus becomes jumbled and robs other cells of nourishment and oxygen. Cells grow and reproduce much faster than normal cells. Cancer cells begin to crowd, push and compress normal cells, growing completely out of control. They take over and cause normal cells to die of starvation and suffocation.

Cancer of the breast—Condition in which breast contains a malignant growth.

Cancer of the cervix—Disease in which cells covering the cervix become cancerous.

Cancer of the endometrium—See *cancer of the uterus.*

Cancer of the placenta—Cancer caused by pregnancy.

Cancer of the uterus—Cancer of the *lining* (endometrium) of the uterus.

Cancer-in-situ—Stage in which cancer is localized; at this stage it may be easy to cure.

Cancerous—Malignant.

Carcinoma-in-situ—Term used for a lesion that has passed from the stage of dysplasia (benign) to neoplasia (cancerous).

Cautery—Burning with electric current, often used in sterilization.

Cellulite—Fat that has become wavy.

Cephalo-pelvic disproportion—Head of baby is too large to safely pass through mother's pelvis.

Cerclage—Band of synthetic material tied around an incompetent cervix to keep it closed until the baby is ready to be born.

Cervical canal—Cervical opening.

Cervical intraepithelia neoplasia (CIN)—Classification system that means abnormal, precancerous cells in the cervix.

Cervical pregnancy—Pregnancy implanted in the cervix.

Cervix—Neck of the uterus.

Cesarean operation—Delivery of a baby though an abdominal incision rather than through the vagina.

Chemical peel—Plastic-surgery process that peels the skin to minimize wrinkles on lips and acne scars on cheeks.

Chlamydia—Sexually transmitted infection.

Choriocarcinoma—Cancerous tumor that grows during pregnancy.

Chronic pain—Pain that is long-lasting.

Classical Cesarean incision—During Cesarean operation, incision made through contractile part of the uterine wall.

Colposcopy—Proceedure in which tissues are examined through the vagina with a colposcope. This allows magnified examination of the cervix and vagina and allows the abnormal areas to be biopsied for diagnosis.

Complete miscarriage—Uterus expels all of the placenta and fetus.

Condylomata—Sexually transmitted warts.

Conization of cervix—Removal of cone of tissue from the cervix when cancer has not spread.

Conization—Cone of tissue cut out with a knife or cautery loop.

Contractile—Area of the uterus involved in uterine contractions during labor.

Corpus luteum cyst—Cyst that usually occurs after ovulation. Normally the area in the ovary that surrounds the egg regresses after ovulation. But when a cyst forms, instead of regression, fluid collects and distends the ovary.

Cryosurgery—Surgery in which a very cold probe (from gases, such as nitrous oxide) is placed on the cervix to cover an abnormal area. Tissue is frozen for 3 to 5 minutes, allowed to "thaw" for a few minutes, then frozen again. "Surgery" works by freezing and killing abnormal tissues.

Culdocentesis—Procedure in which a needle is inserted through the top of the vagina up into the cul-de-sac of the peritoneum to test for the presence of blood in the abdominal cavity.

Cystic—Contains fluid.

Cystoscopy—Examination of the urinary bladder by scope.

D&C—Dilation and curettage.

D&E—Dilatation and evacuation.

DES—Diethylstilbestrol.

Dehiscence—Separation of an incision.

Dermabrasion—Plastic-surgery process in which wrinkles and acne scars are reduced by sanding, like sanding out the rough spots on a piece of wood.

Dermoid—Tumor of the ovaries that contains teeth, hair and other tissues.

Diaphanography—Method of shining a very intense, cool light through the breast and noting any shadow it casts to detect masses in the breast.

Diastasis recti—Wide separation of abdominal muscles.

Diethylstilbestrol—Non-steroidal synthetic estrogen.

Dilatation and curettage—Cervix is dilated, and the inner lining of the uterus is scraped.

Dilatation and evacuation—Cervix is dilated, and a plastic suction curette and ovum forceps are used to empty the uterus.

Direct extensions—Cancer that breaks through the capsule of the organ and spreads to surrounding organs.

Distant spread—Cancer penetrates the walls of blood vessels or lymph channels, which are part of the body's immune system, and are then transported to other organs of the body.

Dyspareunia—Painful intercourse.

Dysplasia—Term used to describe abnormal, non-cancerous changes in cells of the cervix.

Ectasia—Blocked, stretched, swollen or dilated breast ducts.

-Ectomy—To get rid of something by cutting, suctioning or other surgical methods.

Ectopic pregnancy—Pregnancy located in an abnormal place, outside the uterus.

Embolus—Blood clot released from one area—usually a pelvic vein or leg vein—and carried by the bloodstream to another area of the body, such as the lung or brain.

Endocrine therapy—Treatment with hormones.

Endometrial cancer—Cancer of the lining of the uterus.

Endometrial hyperplasia—Thickened or overgrown lining of the uterus, usually due to overstimulation by estrogen and lack of progesterone.

Endometrial polyps—Lining of the uterus that has overgrown enough to hang like thick droplets of paint that "run" on a wall. It is a common cause of increased menstrual flow.

Endometriosis—Condition in which endometrial tissue is located in areas where it should *not* be, such as ovaries, Fallopian tubes, bladder, bowel, lining of the abdominal cavity.

Endometrium—Lining of the uterus.

Epidural anesthesia—Anesthetic placed around the spinal canal.

Ergotrate—Medication given to increase contractions of the uterus and decrease blood loss.

Estrogen—Hormone that causes growth and thickening of the endometrium.

External endometriosis—Endometriosis that encompasses all locations of the endometrial tissue outside the uterine wall.

Fetal distress—When the baby is in trouble during delivery.

Fibroadenoma—Common, benign breast lump that usually appears in young women.

Fibrocystic disease—Breast contains many cysts.

Follicle cysts—Cysts that occur when a woman fails to give off an egg, but the tissue around the egg keeps growing until it becomes a cyst.

Fractional D&C—Specimens obtained by scraping the canal of the cervix and scraping the cavity of the uterus to show where cancer is located.

Gonorrhea—Sexually transmitted infection.

Habitual miscarriage—When three consecutive early pregnancies are lost.

Hematoma—Local swelling or tumor filled with blood.

Hodgkin's Disease—Painless, progressive, sometimes fatal enlargement of the lymph nodes, spleen and general lymphoid tissues.

Human chorionic gonadotropin (HCG)—Hormone present in blood or urine during pregnancy.

Hydatidiform mole—Cystic tumor of the placenta (afterbirth) that may become cancerous.

Hyperpigmentation—Excessive skin discoloration due to iron pigment (from blood) deposited in skin after surgery.

Hysterectomy—Removal of the uterus.

Hysterotomy—Cutting into the uterus; usually refers to removal of an early pregnancy.

IUD—Intrauterine device.

Incompetent cervix—Cervix loses some of the tone necessary to keep it closed during pregnancy.

Incomplete miscarriage—Uterus expels only part of the placenta and fetus and continues to bleed.

Internal endometriosis—Condition in which endometriosis invades wall of the uterus.

Intraductal papilloma—Small, benign tumor in the milk duct.

Intrauterine device—Device placed within the uterus to prevent pregnancy.

Invasive—When cancer cells break through barriers and begin to spread.

Keloid—Piling up of scar tissue.

Laminaria—Narrow strips of Japanese seaweed used to dilate a cervix before D&C or D&E.

Laser—Acronym for "light amplification by stimulated emission of radiation." Laser is used for certain surgical techniques.

Lipo—Fat.

Local anesthesia—Anesthetic placed at the point of the incision.

Local extension—Spread of cancer confined to local area.

Low-cervical Cesarean incision—Incision made vertically or horizontally in the lower uterine segment, which contains little contractile tissue.

Lumpectomy—Removal of a breast lump, leaving all tissue intact.

Lymph nodes—Glands that store lymph fluid.

Malignant—Cancerous.

Mammography—X-ray technique for detection of breast tumors before they can be seen or felt.

Mastectomy—Surgical removal of the breast.

Menstrual extraction—Abortion within 14 days after a missed menstrual period in which contents of the uterus are removed.

Metastases—Sites of spread of additional cancer nests.

Minilaparotomy—Procedure in which a "small" incision is made into the abdomen. It is major surgery on the smallest scale.

Missed miscarriage—When a fetus dies within the first 20 weeks of pregnancy, but the uterus does not expel it.

Myoma—Muscle tumor.

Myomectomy—Removal of a muscle or fibroid tumor.

Neoplasia—Term used to describe abnormal changes in cells of the cervix. Cancerous.

Non-contractile—Area of the uterus not involved in uterine contractions during labor.

Normal cells—Normal cells have a nucleus in the center surrounded by a substance called *cytoplasm*. A normal cell doesn't change into any other type of cell.

Omentum—Apron of fatty tissue that hangs down over the bowel.

Oncologist—Cancer specialist.

Otoplasty—Plastic-surgery procedure that gives ears a different contour or draws them closer to the head.

Outpatient surgery—Surgery performed in one day. The patient goes in, has the surgery and returns home on the same day.

Ovarian cancer—Term for cells of the ovary that have changed their biology so they no longer follow the rules that normal cells adhere to. Cancerous.

PID—Pelvic inflammatory disease.

Paget's Disease—Cancer of the nipple and surrounding area.

Panniculus—Apron of skin that hangs down over the pubic bone when skin is very stretched.

Pap smear—Screening test that helps identify cancer of the cervix.

Paraffin examination—Permanent fixation and staining of biopsied tissue to detect cancer cells.

Partial hysterectomy—Only the body of the uterus is removed.

Pedicle—Cord by which a a tumor hangs.

Pelvic exenteration—Removal of all pelvic organs, plus bladder and rectum.

Pelvic kidney—Kidney that can be felt because it is lower than normal.

Peritoneum—Shiny membrane that lines the abdominal cavity and covers the outside of most abdominal organs.

Pfannenstiel incision—See *bikini incision.*

Phlebitis—Inflammation or clots in the veins of the legs.

Placenta—Source of nourishment for fetus during growth in the uterus. Also called *afterbirth.*

Polycystic ovaries—Ovaries riddled with cysts that causes lack of periods and infertility. Also called *Stein-Leventhal Syndrome.*

Post-partum tubal ligation—Sterilization immediately after delivery of a baby.

Posterior cul-de-sac—Blind pouch in which the peritoneal cavity ends as it extends downward behind the uterus.

Pre-eclampsia—Toxemia of pregnancy.

Presenting part—Part of the baby that comes first during delivery.

Progestin—Hormone that causes the glands in the thickened lining to grow and produce a nutritious, perfect environment to receive a fertilized egg and begin a pregnancy.

Prolapsed cord—When the cord slips down between the presenting part of the baby and the mother's pelvic wall and becomes compressed.

Prophylactic mastectomy—Removal of a breast to avoid the *possibility of cancer.*

Pubic hairline incision—See *bikini incision.*

Punch biopsy—Biopsy done with special hollow forceps that cut out a round piece of tissue when the forceps are closed over a suspicious area. This suspicious area is revealed by staining with iodine and more definitely determined by examination with a colposcope.

Pyelogram—X-ray of the urinary system to see if it there are any abnormalities.

Radiation therapy—Use of radiation in the treatment of cancer.

Radical mastectomy—Removal of the breast, with wide dissection that includes underlying muscles, overlying skin, lymph nodes and fatty tissue.

Rectocele—Hernia or rupture of the rectum into the back wall of the vagina.

Reduction mammaplasty—Surgically reducing size of breasts.

Schiller test—Involves staining the cervix with iodine. Normal cervical tissue contains glycogen, which is readily stained by iodine. Suspicious or cancerous tissues do not take the stain.

Scopolamine—Drug used during surgery that dries up secretions throughout body and decreases the risk of aspirating secretions into the lungs.

Septic miscarriage—Miscarriage complicated by overwhelming infection.

Sigmoidoscopy—Examination of the large intestine just above the rectum.

Simple lumpectomy—Removal of a breast lump.

Simple mastectomy—Surgical removal of the breast.

Skin slough—Death of tissue.

Spinal anesthesia—Anesthetic placed inside the spinal canal.

Stein-Leventhal Syndrome—See polycystic ovaries.

Subacute pain—Less painful.

Subcutaneous mastectomies—Removal of the breast, leaving skin and nipple.

Submammary placement—Breast implant inserted directly under breast tissue, between breast and pectoralis muscle.

Submucous fibroids—Benign muscle tumors that lie beneath the endometrial lining of the uterus and protrude into the cavity of the uterus.

Subpectoral placement—Breast implant inserted beneath pectoral muscle that underlies breast.

Suction lipectomy—Procedure to surgically "spot reduce" areas with fat deposits.

Teratogens—Defect-causing agents.

Teratoma—Dermoid tumor that is malignant.

Thermography—Heat-sensing technique used in detecting early breast cancer.

Total hysterectomy—Body and neck of uterus are removed.

Toxemia of pregnancy—Condition unique to pregnancy. Symptoms include high blood pressure, swelling, albumin in the urine and neurologic changes.

Transverse hysterectomy incision—Incision confined within the pubic hairline.

Transverse lie—Shoulders of baby come first during delivery.

Trochar—Large hollow needle used in many surgerical procedures.

Tubal pregnancy—Most common ectopic pregnancy.

Trophoblastic tumors—Tumors of the placenta.

Theca lutein cysts—Cysts that result from hormones produced in pregnancy. Fertility drugs can cause these cysts in both ovaries.

Ultrasound—High-frequency sound waves used for examination. The wave pattern is recorded as waves are bounced back by structures they encounter.

Ultrasound mammography—Ultrasound test used to detect breast abnormalities.

Uterine myomata—Muscle tumors of the uterus.

Uterine cancer—See *cancer of the endometrium.*

Vacutage—Plastic suction tube used to vacuum the uterus of its lining.

Vaginal hysterectomy—Hysterectomy performed through the vagina.

Vertical hysterectomy incision—Incision extending from the pubic bone to the navel.

Wertheim hysterectomy—Radical hysterectomy.

Index